Carbohydrate Antigens
As
Tumor Markers

Prof.Dr.Sami AlMudhaffar and

Dr .Salwa Hameed Nasir Al-Rubae

Dr. Majid Karbon

Contents

| ChapterTwo:
CA 15-3 in Human Breast Tumor | 47 |

Chapter Four: Kinetic and Thermodynamic Studies of Binding CA15-3 to its antibody

Chapter Five: Characterization of complexes of CA15-3   120

Part A

CA15-3 and CA19-9 in Breast Tumors

Prof.Dr.Sami AlMudhaffar and
Dr .Salwa Hameed Nasir1. Al-Rubae

This Part

Deals with Determination of carbohydrate antigen 15-3 (CA15-3) and carbohydrate antigen 19-9 (CA 19-9) levels in sera of patients with benign and malignant breast tumors , Development of IRMA assay for the determination of CA15-3 and CA19-9 from cytosolic tissues of benign and malignant breast tumors ,Characterization of the binding of 125I-anti CA15-3 antibody with isolated human – CA15-3 in benign and malignant breast tumors, such as those of binding capacity and the effect of various factors (pH, temperature, time, halides, salts, CA15-3 and its antibody concentration) ,Determination of kinetic and thermodynamic parameters of the binding of partially purified CA15-3 with its specific antibody and Spectroscopic studies on (125I-anti CA15-3 antibody / CA15-3) complex in breast tissue .

Further more the level of sera CA 15-3 in patients with benign and malignant breast tumors (preoperative) was measured by Immunoradiometric Assay (IRMA). Data analysis showed, concentrations of CA 15-3 were significantly higher in pre-and post-menopausal malignant breast tumors (P< 0.0001) and significantly lower in benign breast tumors, compared with healthy subjects.

The results obtained revealed higher incidence of CA 15-3 in two groups of malignant breast tumors than those in benign breast tissues and in the supernatant fraction more than the pellet fraction .The binding of 125I –anti CA 15-3 antibodies with CA 15-3 was studied in three groups: benign breast tumor (Fibroadenoma), pre-and post- menopausal malignant breast tumors (IDC). The optimum conditions observed for the binding were as follows:

CA 15-3 in concentration tissue homogenate 100µg. mL-1 for groups II and I while it was 200 µg.mL-1 for group III. 125I -anti CA 15-3 antibody concentrations: 0.175µg.mL-1 for group I and II, whereas it was 0.140 µg.mL-1 for group III. Temperatures of incubation were: 45oC for groups I and III, 15 oC for group II, while time of incubation was 90 min for both group I and III, 30 min. for group II. The optimum pH was 7.0 for group I, 7.6 for group II and 7.8 for group III. The use of different halides was shown to increase the binding between CA 15-3 and 125I –anti CA 15-3 antibody in both group II and III, while inhibition occurred on the binding in group I.

Abbreviations

Ab	Antibody
Ab*	Labeled antibody
Ag	Antigen
(Ab-Ag)	125I-anti CA15-3 antibody / CA 15-3) Complex
B	Bound
Bmax.	Maximal binding capacity
BSA	Bovine Serum Albumin
(B/T) %	Percentage of bound over total
CA15-3	Carbohydrate antigen 15-3
CA19-9	Carbohydrate antigen 19-9
CA27.29	Carbohydrate antigen 27.29
CA125	Carbohydrate antigen 125
CA549	Carbohydrate antigen 549
CAF	Cyclophosphamide Doxorubicin (Adriamycin) 5-Fluorouracil
CEA	Carcino-Embryonic Antigen
Ci	Curi
CMF	Cyclophosphsamide Methotrexate 5-Fluorouracil
cpm	Counts per minute
DCIS	Ductal Carcinoma in Situ
DMSO	Dimethyl sulphoxide
ε	Absorption coefficient
EDTA	Ethylenediammine tetraaceticacid
EG	Ethylene Glycol
ELISA	Enzyme-Linked immunosorbent assay
F	Free
FNA	Fine needle aspiration
h-CA15-3	Human carbohydrate antigen 15-3
His	Histidine
ICR	Iraqi Cancer Registry
IDC	Infiltrating ductal carcinoma

ILC	Infiltrating lobular carcinoma
IRMA	Immunoradiometric Asaay
J	Joule
K	Kelvin
Ka	Affinity constant
Kav	Partition coefficient
Kd	Equilibrium dissociation constant
KD	Kilodalton
KJ	Kilo joule
LCIS	Lobular carcinoma in situ
Mab	Monoclonal antibody
μ	Micro (10^{-6} x)
Max	Maximum
μg	Microgram
μL	Microliter
MCA	Mucin-like carcinoma associated antigen
MRI	Magnetic Resonance Image
MSTI	Molar surface tension increment
λmax	Maximum wavelength
M.Wt	Molecular weight
nm	Nanometer
N.M.R.	Nuclear Magnetic Resonance
P	Probability
PEG	Polyethylene glycol
P53	Tumor suppressor gen
PR	Progesterone receptor
PAGE	Polyacrylamide gel electrophoresis
RIA	Radioimmuno assay
r.p.m	Round per minute
RRA	Radio active iodine ablation
SD	Standard deviation
Ser	Serine
SDS - PAGE	Sodium dodecyle sulfate – poly acrylamide gel electrophoresis
T	Total

Thr	Threonine
TNM	Tumor, Node, Metastasis, Staging System
TPA	Tissue polypeptide antigen
TPS	Tissue polypeptide specific antigen
Trp	Tryptophane
Tyr	Tyrosine
UV	Ultraviolet
WHO	World Health Organization

1. The level of CA15-3 was determined in sera of (16) premenopausal malignant breast tumors patients, (12) postmenopausal malignant breast tumors patients, and (20) benign breast tumors patients matched with one group of (10) healthy women as control by Immunoradiometric Assay (IRMA). The data obtained demonstrated highly significant increase ($P<0.0001$) in patients with malignant breast tumors, whereas slightly increase ($P<0.05$) in patients with benign breast tumors when matched with normal women.

2. A modified Imunoradiometric Assay (IRMA) was used for determination of cytosolic carbohydrate antigen 15-3, using 125I-anti CA15-3 antibody and found to be suitable for the assessment of those antigens in benign and malignant breast tumors. The data revealed an increment of CA15-3 in the cytosolic fraction in comparison to the nuclear fraction.

3. CA 15-3 was isolated from cytosolic of human benign and malignant breast tumors homogenate by gel filtration techniques. The binding characteristics of the partially purified CA15-3 from benign and malignant breast tumors homogenate with 125I-anti CA15-3 antibody were investigated.

4. Kinetic parameters of the binding 125I-anti CA15-3 antibody with partially purified CA15-3 from benign and malignant breast tumors homogenate were determined at five different temperatures, the results indicated that the binding reaction was time and temperature –dependent process. However the time – course data for the binding followed the pseudo –first order kinetic.

5. The thermodynamic studies of the 125I-anti CA15-3 antibody binding to the partially purified CA15-3 from benign and malignant breast tumors were studied. The thermodynamic parameters of the standard state (ΔG_o, ΔH_o, ΔS_o) and the transition state (ΔG^*, ΔH^*, ΔS^*) and activation energy (E_a) were determined.

6. The complex formed (125I-anti CA15-3 antibody / CA15-3) of partially purified CA15-3 from benign and malignant breast tumors and 125I-anti CA15-3 antibody, were investigated by UV methods. Different factors affecting the absorption band were extensively studied, such as pH, solvent perturbation, and denaturation agents. The heat stability and spectroscopic titration were also studied.

7. The level of CA19-9 was determined in sera of (10) premenopausal malignant breast tumors patients, (10) postmenopausal malignant breast tumors patients, and (10) benign breast tumors patients matched with one group of (10) healthy women as control by Immunoradiometric Assay (IRMA). The data obtained demonstrated significant increase ($P<0.05$) in patients with benign and premenopausal malignant breast tumors, whereas highly significant increase ($P<0.005$) in patients with postmenopausal malignant breast tumors when matched with normal women.

8. An Immunoradiometric Assay (IRMA) for the determination of cytosolic CA19-9 was developed, using 125I-anti CA19-9 antibody and found to be suitable for assessment of those antigens in benign and malignant breast tumors. The data revealed an increment of CA19-9 in the cytosolic fraction in comparison to the nuclear fraction.

Chapter one

1.1 Introduction

The breast is constantly responding to changes in hormonal, nutritional, genetic, psychological, and environmental stimuli such as radiation that cause continual cellular changes (1). As a result of these changes, breast tumors (abnormal breast tissue) may develop either benign (noncancerous) or malignant (cancerous) (2). The major significance of the benign processes less in the need to separate them from malignancies. The World Health Organization (WHO) classifies tumors of the breast (1981) according to histological aspects (3) (Table 1.1).

Table (1.1): Histological classification of breast tumors (3)

I. Epithelial Tumors	
A. Benign	
1.	Intraductal papilloma
2.	Adenoma of the nipple
3.	Adenoma
a.	Tublar
b.	Lactating
B. Malignant	
1.	Non invasive
a.	Intraductal carcinoma
b.	Lobular carcinoma
2.	Invasive
a.	Invasive ductal carcinoma
b.	Invasive lobular carcinoma
3.	Paget's disease of the nipples
II. Mixed Connective Tissue and Epithelial Tumors	
a.	Fibroadenoma

Table (1.1): Continued.

b.	Phyllodes tumor (cystosarcoma phyllodes)
c.	Carcinosarcoma
III. Miscellaneous Tumors	
a.	Soft tissue tumors
b.	Skin tumors
c.	Tumors of haemopcietia and lymph tissues
IV. Unclassified Tumors	
V. Mammary Dysplasia / Fibrocystic Change	
VI. Tumor like Lesion	
a.	Duct ectasia
b.	Inflammatory pseudotumors

1.2. Benign Breast Tumors

1.2.1. Fibroadenoma

This is the most common benign tumor of the female breast. It is a new growth composed of both fibrous and glandular tissue (4). These tumors are commonly found in younger women between the ages 20-35 years (5). It increases in size, during pregnancy (6). It is less likely to develop after menopause. An epidemiological study suggests that fibroadenoma represents a long-term risk for breast carcinomas and that risk is increased in women with ductal hyperplasias, or a family history of breast carcinoma (7).

1.2.2. Fibrocystic disease

This is an ill-defined condition of the breast where palpable lumps can be felt and is usually associated with pain and tenderness that fluctuates with the menstrual cycle (8). Fibrocystic changes are the most common, occurring in approximately 60% of premenopausal women. Women with this disease usually have a freely movable, palpable mass, at time it may cause pain, particularly when women are in the premenopausal phase of the menstrual cycle, however, breast pain can be caused by lesions other than fibrocystic changes. The palpable lesion may appear to increase and decrease is size cyclically; usually achieving its maximum size in the premenstrual phase of the menstrual cycle. Cystic disease is frequently accompanied by varying degrees of epithelial hyperplasia in adjacent ducts and lobules (9). In patients

17

who have one particular form of fibrocystic disease (the proliferate form), the incidence of cancer increased very slightly (10).

1.3. Malignant Breast Tumors

1.3.1. Incidence

Breast cancer is the most common malignant tumors in women (11), and it is the leading malignancy affecting women in North America and Europe. In 2000, approximately 184200 new cases of invasive breast cancer were diagnosed in the United States. The number of noninvasive breast cancer is hard to verify, but it probably account for and an additional 20000 to 30000 new cases; thus, the number of invasive and noninvasive breast cancer treated in 2000 approximately 200000 (12).

In Iraq, according to the results of Iraqi Cancer Registry (ICR), breast cancer accounting for (31.11%) and remained the commonest tumors in the year 2000 (13-15), it was also shown that breast cancer was the first among the commonest ten cancers in Iraq. Figure (1.1) represents the population of breast cancer in Iraq for the last nine years. As shown in the same figure, the population of breast cancer increased more than double in the last nine years (16).

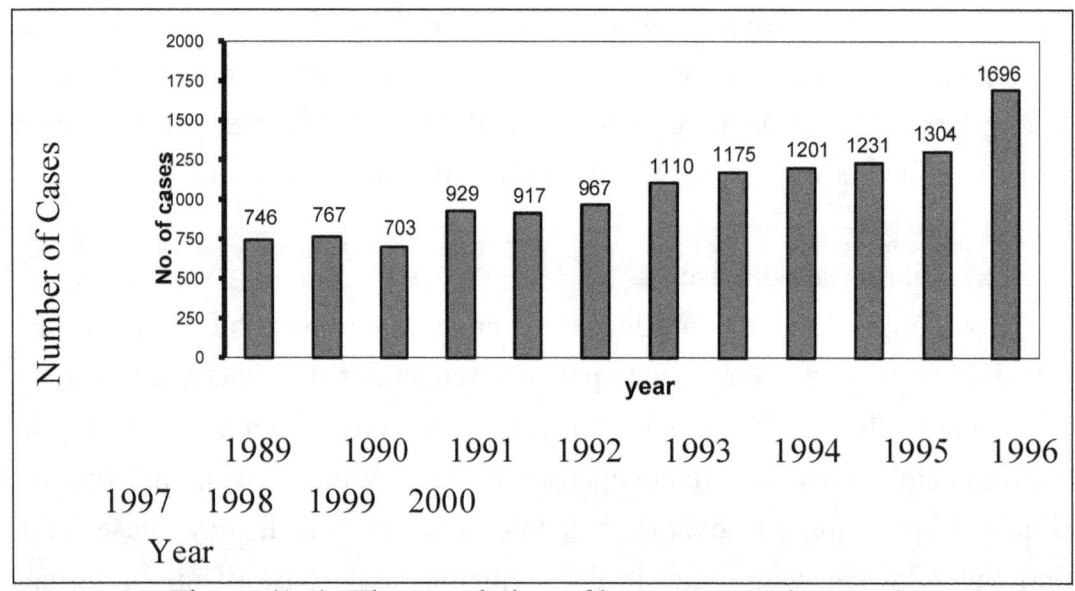

Figure (1.1): The population of breast cancer in Iraq through (1989-2000)(13-16).

1.3.2. Etiology and Risk Factors in Breast Cancer

Numerous risk factors have been associated with the development of breast cancer, such as genetic, environmental, hormonal, and nutritional.

Despite all available data on breast cancer risk factors, 75% of women with this cancer have not exposed to any risk factors (17).

1.3.2.1. Genetic Factors

Breast cancer is the result of mutations in one or more critical genes. Two genes in women on chromosome 17 have been implicated. The most important gene is called BRCA-1; the other is the P53 gene. A third gene is BRCA-2 on chromosome 13 (11).

1.3.2.2. Increasing Ages

Breast cancer is uncommon before age 25 years, but then there is a steady rise to the time of menopause, followed by a slower rise throughout life. The average age at the diagnosis is 64 years (4).

1.3.2.3. Family History

The overall relative risk of breast cancer in women with a positive family history in a first –degree relative (mother, daughter, or sister) is 1.7. Premenopausal onset of the disease in a first–degree relative is associated with three-fold increase in breast cancer risk, whereas postmenopausal diagnosis increases relative risk by only 1.5. When the first degree has relative bilateral disease, there is fivefold increase in risk. The relative risk for a woman whose first-degree relative developed both bilateral and premenopausal breast cancer is nearly nine. No increased risk has been demonstrated when only a second-degree relative (aunt, cousin, or grandmother) has had breast cancer (17).

1.3.2.4.Proliferative Breast Disease

The diagnosis of certain condition after breast biopsy is also associated with an increased risk for the subsequent development of invasive breast cancer(17) . Women with proliferative disease of the breast with a typical hyperplasia (atypia) are at increased risk for developing breast cancer (five-fold increase), however. The risk for atypia is greater in patient with a strong family history of breast cancer (11-fold increase) (11) .

1.3.2.5. Personal Cancer History

A personal history of breast cancer is significant risk factor for the subsequent development of a second, new breast cancer. This risk has been estimated to be as high as 1% per year from the time of diagnosis of the initial cancer. Women with a history of endometerial, ovarian, or colon cancer also have a higher likelihood of developing breast cancer than those with no history of these malignancies (17).

1.3.2.6. Menstrual and Reproductive Factors

Early onset of menarche (<12 years old) has been associated with a modest increase in breast cancer risk (two fold or less). Women who undergo menopause before age 30 have a twofold reduction in breast cancer risk when compared to women who undergo menopause after age 55. A first full-term pregnancy before age 30 appears to have a protective effect against breast cancer, whereas a late first full-term pregnancy or nulliparity may be associated with higher risk, There is also suggestion that lactation protects against breast cancer development (17).

1.3.2.7. Environmental Factors

Women exposed to therapeutic radiation or after atom bomb exposure have a higher rate of breast cancer. Risk increases with younger age and higher radiation doses (4). Radiation is believed to cause 1-2% of all cancer deaths(18,19). In respect to pollution studies, which have shown that there is a well-established correlation between many pollutants and cancer, it has been estimated, that 1% of cancer deaths is due to air, water and land pollution (20).

1.3.2.8. Hormonal Influences

Endogenous estrogen excess, or more accurately, hormonal imbalance, clearly plays a significant role. Many risk factors mentioned-long duration of reproductive life, nulliparity, and late age at first child-imply increased exposure to estrogen peaks during the menstrual cycle (4).

1.3.2.9. Dietary Factors

Diets that are high in fat have been associated with an increased risk factor for breast cancer (21). It has been suggested that differences in dietary fat content may account for the variations in breast cancer incidence observed among different countries. Sala et.al, illustrated that certain macronuterients and food such as protein, carbohydrate and meat intake influence of risk of breast cancer through their effects on breast tissue morphology (22). Data from prospective studies have confirmed that the relationship exists between alcohol intake and risk of developing breast cancer (23). Alterations in endrogenous estrogen levels secondary to obesity may enhance breast cancer risk (17).

1.3.2.10. Lactation

In the search of practical methods to prevent breast cancer, lactation has strong evidence as a potentially modifying factor especially at early age and for long period. There is a significant reduction in the risk of breast cancer associated with lactation for more than two years. This effect appeared to be limited to premenopausal women (24). Lactation may reduce the risk of breast cancer by interrupting ovulation or by modifying pituitary and ovarian hormone secretions. Direct physical changes in the breast that accompany milk production may also contribute to prevent the effect (25).

1.3.3. Histopathology of Breast Cancer

Most cancer of the breast is a carcinoma of the epithelial cells that line breast ducts and lobules. Rarer forms of cancer occurring in the breast arise from the stromal cells that surround the epithelial glands (12). Breast cancer is a complex, devastating diseases and the most frequently diagnosed cancer in women. It is the single leading cause death for women of age 20-59 years (26).

There are a various type of breast carcinomas according to (WHO) classification (3) :

1.3.3.1. In Situ Carcinoma (Non-Spreading Type)

A. Ductal Carcinoma In Situ (DCIS)

The malignant cells in this disease are confined to the ductal basement membrane (27). DCIS usually occurs without forming a mass because there is no scirrhous component (11).   DCIS is also known as intraductal carcinoma.

B. Lobular Carcinoma In Situ (LCIS)

LCIS is composed of smaller lobular or acinar cells and fills the terminal breast lobule with a homogenous proliferation; most clinicians currently regard LCIS as a risk factor for the development of invasive breast cancer. LCIS is usually not treated, but affected women are placed under frequent   surveillance (28,29).

1.3.3.2. Infiltrating Carcinoma (Invasive Carcinoma)

A. Infiltrating Ductal Carcinoma (IDC)

Most invasive carcinoma of the breast is ductal in origin (11). Infiltrating (invasive) breast carcinoma differs from intraductal carcinoma (ductal carcinoma in situ) by the presence of stromal invasion, through which tumor cells spread not only locally but also regionally and distantly via vascular lymphatic space (30).

B. Infiltrating Lobular Carcinoma (ILC)

This type is rare, from about (5%-10%) of breast cancer. It is begins in the milk-secreting glands of the breast. It is often multicentirc, several areas of thickening may occur in one or both breasts. It is characterized by the presence of small and relatively uniform tumors cell growing singly around lobules involved by in situ lobular neoplasia (31).

1.3.4. Staging System of Breast Cancer (11)

The standard staging system for breast cancer is the TNM system table (1.2). The TNM classification devised by the International Union Against Cancer (UICC) and accepted by the American Joint Commission on Cancer Staging a world standard (32). Another system is the Colombia Clinical Classification (CCC), formulated by Haagensen and Stout (33). Although this system was a valuable precursor and is easier to remember than the TNM, it is a less precise classification where stage A represents a tumor confined to the breast; stage B include tumors with clinical axillary lymph node enlargement; stage C represents the presence of grave prognostic sings in the breast; and stage D indicates metastatic disease. The TNM based on the clinical features of tumor (T), the regional lymph nodes (N), and the presence or absences of distant metastases (M) (34). The purposes of staging are the following (23):

- Plane a therapeutic strategy that most appropriate for the patient.
- Allow for more intelligent prognostication of the disease statues of the patient.
- Permit comparison of therapeutic results obtained from different sources by different means.

Table (1.2): TNM System and Stage Grouping (35).

T	Primary tumor
TO	No evidence of primary tumor
Tis	Carcinoma in situ
T1	Tumor 2 cm or less in greatest diameter
T2	Tumor more than 2 cm but less than 5 cm in greatest diameter
T3	Tumor more than 5 cm in greatest diameter
T4	Tumor of any size with direct extension to chest wall or skin
N	Regional lymph nodes

Table (1.2): Continued.

N0	No regional lymph node metastases
N1	Metastasis to movable ipsilateral axillary lymph node(s)
N2	Metastasis to ipsilateral lymph node(s) fixed to one another or to other structures
N3	Metastasis to ipsilateral internal mammary lymph node(s)
M	Distant metastasis
Mo	No distant metastasis
M1	Distant metastasis (including metastasis to ipsilateral supraclavicular lymph nodes)

Stage 0	Tis	No	Mo
Stage I	T1	No	Mo
Stage IIA	T0	N1	Mo
	T1	N1	Mo
	T2	N0	Mo
Stage IIB	T2	N1	Mo
	T3	N0	Mo
Stage IIIA	T0	N2	Mo
	T1	N2	Mo
	T2	N2	Mo
	T3	N1/N2	Mo
Stage IIIB	T4	Any N	Mo
	Any T	N3	Mo
Stage IV	Any T	Any N	M1

1.3.5. Treatment of the Breast Tumors

The goal of any oncologic treatment is to maximize the cure and at the same time optimize the quality of life (36).

1.3.5.1. Surgical Therapy

Surgical treatment represents most frequently used and the most successful sign method of cancer therapy currently available. More patients are cured of cancer by surgery than by any other therapeutic modality (37).

1.3.5.2. Conservation Breast Cancer Surgery

It is aimed at removing the tumor plus a rim of at least (1 cm) of normal breast tissue. This is commonly referred to as a wide local excision or lymphectomy (38).

1.3.5.3. Mastectomy

Removal of all breast tissue, choice may not be offered if the lesion is too large, multi-focal, and lobular or, in the surgeon's opinion, so close the nipple that it is likely to cause distortion (39).

1.3.5.4. Radiotherapy

Palliative radiotherapy may be advised for locally advanced cancers with distant metastasis in order to control ulceration, pain, and other manifestation in the breast and regional nodes (40). Radiotherapy is especially useful in the treatment of the isolated bony metastasis, chest wall recurrence and brain metastasis (41,42).

1.3.5.5. Chemotherapy

Breast cancer is responsive to all major classes of cytoxic drugs: alkylating agents, antimetabolites, mitotic inhibitor, and the antitumor antibiotic(43). Among the most active are alkylating agent including cyclophosphamide and thaitepa, and anthracyclines such as doxorubicin. The antimetabolites methotrexate (MTX) and 5–flourouracil (5-FU) are also active. Numerous combination of chemotherabutic agents have been evaluated in the treatment of metastatic breast cancers such as: CMF, CAF (44-47).

1.3.5.6. Endocrine Therapy

Hormonal therapy is the initial treatment of metastatic disease in patients with ER or PR positive tumors. Tamoxifen, a nonsteroidel antiestragon was approved first for the treatment of metastic breast cancer over 20 years ago, is usually the first agents of choice because of its favorable toxicity profile.(48,49)

1.3.6. Detection and Diagnosis (50)

Although an accurate history and clinical examination are still the most important method of detecting breast disease, there are a number of investigations that can assist in the diagnosis as follows:

1.3.6.1. Self Examination

All women over age 20 should be advised to examine their breast monthly–premenopausal women should perform the examination 7-8 days after the menstrual period. The breast should be inspected initially while standing before a mirror with the hands at the side, overhead, and pressed firmly on the hips to contract the pectoralis muscles. Masses asymmetry of breasts and slight dimpling of the skin may become apparent as a result of these maneuvers. Next, in a supine position, each breast should be carefully palpated with the fingers of the opposite hand. Some women discover small breast lumps more readily when their skin is moist while bathing or showering. Most women do not practice self-examination, and its value is controversial. Clearly, however, it is not harmful, it is inexpensive, and it may be beneficial (35).

1.3.6.2. Mammography

Soft tissue x-rays are taken by placing the breast in direct contact with ultrasensitive film and exposing it to low-voltage, high-amperage x-rays. The dose of radiation in approximately 0.1 Gy and therefore mammography is a very safe investigation (50).

1.3.6.3. Ultrasound

Ultrasound is particularly useful in young women with dense breasts in whom mammograms are difficult to interpret, and in distinguishing cysts for solid lesions. It can also be used to localize impalpable breast lumps (50).

1.3.6.4. Magnetic Resonance Imaging (MRI)

MRI is of increasing interest to breast surgeons in a number of settings, it can be useful to distinguish scar from recurrence in women who have had previous breast conservation therapy for cancer (although it is not accurate within 9 months of radiotherapy because of abnormal enhancement); it is the gold standard for imaging the breast of women with implants; it may prove useful as a screening tool in high-risk women; and it is being evaluated in the management of the axilla in both primary breast cancer and recurrent disease (50).

1.3.6.5. Needle Biopsy/Cytology

Histology can be obtained by using a fine needle such as a trucut or corecut biopsy device under local anesthesia. Cytology is obtained by using a 21 or 23 gauge needle and 10 mL syringe with multiple passes throughout the lump without releasing the negative pressure in the syringe. The aspirate is then smeared on to a slid, which is air-dried. Fine needle aspiration cytology (FNAC) is the least invasive technique to obtain a cell diagnosis and is very accurate if both operator and cytologist are experienced. However, false negatives do occur mainly through sampling error, and invasive cancer cannot be distinguished from in situ disease (50).

1.3.6.6. Triple Assessment

In any patients who presents with a breast lump or other symptoms suspicious of carcinoma, the diagnosis should be made by a combination of clinical assessment, radiological imaging and tissue sample taken for either cytological or histological analysis (50).

1.4. Tumor Markers
1.4.1. Definition of Tumor Marker (51)

A tumor marker is a substance present in or produced by a tumor or by the tumor's host in response to the tumor's presence that can be used to differentiate a tumor from normal tissue or to determine the presence of a tumor based on measurement in the blood or secretions. Such a substance can be found in cells, tissue or body fluids. It can be measured qualitatively or quantitatively by chemical, immunological, or molecular biological methods to identify the presence of a cancer.

Tumor markers are the biochemical for immunological counterparts of the differentiation state of the tumor. In general, tumor markers represents re-expression of substances produced normally in embryoginically closely related tissues. Few markers are specific for a single individual tumor (tumor-specific markers); most are found with different tumor of the same tissue type (tumor-associated markers). They are present in higher quantities in cancer tissue or in blood from cancer patients than in benign tumors or in the blood of normal subjects (51).

1.4.2. Routes of Tumor Markers Production

Benign tumors are generally well differentiated. The cells in a benign tumor are similar to the cells of the normal tissue, and the tumor markers produced are the products found in the normal tissue. They may be found in increased amounts in the circulation depending on the size of the tumor.

Malignant tumors may produce substance may associated with normal cell, or they may be different. As a zygote is transformed into an embryo, which then evolves into a fetus, the rapidly dividing cells became differentiated into specialized tissues by selective gene expression. The genes expressed are responsible for the production of hormones, enzymes, receptors, structural proteins, and cell metabolism. When a normal cell is transformed into tumor cell, gene expression changes. The affected cell may lose its ability to synthesize some specific cell products, or it may manufacture greatly increased amounts. The cell may be less specialized than the tissue it evolved from and assume the characteristics of the less well-differentiated cells of the embryo, synthesizing proteins found in the embryo but not in a normal adult. Cell proliferation rates change as the metabolic rate of the cells increases. After the cell is transformed, it loses growth control and begin to divide rapidly. The cells lose contact inhibition and invade the primary site. They then invade the adjacent organs and blood and lymph system, which may carry the cells to distance organs. The cell may then lodge in a capillary bed and begin to invade the new site. As this invasion process takes place, new proteins are produced that actively aid in the invasion. These proteins can also be used as markers. (52)

1.4.3. Classification of Tumor Markers

Tumor markers may be classified into chemical and genetic tumor markers. (52)

1.4.3.1. Chemical Tumor Markers

Table (1.3) summarizes the chemical tumor markers classified according to biochemical characteristics, and their associated malignancy. The table shows the low specificity of tumor marker for cancer (52).

Table (1.3): Chemical tumor markers (51).

Marker	Example	Associated Malignancy
Enzyme	Alcohol	Liver
	Alkaline phosphatase	Bone, Liver, Leukemia, Sarcoma
	Alkaline phosphatase Placental	Ovarian, Lung, trophoplastic gastrointestinal, seminoma, Hodgkin's
	Amylase	Pancreas, Various
	Aryl Sulfatase B	Colon, breast
	Galactosyi transferase	Colon, bladder, gastrointestinal, Various
	Neuron-Specific enolase	Lung (small-cell), neuroblastoma, carcinoid, melanoma, Pheochromocytoma,
	Prostate-specific antigen (PSA)	Prostate Various (Large bowel. Lung, ovarian)
	Telomerase	Colorectal, Breast, etc.
	Sialyl transferenase	Colon, Breast, Lung
Hormone	ACTH	Gushing's syndrome, lung (small – cell)
	Antidiuretic hormone	Lung (small - cell) adrenal cortex,
	Calcitonin	Medullary thyroid
	Growth hormone hCG	Pituitary adenoma, renal, lung, Embryonal choriocarcinoma testicular
	Human placental	Trophoblastic, gonads, lung, breast
	Parathyroid hormone	Liver, renal, breast, lung, various
	Prolactin	Pituitary adenoma, renal, lung. Breast
	Vasoactive intestinal	Pancreas, bronchogenic,
	Peptide 5	Pheochroinocytom neuroblastoma

Table (1.3): Continued.

Oncofetal Antigen	□-Feto protein	Hepato cellular, germ line (non-
	□-oncofeta antigen	Colon
	Carcino fetal ferritin	Liver
	CEA	Colorectal, gastrointestinal,

	Pancreatic oncofetal	Pancreatic
	Sequamous cell antigen	Cervical, lung, skin, head and neck
	Tennessee antigen	Colon, gastrointestinal, bladder
Mucin	CA 125	Ovarian, endometrial
	CA 15-3 (Episialin)	Breast, Ovarian
	CA 27-29	Breast
	MCA	Breast, ovarian
	Du-PAN-2	Pancreatic, ovarian, gastrointestinal,
Blood group related antigen	CA 19-9	Pancreatic, hepatic; gastrointestinal
	CA 19-5	GastrointestinaT, pancreatic, ovarian
	CA50	Pancreatic, colon, gastrointestinal
	CA 27.4	Ovarian, breast, colon,
	CA 242 1	Ovarian, breast, colon,
Protein	□2-Microglobulin	Multiple myeloma, □-cell
	C-peptide	Insulinoma
	Ferritin	Liver, lung, breast, leukemia
	Immunoglobuin	Multiple myeloma, lymphomas
	Melanoma associated antigen	Melanoma
	Pancreas associated	Pancreatic, stomach
	Pregnancy specific	Trophopiastic, germ cell
	Prothrombin precursor	Meato cellular
	Tumor associated trypsin	Ovarian
Others	Estrogen and progesteron	Breast
	Catecholamine	Neuroblastoma, pheochromocytoma
	Hydroxy proline	Bone metastasis (breast) multiple
	Lipid-associated sialic	Gastrointestinal, lung. Rheumatoid
	Polyamine	Brain, various

1.4.3.2. Genetic Tumor Markers (51)

Two classes of genes are implicated in the development of cancer: Oncogenes (Cell activation genes–table 1.4) and suppressor genes (genes involved in the recognition and repair of damaged DNA-table 1.4). Oncogenes are derived from proto-oncogenes, which may be activated by dominate mutations. The type of mutation could be point mutation, insertion, deletion, translocation, and inversion. Most oncogenes code for proteins that function at the same stage of activation of cells for proliferation, and there activation leads to cell division. Most oncogenes are associated with hematological malignancies, such as Leukemia and to a lesser extent, solid tumors.

The other class of tumor genes the suppressor genes has been isolated from mostly solid tumors. The oncogenicity of suppressor genes is derived from the loss of the gene rather than their activation, as with oncogenes. The major tumor suppressor gene, P53, functions to repair damaged DNA by apoptosis (programmed cell death).

Repair is mediated by activation of the production of P21, which blocks the cell cycle in late G1 to allow repair to take place. The loss of function of this gene may result in the inability of the DNA repair process and lead to the development of tumorgensis.(53)

The exciting promise of using detection of oncogenes and suppressor genes, for the diagnosis, determining the prognosis, and predicting the response to chemotherapy remains to be realized. However, oncogenes detection remains an experimental approach to human cancer, with great expectations not yet fulfilled. The ability to develop cancer by detection of mutations in tumor suppressor genes raises ethical questions that remain to be resolved.

Table (1.4): Classification of genetic tumor markers (52) .

Marker	Example	Associated Malignancy
Oncogene	N-ras mutation	Acute myeloid leukemia neuroblastoma
	K-ras mutation	Leukemia, lymphoma
	C-myc	b-and T-cell lymphoma., small cell
	C-erb B-2	Breast, ovarian, gastrointestinal
	C-abllber	Chronic myelocytic leukemia
	N-myc	Neuroendocrine
	bcL-2	Leukemia, iymphoma
Suppressor Gene	VHL mutation	Kidney
	APC mutation	Colorectal

	PI 6 (cd Kn2)	Bladder, glioblastoma, melanoma
	WT1 mutation	Wilms', tumor
	Loss of	Wilms', breast, hepatoblastoma
	BRCA2, PB1	Breast
	RB1 mutation	Retinoblastoma, osteosarcoma small-
	PI 6 E-cadheim	Breast
	BRCA1 mutation	Neurofibromatosis 1 Melanoma, breast
	P53 mutation	Breast, colorectal, lung, liver, renal cell,
	DCC mutation	Colorectal
	NF2 mutation	Neurofibro matosis2, meningioma

1.4.4. Clinical Applications of Tumor Mrkers (54)
The potential uses of tumor markers are summarized in table (1.5). In general, tumor markers may be used for diagnosis and prognosis of carcinomas and for monitoring the effects of therapy as well as targets for localization and therapy. Ideally, a tumor marker should be produced by tumor cells and be detectable in body which fluids should not be present in healthy people or in benign conditions. Therefore, it could be used for screening for the presence of cancer in symptomatic individuals in general population.

Most tumor markers are present in normal, benign, and cancer tissues. They are not specific enough to be used for screening cancer. In situations where the incidence of cancer is high among certain populations, screening might be possible.

Table (1.5): Clinical Usefulnees of tumor markers (55).

	Biochemical properties	Molecular weight	Primary clinical applications
Alpha-fetoprotein (AFP)	Glycoprotein, 4% carbohydrate; considerable	~70 KD	Diagnosis and monitoring of primary hepatocellular carcinoma and germ

	homology with albumin		cell tumors. Prognosis of germ cell tumors.
Cancer antigen 125 (CA 125)	Mucin identified by monoclonal antibodies	~200 KD	Monitoring ovarian carcinoma. Prognosis after chemotherapy
Cancer antigen 15-3 (CA 15.3, BR 27.29)	Mucin identified by monoclonal antibodies	>250 KD	Monitoring breast cancer
Cancer antigen 72.4 (CA 72.4)	Glycoprotein identified by monoclonal antibodies	~48 KD	Monitoring gastric carcinoma
Cancer antigen 19-9 (CA 19-9)	Glycolipid carring the Lewisa blood group determinate	~1,000 KD	Monitoring pancreatic carcinoma
Carcinoembri-yonic antigen (CEA)	Family of glycoproteins, 45%-60% carbohydrate	~180 KD	Monitoring gastrointestinal and other adenocarcinomas
CYFRA 21-1	Fragments of cytokeratin	~30 KD	Monitoring bladder and lung carcinoma
Estrogen receptor	Nuclear transcription	65 KD	Predicting response to endocrine therapy in breast cancer

Table (1.5): Continued.

Human chorionic gonadotrophin (hCG)	Glycoprotein hormone consisting of tow non-	~36 KD	Diagnosis and monitoring non-seminomatous germ cell tumors ,

			choriocarcinomas , hydtidiform moles , seminomas. Prognosis of germ cell tumors.
Neuron specific enolase (NSE)	Dimer of the enzyme enolase	~87 KD	Monitoring small cell lung carcinoma , neuroblastoma , apudoma.
Placental alkaline phosphatase (PLAP)	Heat-stable isoenzyme of alkaline phosphatase	~86 KD	Monitoring of germ cell tumors (seminomas)
Progestero ne receptor	Nuclear transcription factor	A from: 94 KD B from: 120 KD	Predicting response to endocrine therapy in breast cancer .
Prostate specific antigen (PSA)	Glycoprotein serine protease	~36 KD	Diagnosis , screening and monitoring prostatic carcinoma
Squamous cell carcinoma antigen (SCC)	Glycoprotein sub-fradion of tumor antigen T4	48 KD	Monitoring squamous cell carcinomas
Tissue polypeptide antigen (TPA)	Fragments of cytokeratin 8,18 and 19	~22 KD	Monitoring bladder and lung carcinoma
Tissue polypeptide specific antigen (TPS)	Fragment of cytokeratins 18	~22 KD	Monitoring metastatic breast carcinoma

1.4.5. Tumor Markers in Breast Cancer (56)

Several tumor markers have been investigated for one or more clinical use in breast cancer (Table 1.6).

Tumor-associated antigens (TAAs) that have been associated with breast cancer include carcinoembryonic antigen (CEA); tissue polypeptide antigen (TPA), tissue polypeptide-specific antigen (TPS), gross cystic disease protein (GCDP); prostate specific antigen (PSA); and the products of the MUC-1 gene. The MUC-1 gene encodes a cell-associated mucin-like protein. Secretary epithelial cells such as breast epithelial cells express this antigen. Several assays detect the MUC-1 gene products, but they are not identical. These proteins have been identified by monoclonal antibodies to breast cancer cell lines, breast cancer tissue, or human milk fat globule membranes. Assays that detect circulating MUC-1 products include CA 15-3, CA 27-29, CA 549, breast cancer mucin (BCM), mammary serum antigen (MSA), and mucin-like carcinoma-associated antigen (MCA) (57).

The results obtained with these assays may not be identical, presumably due to reactivity of different antibodies to different epitopes, and/or different sensitivities and specificities that result from different assay configurations (46).

More recently, markers of tumor biology have been investigated in breast cancer (Table 1.6), and molecules related to angiogenesis, adhesion, invasion, and metastases. Several, but not all of these are indeed, detected with immunologic assays, and could arguably be designated as TAAs.

Table (1.6): Tumor markers that have been investigated in breast cancer(56)

Tumor-associated antigens
Carcinoembryonic antigen (CEA)
Products of or related to products of the MUC-1 gene
CA 15-3

CA 27-29
CA 549
Breast cancer mucin (BCM)
Mammary serum antigen (MSA)

Table (1.6): Continued.

Mucinous carcinoma antigen (MCA)
Tissue polypeptide antigen (TPA)
Tissue polypeptide-specific antigen (TPS)
Gross cystic disease protein (GCDP)
Prostate-specific antigen (PSA)
Markers of tumor biology
Extra-ceullular domain (ECD) of c-erbB-2/HER2/neu
Molecules of adhesion and invasion
E-selectin
Soluble urokinase plasminogen activator receptor (SuPAR)
Intercellular adhesion molecule-1 (ICAM-1)
Molecules associated with angiogenesis
Vascular endothelial growth factor (VEGF)
Basic fibroblast growth factor (bFGF)
Hepatocyte growth factor (HGF)
HUVEC assay

Antibody response against TAAs
c-erbB-2/HER2/neu
P53

There are several tumor markers correlate with the incidence of breast cancer, but the most important markers are:

1.4.5.1. CEA

Carcinoembryonic antigen is a marker for breast carcinoma (59), lung, gastrointestinal and colorectal (60). CEA is one of the older oncofetal protenis in use. CEA is a large family of related cell-surface glycoproteins with a high molecular mass of 150 to 300 KD, it contains 45 to 55% carbohydrate with increase expression found in a variety of malignancies, including breast cancer(61) .CEA is not recommended for screening, diagnosis, staging or routine surveillance of breast cancer patients following primary therapy (62).

1.4.5.2. TPA

Tissue polypeptide antigen is not a specific tumor marker (63). Antibodies that react with cytokeratin 8,18 and 19 identify it. TPA is a heterogeneous group of molecules with molecular weight range 20-45 KD (64). Both normal and   cancerous cells produce TPA; it is useful in the monitoring of metastic diseases(54).

1.4.5.3. TPS

Tissue polypeptide-specific antigen (TPS) is a new tumor marker defined by monoclonal antibody against the soluble tissue polypeptide antigen (TPA) (65). First described as specific tumor marker by Bjorklund in 1957 (63). In breast cancer patients TPS was especially useful in monitoring response to treatment and effectiveness of therapy in metastatic disease (66).

1.4.5.4. CA 549

CA 549 is an acidic glycoprotein and it is a marker for breast carcinoma. CA 549 is not useful in detecting early breast carcinoma but it is useful is detecting recurrence of breast cancer in patients after initial therapy followed by adjuvant therapy (67).

1.4.5.5. CA 27.29

CA 27.29 is detected by a monoclonal antibody B 27.29 (68), this is produced against antigen in ascites of patients with metastatic breast carcinoma. CA 27.29 test above 37.7 KU.L-1 were considered positive, its most useful in monitoring metastatic breast carcinoma (69).

1.4.5.6. CA 125

CA 125 is a high-molecular mass (>200 KD) glycoprotein recognized by the monoclonal antibody OC 125. The level of CA 125 is measured quantitatively by using immunoradiometric assay (70). In healthy population, the upper limit of CA 125 level is 35 KU.L-1. CA 125 is elevated in ovarian carcinoma, endometerial, pancreatic, Lung, breast, colorectal and other gastrointestinal tumors (71,72). CA 125 is useful to detecting residual disease in cancer patients following initial therapy (73).

1.4.5.7. Mammary Antigen

Several new antigens have been recognized by monoclonal antibodies. Which have been identified in patients with breast cancer (74). They have been proposed as "tumor markers":

- MCA

Mucin-like carcinoma associated antigen (MCA) is a mucin glycoprotein with a molecular mass of 350 KD. MCA was identified on the surface of a breast carcinoma cell line by the monoclonal antibody b-12 (54). MCA level is elevated in 60% of metastatic breast cancer patients (75) .

- MAM-6

MAM-6 an epithelial membrane antigen present on ductal and alveoli epithelial cells that is detected by monoclonal antibody raised against human milk-fat globule membranes (76). Partial characterization of the antigen by

SDS-PAGE showed that the antigen is a polymorphic epithelial sialomucin with a molecular mass over 400 KD (77).

- MSA

Mammary serum antigen (MSA) was detected by an antibody raised against a whole cell suspension of intraductal breast cancer (74).

1.4.5.8. Galectin-4

A protein Galectin-4 is expressed in non-invasive and invasive breast cancer but not in normal cell. An anti-Galectin-4 antibody was able to detect the presence of Galectin-4 very specifically. Galectin-4 is specific diagnostic marker of breast cancer whose patterns of expression at early stages of disease could identify those patients with a high risk of progression to aggressive cancer (78).

1.4.5.9. Cathepsin-D

Cathepsin-D is a glycoprotein with molecular weight M.wt: 52 KD. It was discovered in 1979 in the culture medium of hormone dependent human breast cancer. It is a precursor to lysosomal acidic protease. This proteolytic enzyme can react against basement membranes (79).

Cathapsin-D may facilitate cellular actions such as migration, metastasis, and an invasion of other tissues. Estrogen has been shown to stimulate secretion of this tumor marker in certain hormone-dependent breast cancer cell lines. This antigen has been found to have potential application in breast cancer prognosis as its concentration appears to be related to the patients overall change for survival (80,81).

1.5. Carbohydrate Antigen 15-3 (CA 15-3)

CA 15-3 is a breast-associated antigen identified on the apical side of alveoli and ducts of mammary glands and as a circulating antigen (82). Distinct epitopes of this high molecular-weight mucin-like glycoprotein of 300-400 KD(83-85), which carbohydrate side chain account for about 50% (86).

Also known as polymorphic epithelial mucin (87) (PEM), epithelial membrane antigen (88) (EMA) or episialin (89). CA 15-3 can be identified by two monoclonal antibodies DF3 and 115 D8, in a double-determinate or sandwich-type immunoassay (90). The 115 D8 antibody was prepared against human milk-fat globulin membrane (91) while the DF3 antibody was raised against a membrane-enriched fraction of a human breast carcinoma (92).

1.5.1. Structure of CA 15-3

CA 15-3 (Episialin) is synthesized as transmembrane molecule with a relatively large extracellular domain and cytoplasmic domain of 69 amino acids(93). The extracellular domain mainly consists of region of nearly identical repeats population, leading to substantial differences in molecular weights of the CA 15-3 molecules from different individuals (94).

The repeats together with adjacent degenerated repeats contain many serins and threonines that are potential attachment sites for O-liked glycans and constitute the mucin-like domain, which comprises more than half of the polypeptide backbone. The mucin domain of CA15-3 contains many prolines and other helix-breaking amino acids, resulting in a molecule with an extended structure and many β-turns (95). The extended structure is very rigid as aresult of the numerous O-linked glycans attached to the molecule (96). The CA15-3 extends 200 to 500 nm above the cell membrane (97).

1.5.2. CA 15-3 Expression

- CA 15-3 Expression in Normal Tissues

CA 15-3 is predominatly found at the apical side of epithelial cells lining the acini alveoli, or lumens in various organs, i.e. in the mammary glands, salivary glands, sebacious glands, sweat glands, esophagus, stomach, pancreas, bile ducts, lungs, kidney, bladder, prostate, uterus, and rete testis (98-100).

- CA 15-3 Expression In Malignant Tissues

Relative to the expression levels of CA 15-3 found in normal tissues, CA15-3 is often overexpressed several-fold in many types of carcinomas derived from these tissues (101). In these tumors, polarization of the cells is often lost, resulting in the presence of CA 15-3 at the entire cell surface. High levels of CA 15-3 are also detected on carcinoma cells present in pleural effusions on ascites from patients with breast or ovary carcinoma and on many breast carcinoma cell lines.

1.5.3. Biosynthesis of CA 15-3

CA15-3 is synthesized as a large single polypeptide, in most cell lines approximately 200 KD or more (102,103). This precursor is rapidly cleaved by proteolysis in a small moiety, which contains the transmembrane and cytoplasmic domains, and a larger part, which comprises most of the extra cellular domain. Both moieties remain non-covalently associated (104). This proteolytic processing step occurs in the endoplasmic reticulum and may be essential for further maturation. CA 15-3 is mainly processed by adding numerous O-linked glycans, which increases the apparent molecular weight on SDS-polyacrylamide gels to more than 400 KD. The extensive glycosylation protects the molecule against proteolytic degradation, since the precursors without O-linked sugars are degarded rapidly, while the mature molecule is extremely resistant to the action of proteases. The glycosylation also determines the rigidity of the molecule. The last step in the processing of CA15-3 is the addition of sialic acid to the glycans, which increases the mobility of the molecule on SDS-gels (96).

The early proteolytic cleavage step is not directly responsible for the release of CA15-3 for the membrane, which suggests that CA15-3 is most likely released from the membrane by a second proteolytic cleavage step after arrival at the cell surface. The second proteolytic cleavage seems to be a slow and probably a random process, allowing the mucin to remain associated with the cell surface with a half-life of 16-24 hrs (96).

1.5.4. Methodology

The CA 15-3 test from all sources uses both DF3 and 115-D8 antibodies. Serum is initially incubated with a polystyrene bead to which 115-D8 antibody has been attached. This antibody binds to antigenic sites on the glycoprotein, pulling it out of solution. The beads are then washed to remove unbound meterial and incubated with the radioiodine (125I)-labeled DF3 antibody. The radiolabeled DF3 antibody binds its antigenic sites and then the amount of radioactivity is quantitated (105). This is called Immunoradiometric Assay (IRMA).

1.5.5. Biology of CA15-3

- CA15-3 and Cell Adhesion

Similar to mucins in mucus, membran-associated mucins might act as barrier molecules to protect cells against toxic substances, as in pancreatic and bladder ducts. The high densities of CA15-3, due to its extended and relatively rigid structure, might also interfere with the function of the adhesion molecules. In this way, CA15-3 might prevent interactions between opposing apical membrane of polarized normal cells and facilitate the formation and maintenance of the ducts during development (106,107).

In carcinomas, the combination of overproduction and loss of polarization of CA15-3 expression might reduce cell adhesion and facilitate the invasion of tumor cells because CA15-3 might now interfere with the function of molecules required from tissue integrity (104).

- CA15-3 and Immune System

The putative function of CA15-3 in tumor progression may not only be restricted to inhibition of adhesion which will probably result in an increased invasive potential of cells, but CA15-3 overexpression may well be critical to the survival of tumor cells during dissemination (108). A completely different aspect of CA15-3 is its ability to act as a tumor-specific antigen. The underglycosylation of CA15-3 in various tumor cells exposes the protein backbone, leading to the generation of novel epitopes. This could elicit an immune response (109-112).

1.5.6. Clinical Application

In healthy subjects, the upper limit of CA 15-3 concentration is 25 (KU.L-1). At this level, (5.5%) of 1050 normal subjects, (23%) of patients with primary breast cancer, and (69%) of those with metastatic breast cancer show elevated CA 15-3 levels (113).

Elevated CA15-3 levels are also found in other malignancies, including pancreatic (80%), lung (71%), breast (69%), ovarian (64%), colorectal (63%) and liver (28%) cancer. It is also reported to be elevated in benign diseases, although with less frequency (e.g., in benign liver [42%] and benign breast diseases [16%]).

CA15-3 should be used to diagnose primary breast cancer, because the incidence of elevation (23%) is fairly low. CA 15-3 is most useful in monitoring therapy and disease progression in metastatic breast cancer patients. A significant change must be at least (25%) and correlates with disease progression in (90%) of patients, with its regression in (78%). No change correlates with disease stability in (60%). CA 15-3 could replace CEA in metastatic breast cancer owing to its sensitivity and specificity.

1.6. Carbohydrate Antigen 19-9 (CA 19-9)

1.6.1. Marker Definition

CA 19-9 is a carbohydrate antigen identified as a glycolipid-that is, sialylated lacto-N-fucopentose II ganglioside, which is a sialylated derivative of the Lewis a blood group antigen and is denoted as Le a (114). CA19-9 is synthesized by normal human pancreatic and biliary ductular cells and by gastric, colonic, endometerial, kidny, salivary gland, sweat gland and present in ductal epithelium of breast (115-117). In serum it exists as a mucin, a high-molecular weight (200-1000 KD) glycoprotein complete (54). The monoclonal antibody against CA19-9 was developed from a human colon carcinoma cell line, SW-1116 by Koprowski and associates (118).

Monoclonal antibody 19-9 derived from spleen cells of a mouse immunized with human colon adenocarcinoma cell line SW-1116 (119). The epitope of this antibody is carbohydrate with the sugar sequence

NeuNAcα 2-3 Gal β 1-3 GlcNAc β 1-3 Gal…

4

|

Fuc α 1

As described by Magnani et.al. (119).

1.6.2. Methodology

CA 19-9 is measured with a double monoclonal immunoradiometric assay, using monoclonal antibodies raised against the SW-1116 cell line (120). The antibody reacts with CA19-9 found at low concentrations in sera from healthy individuals, but frequently increased in sera from patients with adenocarcinomas (120). The upper limit of normal for healthy subjects has been defined by the cutoff value of 37.0 (U.mL-1) (121). CA 19-9 has become an established marker for pancreatic cancer (121-123), but it must still be regarded as a research test for colorectal cancer.

Another methods to determinate CA 19-9 were enzyme-linked immunosorbent assay. Both the capture and the enzyme-conjugated antibody use the CA 19-9 monoclonal antibody. It should be noted that this antibody is useless for cancer diagnosis when a patient is lacking the enzyme for the synthesis of sialyl Le a. In Japanese, about 5-10% of the population lacks this enzyme. Determination carbohydrate antigen CA 19-9 levels in serum were also measured by radioimmunoassay (RIA) (125). Immunohistochemical technique used for the distribution of CA19-9 in tissues using an immunoperoxidase assay (126).By this technique the CA 19-9 can be detected not only in cancerous tissues but also in non cancerous normal tissues.

1.6.3. Screening

Numerous studies have addressed the potential utility of CA 19-9 in adenocarcinoma of the colon and rectum.

The reported incidence of elevated serum CA 19-9 in colorectal cancer ranges from 20% to 40% (127,128). The incidence of elevated CA 19-9 in stage-related, with the highest sensitivity occurring in patients with metastases (129-131). However, the sensitivity of CA 19-9 was always less than that of the CEA test for all stages of disease (127-130). The false-positive rate (>37.0 U.mL-1) is 15% to 30% in patients with non-neoplastic diseases of the pancreas, liver and biliary tract (131). Consequently, CA 19-9 cannot be used for screening asymptomatic populations.

1.6.4. Monitoring Response to Treatment

Kouri et.al.(132) compared CEA and CA 19-9 for predicting response to chemotherapy in 85 patients. Decreases in CEA more accurately reflect the response to therapy than did the decreases of CA 19-9. The pretreatment CA 19-9 value was, however, an important prognostic factor. Median survival was 30 months for patients with normal CA 19-9 values and 10.3 months for patients with elevated CA 19-9 values. CA 19-9 used to examined the serum levels and immunohistochemistry during the clinical course of female patient treatment with idiopathic interstitial pneumonia (IIp) that had elevated serum levels of CA 19-9 (133).

1.6.5. Clinical Application

Elevated levels (>37 U.mL-1) were seen in patients with pancreatic (80%), hepatobiliary (67%), gastric (40-50%), hepatocellular (30-50%), colorectal (30%), and breast (15%) cancer. Pancreatits and other benign gastrointestinal diseases show a 10 to 20% elevation; however, the levels are usually lower than 120 (U.mL-1). CA 19-9 levels correlate with pancreatic cancer staging (54). CA19-9 is useful in monitoring pancreatic and colorectal cancer. Elevated levels can indicate the recurrence before clinical finding by 1 to 7 months (134). Unfortunately, early detection of relapse may not be useful because of the lack of effective therapy for pancreatic cancer.

ntroduction

The role of tumor markers in breast cancer is to enhance the clinicians, ability to provide more effective management of the disease (135). Serum CA15-3 concentration was determined by using sandwich enzyme immunoassay of a double monoclonal antibody (136,137), automated chemiluminescent immunoanalyzer (138), immunoradiometric assay (139) and radioimmunoassay(140), in women with benign breast tumor and breast cancer.

CA 15-3 has been used in management of patients, with breast cancer. CA 15-3 has been evaluated for its ability to determine diagnosis, prognosis, monitor therapy and predict recurrence of breast cancer following curative surgery and radiation therapy (141,142). Low incidences of CA 15-3 elevation in early stage cancer (stage I and stage II) have been observed (143).

Incidence of abnormal values of CA 15-3 in stage III and stage IV, and a very high CA 15-3 level have been correlated with metastases of breast cancer(144).

Therefore the development of immunoradiometric was planned to carry out the determination of the optimum conditions of 125I-anti CA 15-3 antibody binding with CA 15-3 in breast tumor tissue homogenate, hence determination of CA 15-3.

Chapter Two

CA15-3 in Breast Tumors

Materials and Methods

2.1. Materials

2.1.1. Chemicals

All chemicals and reagents used in this study were of analytical grade, tabulated in the following table.

Table (2.1): Chemicals used and Companies.

Chemicals	Company
1. Immunoradiometric assay kit for CA 15-3 level	Diasorin Inc. (USA)
2. Bovine serum albumin (BSA) , urea , $ZnCl2,CaCl2,NH4Cl$, NaBr, ethylendiamine-tetraaceticdisodium salt (EDTA).	Fluka: (Switzerland)
3. $CuSO4.H2O$, NaK-tartarate glycine, $NaOH,HCl$, $NaCO3,NaF,NaCl,NaI,Na2HPO4$, $NaH2PO4$.	BDH,limited,Poole (UK)
4.Folin-Ciolteau	E.Merck AG. Dastmstapt
5.Blue dextran (2000),sepharose CL-4B.	Pharmacia fine chemicals (Sweden)

2.1.2. Instruments

Table (2-2): Instruments used and Companies.

Instruments	Company
1.Gamma counter type 1270-rack gamma II 2. Spectrophotometer ultraspace type 4050	LKB
3. UV-210 a double beam spectrophotometer	Shimadzu
4.pH-meter	Pye-Unicam
5.Cooling centrifuge; with a maximum speed 5000 r.p.m.	Hettich
Cooling centrifuge type 202-MK; with a maximum speed 13500 r.p.m.	Sigma
7.Memmert water bath, memmert incubator	West Germany

8. SM-shaker	England
9. Combicold rack	LKB

2.1.3. Patients

Three groups of breast tumors patients were included in this study.

Group I   : Consisted of 40 patients with benign breast tumors

Group II : Consisted of 32 premenopausal patients with breast cancer.

Group III : Consisted of 15 postmenopausal patients with breast cancer.

Group IV : Consisted of 10 controls.

All patients were admitted for treatment to (Saddam Medical City, Baghdad Teaching Hospital),(University Hospital, Saddam College of Medicine), (Nursing Home Private Hospital) and (Al-Arabi Private Hospital).

Patients suffered from any disease that may interfere with this study were excluded. All surgical operation of breast tumors were carried out under the supervision of the following surgeons:

Dr. Saab Sedeq, Dr.Munthir Al-Aubaidi, Dr.Azam Qanbar Agha, Dr. Abd Al-Salam Al-Tai, Dr. Zuhair Abid Al-Hadi.

The host information of all patients and normal healthy subjects is summarized in table (2-3).

Table (2.3): The host information of breast tumors patients and healthy subjects studied.

Group	Patients	No.	Age	Type of tumor	Metastases
I	Benign breast tumor	40	18-42	23 fibroepithelial tumor (fibroadenoma)	–
				17 fibrocystic changes (adenosis)	–
II	Premenopausal malignant	32	34-52	22 Infiltrative Ductal	2 lymph

	breast tumor			carcinoma 10 Ductal carcinoma	nodes
III	Postmenopausal malignant breast tumor	15	55-73	Infiltrative Ductal carcinoma	4 lumph nodes
IV	Control	10	25-40		

2.1.4. Preparation of Blood Samples

Five milliliters of blood samples were obtained from patients by venipuncture just before surgery. Ten physically normal age volunteers were used as controls. Blood samples were left for 20 min. at room temperature. After coagulation, sera were separated centrifugation at 3000r.p.m for 10 min., and then sera were aspirated and stored at –20oC until time analysis. The samples were not thawed and refrozen before testing.

2.1.5. Collections of Specimens

The tumors tissues were surgically removed from breast tumor patients by either mastectomy (cancer patients) or lumpectomy (benign tumor patients). The specimens were cut off and immediately rinsed with ice-cold isotonic saline solution. They were collected individually in plastic receptacle and stored at –20 oC until homogenization.

2.1.6. Preparation of Phosphate–Buffered Saline

Phosphate –buffered saline (PBS) 0.15 M, pH 7.2 was prepared as following:

A: Disodium basic phosphate (0.15M); 21.2940g Na_2HPO_4 and 9.0g of NaCl were dissolved in a final volume 1L deionized distilled water.

B:.Monobasic sodium phosphate (0.15M) 17.9970g of NaH_2PO_4 and 9.0g NaCl were dissolved in a final volume 1L deionized distilled water.

Phosphate buffer saline pH 7.2 was prepared by mixing a volume of solution A with appropriate amounts of solution B to obtain the required pH.

2.1.7. Preparation of Breast Tumors Tissues Homogenates

The frozen tissue were weighed, sliced finely and scalped in petri dish standing on ice bath, and then homogenized with fivefold volumes of PBS buffer pH7.2, using manual homogenizer (145). The homogenate was filtered through four layers of nylon gauze in order to eliminate fibers connective tissues, and then centrifuged at 4000 r.p.m for 45 min. at 4 oC in order to precipitate the remaining intact cells and the intact nucleus. The supernatant fraction at this speed was separated, divided in aliquots and freezed-20 oC until use.

2.1.8. Statistical Analyses

Students' t-test was used to determine if the mean values of studied parameters were significant different in the individual groups included in this work. $P < 0.05$ were considered significant (146).

2.2. Methods

2.2.1. Protein Determinations

Total homogenate protein content was determined by the method of Lowry (147), using bovine serum albumin (BSA) as the standard.

Figure (1.1) represents the standard curve of protein, which was constructed by plotting the absorbance at 600 nm against standard protein concentrations

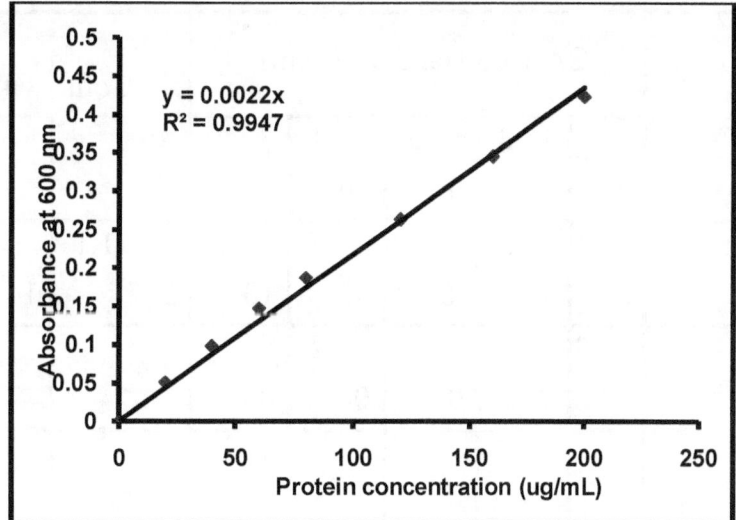

Figure (2.1): Standard curve of protein concentration. (All other details are explained in the text).

2.2.2. Determination of CA 15-3 Levels in Sera of Breast Tumors Patients

51

Reagents

The following reagents provided in the CA15-3 IRMA kit from Dia–Sorin-U.S.A. were used:

• Tracer: two vials each one contained 1.0 µ Ci/mL (37.1 KBa /mL). CA15-3 antibody labeled with 125I in 10 mL / Tris buffer with protein stabilizer and preservative.

• CA15-3 standards: The vial contained 100 mL, which represented 0 U.mL-1. There are four vials, 1.2 mL in each vial with different concentrations of human CA15-3 (25, 50, 100, 200) U.mL-1 in Tris. buffer with protein stabilizer and preservative.

• One bottle contained 100-coated beads, Anti-CA15-3-mouse, monoclonal.

• One vial contained 0.5mL CA15-3 control, CA15-3 in re-calcified human plasma with preservative.

Procedure

The assay protocol is described in table (2.4).

Table (2.4): IRMA protocol of serum CA 15-3 (U.mL-1) (All other details are explained in the text).

	CA 15-3 standard (U.mL-1)					Cont rol	Unknown samples	
	0	25	50	100	200		1	2-etc.
Reaction trays no.	1.2	3.4	5.6	7.8	9.10	11.12	13.14	15.16-etc.
Standard (µL)	200	200	200	200	200	–	–	–
Control serum or samples (µL)	–	–	–	–	–	200	200	200
125I-anti CA15-3	200	200	200	200	200	200	200	200

The specimens and reagents must be brought to room temperature (20-30 oC) before opening. The reaction trays and data sheets were marked.

First Incubation

The specimens and the control were diluted to (1:15) prepared by adding 20 µL of specimen or control to 1000 µL CA15-3 standard, 0 U.mL-1 in a tube marked proper identification of specimen. Two hundred microliters of diluted specimen and control were pipette to their assigned wells. Two hundred microliters of each standard was pipette to its assigned well (standards are not to be diluted). One bead was dispensed into each well and the adhesive cover sealer was applied. After incubation for 2hrs at room temperature, the adhesive cover sealer was removed and the liquid was aspirated, then each bead was washed three times with 5 mL distilled water.

Second Incubation

Two hundred microliters of 125I-antiCA15-3 was pipetted on each bead. The adhesive cover sealer was applied again. After incubation time for 3hrs at room temperature, the cover was removed and the liquid was aspirated from wells, then the beads were washed as it is above. The beads were transferred to the counting tubes, and then the tubes were counted for 1 min.

Calculations

The standard curve was constructed by plotting counts per min. (Y axis) versus concentration for CA15-3 standard (X axis), figure (2-2). Then the points were connected with straight-line segments.

The CA15-3 concentration of specimens and control were determined directly from the standard curve.

2.2.3. Preliminary Test of CA 15-3 Binding to 125I -Anti CA15-3 Antibody in Breast Tumor Homogenate

Reagents

Phosphate buffered saline 0.15 M; pH 7.2 was prepared as described in section (2.1.6).

Procedure

The supernatant and pellet were centrifuged and detected by using ordinary tubes. In order to detect CA 15-3, 100 µL of the supernatant breast homogenate having (900µg protein) were incubated with 50 µL (0.35 mg.mL-1) of 125I -anti CA15-3.The volume of reaction was completed to 500 µL with PBS buffer pH7.2, then incubated at 37 oC for 2hrs. The assay tubes were centrifuged at 4000 r.p.m. for 45 min. at 4 oC.

The supernatant was discarded, the rim at each tube was swabbed with cotton, and then gamma counter counted the complex formed for one minute. The pellet of CA 15-3 was estimated by dissolving the sediment in PBS-buffer pH 7.2 with the ratio 1:5 (weight: volume) shaking was then carried out. Hundred microliters of the supernatant fraction of the sediment having (540 µg.mL-1 protein) was added to 50 µL (0.35 mg.mL-1) of 125I -anti CA 15-3 antibody. The same steps mentioned in this experiment were followed to determine the radioactivity of the complex formed. For total count two additional tubes with 50µL of 125I –anti CA 15-3 antibody were counted in gamma counter.

Calculations

1. The counted radioactivity in each tube (expressed in c.p.m.) represents the bound fraction (B), (i.e., 125I antiCA15-3 antibody/CA 15-3 complex).

2. The counted radioactivity in the tubes containing 125I-anti CA15-3 antibody only represents the total count (T).

3. The (B/T) ratio for each tube counted as follows:

$$(B/T)\% = \frac{Sample \ Counts \ (B)}{Total \ Counts \ (T)} \times 100$$

2.2.4. Factors Effecting of 125I-Anti CA-3 Antibody Binding to CA 15-3 in Breast Tumors Homogenates

2.2.4.1. The Effect of Different Amounts of Protein Concentration of the Tumor Homogenate on the Binding with 125I-Anti CA 15-3 Antibody

Reagents

All reagents prepared as described previously in sections (2.1.6) and (2.2.3).

Procedure

1. Fifty microliters (0.35 mg.mL-1) of 125I -anti CA 15-3 antibody were added to 100μL of the supernatant (benign Fibroadenoma, pre-and post-menopausal malignant breast tumors (IDC) respectively) containing increasing amounts of protein (50, 100, 150, 200, 250 μg.mL-1) then completed to a final volume of reaction to 500 μL with 0.15 M PBS pH 7.2.

2. The assay tubes were then incubated for 2 hrs at 37oC.

3. Two additional tubes, containing 50μL (0.35 mg.mL-1) of 125I –anti CAB-3 antibody only, for total counts were set-aside until counting.

4. At the end of incubation, the assay tubes were centrifuged at 4000 r.p.m for 45 min at 4oC.

5. The supernatant were decanted, the rims at the tube were swabbed with cotton piece.

6. The radioactivity of the complex were counted using gamma counter.

Calculations

1. The B/T percent were determined according to section (2.2.3).

2. The percent of binding values B/T were plotted versus the increasing amount of protein of the breast tissue homogenate.

2.2.4.2. The Effect of 125I -Anti CA15-3 Antibody Concentration on the Binding

Reagents

All reagents prepared as described previously in section (2.1.6) and (2.2.3).

Procedure

1. Fifty microliters of increasing concentration (0.070,0.140,0.175,0.350, 0.701 mg.mL-1) of 125I -anti CA 15-3 antibody were added to 100μL of

homogenate (benign breast tumor (Fibroadenoma), pre-and post-menopausal malignant breast tumors) (IDC) containing (100, 100, 200 µg.mL-1 protein) respectively.

2. The volume of reaction was made up to 500 µL with PBS pH 7.2.

3. Steps 2,3,4,5 and 6 of the experiment (2.2.4.1) were repeated.

Calculations

1. The same mathematical equation mentioned in section (2.2.4.1) was used to calculate (B/T)%.

2. Values of (B/T)% were plotted versus concentration of labeled antibody (125I -anti CA15-3 antibody).

2.2.4.3. The Effect of pH on the Binding

Reagents

All reagents prepared as described previously in section (2.1.6) and (2.2.3).

Procedure

1. One hundred microliters of human homogenate (benign breast tumor (Fibroadenoma), pre-and post-menopausal malignant breast tumors (IDC)) containing (100,100,200, µg.mL-1 protein) were added to 50µL (0.175, 0.175,0.140mg.mL-1) of 125I -anti CA15-3 antibody respectively.

2. Each mixture was completed to 500 µL with PBS of different pH ranging (6.8-8.0).

3. Step 2,3,4,5 and 6 of the experiment (2.2.4.1) were repeated.

Calculations

1.Values of (B/T) % were calculated as described in section (2.2.4.1).

2. (B/T)% were plotted against their corresponding pH.

2.2.4.4. Time Course of the Binding of 125I -Anti CA15-3 Antibody to CA 15-3 in Breast Tumors Homogenates

Reagents

All reagents prepared as described previously in sections (2.1.6) and (2.2.3).

Procedure

1.   One hundred microliters of homogenate (benign breast tumor (Fibroadenoma), pre-and post-menopausal malignant breast tumors (IDC)) containing (100,100,and 200 μg.mL-1 protein) were incubated with 50μL of 125I -anti CA15-3 antibody concentration (0.175,0.175 and 0.140 gm.mL-1).

2.   The volume of reaction was made up to 500 μL with PBS pH (7.0,7.6 and 7.8).

3.   All tubes were incubated at 37oC at different time intervals (30, 60, 90, 120, 150 and 180) min.

4.   Step 3,4,5,6 of the experiment (2.2.4.1) was repeated.

5.   To determine the time course of CA 15-3 binding to 125I –anti CA 15-3 antibody at different temperatures. Steps 1, 2, 3 and 4 in the same experiment were repeated at different temperatures (5, 15, 25, 45°C).

Calculations

1. The values of (B/T)% were calculated as described in section (2.2.4.1) at each time and temperature used.

2. The values (B/T)% was plotted against the time of incubation at different temperatures.

2.2.4.5. The Effect of Different Halides on the Binding

Reagents

1. Phosphate buffer (PB) were prepared as described in section (2.1.6) without the addition of NaCl .

2. Halid reagents were prepared in concentration of 0.01M PB at pH (7.0, 7.6 and 7.8) individually, by dissolving each of 0.021gm of NaF, 0.0292gm of NaCl, 0.0515 gm of NaBr, and 0.075gm of NaI in a final volume 50μL of PB and the pH was adjusted.

3. The breast tumors homogenates (benign breast tumor (Fibroadenoma)) were prepared as described in section (2.1.7), except using PB-buffer instead of PBS at the same pH and concentration carried out the homogenization.

Procedure

1. One hundered microliters of each group homogenate (benign breast tumors (Fibroadenoma) and pre-post menopausal malignant breast tumors (IDC)) containing (100,100 and 200 µg.mL-1 protein) were incubated with 50 µL of 125I -anti CA 15-3 antibody concentration (0.175,0.175 and 0.140 gm.mL-1). The volume was made up to 500 µL with PB pH (7.0, 7.6 and 7.8) containing 0.01 M of the following halides: NaF, NaCl, NaBr and NaI in each assay tube. (A sample without the addition of any salt was used as a control).

2. The assay tubes were then incubated for 90min. at 45, 15 and 45°C for the three groups individually.

3. Steps 3, 4, 5 and 6 of the experiment (2.2.4.1) were repeated.

Calculations

1. The values of (B/T) % were calculated as described in section (2.2.4.1).

2. (B/T)% was plotted against halides concentrations.

2.2.4.6. The Effect of Monovalent and Divalent Cations on the Binding

Reagents

1. PB was prepared as described in section (2.1.6) without addition of NaCl.

2. Monovalent and divalent cations salts were prepared in concentration of (0.025 M) PB at pH (7.0,7.6 and 7.8) individually, by dissolving each of 0.0931gm of KCl, 0.0668gm of NH4Cl, 0.2541 gm of MgCl2.6H2O, 0.1388 gm of CaCl2.2H2O, 0.2474gm of MnCl2.4H2O, 0.3150 gm of CuSO4.5H2O and 0.1703gm of ZnCl2, in a final volume 50 mL of PB and the pH was adjusted.

Procedure

1. The same steps mentioned in section (2.2.4.5) were followed to determinate the effect of monovalent and divalent of CA 15-3 in the tissues homogenates of (benign breast tumors (Fibroadenoma) and pre-and postmenopausal malignant breast tumors (IDC)) with 125I -anti CA 15-3 antibody, except the PB buffer containing (0.025M) of the following salts:

KCl, NH4.Cl, MgCl2.6H2O, CaCl2.2H2O, MnCl2.4H2O, CuSO4.5H2O, ZnCl2.

2. A sample without the addition of any salt was used as control.

Calculations

1. The values of (B/T)% were calculated as described in section (2.2.4.1)

2. (B/T)%was plotted against monovalent and divalent cations salts concentrations.

2.2.4.7. Recovery of CA 15-3

Reagents

1. All reagents are described previously in section (2.1.6) and (2.2.3).

2. Standard concentration of CA 15-3 200 U.mL-1 was used.

Procedure

Known concentration of CA15-3 (200 U.mL-1) was added to the three groups of tissues homogenates (benign breast tumors (Fibroadenoma), and pre-and post-menopausal malignant breast tumors (IDC)). The experiment was carried out at optimum conditions that were obtained in experiments of (2.2.4). The CA15-3 was determined according to the experiment in section (2.2.3).

Calculations

1. The bound (c.p.m) of the reaction mixture (standard CA 15-3 was added to tissue homogenate) with 125I -antiCA15-3 antibody, represent the measured value.

2. The bound (c.p.m.) of CA 15-3 in tissue homogenate with 125I – antibody CA 15-3 antibody only , represent the expected value.

3. The recovery % (yield%) was calculated as follows:

$$Recovery\% = \frac{Measured\,values}{Expected\,values} \times 100$$

2.3. Results and Discussion

Human breast tissues in this study were classified according to type of breast tumors (benign and malignant) and the malignant breast tumors were again classified into sub groups (premenopausal and postmenopausal). Each type was examined histologically according to WHO classification. Homogenization was carried out in a cold medium (i.e.4°C) to avoid protein denaturation (148,149), by proteolytic enzymes (150). The filtration of the tissue homogenate through several layers of nylon gauze was used to remove any suspended pieces unhomogenized fragments and blood vessels.

Determination of CA 15-3 Levels in Sera of Breast Tumors Patients

CA 15-3 levels in sera of patients with benign breast tumors (group I) and pre and post-menopausal malignant breast tumors (group II and group III) were measured by IRMA method. These three groups were matched with a group of control subjects.

Table (2.5) summarizes the groups and the mean concentrations of CA15-3 for the control women and patients with benign breast tumors and pre-and post-menopausal malignant breast tumors.

Table (2.5) showes that CA15-3 levels in three different groups (benign breast tumors and pre-and post-menopausal malignant breast tumors) were significantly elevated ($p<0.05$) for benign breast tumors and highly significantly elevation ($p<0.0001$) for pre-and post menopausal malignant breast tumors respectively, as compared with the control.

The mean serum CA15-3 level of the control was found to be (17.26 ± 4.06 U.mL-1) as shown in table (2-5), and the cutoff values was (25 U.mL-1) that obtained from (mean +2 SD). This cutoff value is in agreement with Geraghty J.G(151), other study obtained that cutoff value of 40 U.mL-1 (152), 22 U.mL-1 (153), 30 U.mL-1 (154).

It has shown that widely different cutoff value which was described ranging from 20-40 U.mL-1 in different reference (155-159).

According to Bon et al (160) the upper limit of CA 15-3 of normal may be method-dependent. No association between the CA 15-3 and either age or menopausal status was found in the control group. Therefore , the cutoff values do not require adjustments related to these variables. These results were in agreements with Gion M.et.al. (68). Figure (2.3) shows the distribution of the individual values of CA15-3 in sera of patients with benign breast tumors and pre-and post menopausal malignant breast tumors and control, were determined by using the standared curve in figure (2-2).

It was found that the mean of serum CA 15-3 concentration in 20 patients with benign breast tumors was 21.9 ± 6.6 U.mL-1 (mean $\pm$ SD). These results are in agreement with Hayes D.F. et.al (161). The results show there was highly significant correlation between serum connections of CA15-3 in both groups pre-and post-menopausal status with control, while it was significantly lower in benign breast tumors status.

This is in agreement with Ichihara S. et.al (162). Therefore all of the cases used in the binding studies were concentrated to this type of carcinoma (IDC) and this type is the common type of breast cancer. In Iraq very high levels of CA15-3 advanced disease and the value 5 to 10 times of normal suggest the presence of metastasis. Increasing numbers of metastatic sites correlate with increasing CA15-3 levels (163,164).

These findings suggest that higher levels of CA15-3 represent the breast cancer extent and reflect the cell differentiation and aggressiveness of the tumor. Therefore, it could be concluded that the determination of CA15-3 before surgical operative may be useful as a prognostic factor in breast cancer.

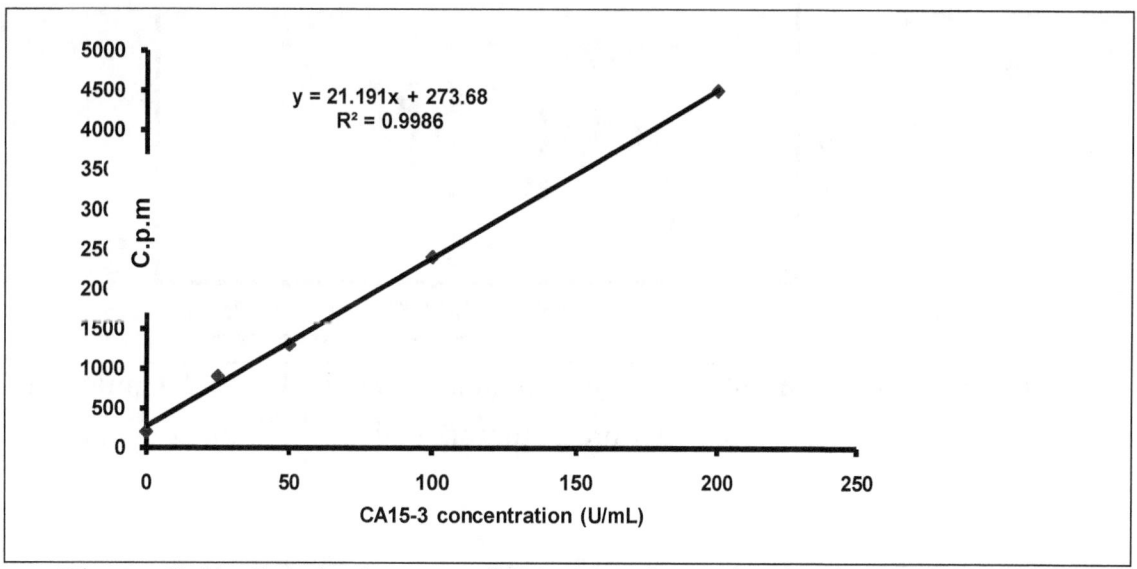

Figure (2.2): Standard curve of CA 15-3 determination in human sera by IRMA method.(All other details are explained in the text).

Table (2.5): Sera CA15-3 levels (U.mL-1) in patients with benign and malignant breast tumors. (All details are explained in the text).

Group	Patients	No. of cases	Age range (Year)	Sera CA15-3 U.mL-1 (mean ± SD)	P values
I	Benign breast tumors	20	18-42	21.9 ± 6.6	P<0.05
II	Premenopausal malignant breast tumors	16	34-52	37.3 ± 6.8	P<0.0001
III	Postmenopausal malignant breast tumors	12	55-73	60.3 ± 10.9	P<0.0001
IV	Control	10	25-40	17.3 ± 4.06	--

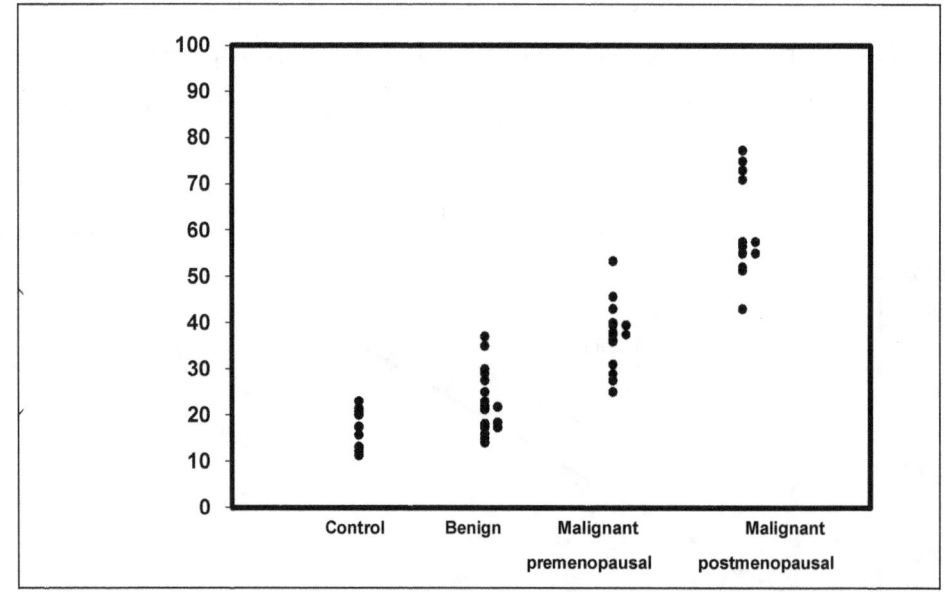

Figure (2.3): Distribution of the individual value of CA15-3 U.mL-1 in the sera of benign and malignant breast tumors patients. (All other details are explained in the text).

Binding Studies of 125I-Anti CA15-3 Antibody with CA15-3 in Benign and Malignant Breast Tumors Homogenates

Preliminary Test of the Binding of 125I-Anti CA15-3 Antibody with CA

Supernatant and pellet formed at speed (4000 r.p.m.) in three groups of human breast tumor homogenate (benign breast tumors, pre-and post-menopausal malignant breast tumors) were used in this experiment. In each fraction CA 15-3 was detected through the incubation of 125I-anti CA15-3 antibody with supernatant fraction and pellet individually for 2hrs at 37°C in PBS buffer as a medium to complete the reaction. The separation of the bound antibody from the unbound was carried out at 4000 r.p.m. for 45 min. to precipitate the (125I-anti CA15-3 antibody/CA15-3) complex formed. Preliminary experimental conditions used in Table (2.6), which is show, the amount of binding B/T% in both fractions. The data revealed that CA15-3 was higher in incidence according to B/T%.

Table (2.6): Incidence of CA15-3 in supernatant and pellet fractions in three different breast homogenate.

Groups	(B/T)%		CA15-3 U.mL-1 in supernatant fraction kit
	Supernatant Fraction	Pellet Fraction	
Benign	6.20	3.40	90
Premenopausal	8.04	5.53	356
Postmenopausal	6.31	4.64	144

B/T% in supernatant is more than in pellet fractions of this speed (4000 r.p.m.). According to these results supernatant fractions was collected and the pellet was then discarded. The CA15-3 levels in the supernatant of breast tumors homogenate were determined according to IRMA method.

In general, results show that CA15-3 concentration in pre-and post-menopausal malignant breast tumors homogenates is more than benign breast tumors homogenates. These results are in agreement with the result obtained from B/T% from IRMA developed method.

From these results, it can be said that developed method was useful for determination CA15-3 in breast tumors homogenate using 125I-anti CA15-3 antibody.

Factors Effecting of 125I-Anti CA15-3 Antibody Binding to CA15-3 in Breast Tumors Homogenates

The Effect of Different Amounts of Protein Concentration of the Tumor Homogenate on the Binding with 125I-Anti CA 15-3 Antibody

To obtain the optimum protein of homogenate for the binding of CA15-3 with 125I-anti CA15-3 antibody, the supernatant homogenate containing increasing amount of CA15-3 in the presence of fixed amount of 125I-anti CA15-3 antibody as it was mentioned in section of (2.2.4.1).

Figure (2.4) represents the quantitative precipitation curve in which the amount of (125I-anti CA15-3 antibody/CA15-3) complex in three groups (benign breast tumors and pre-and-post menopausal malignant breast tumors) was plotted as a function of CA15-3 concentration.

As shown in this figure, in the first phase of the reaction no precipitate was formed. The amount of precipitate increased until a point of maximum binding was reached. After this point as the amount of CA15-3 increased the amount of precipitate diminished; thus the increase in protein concentration which would increase the number of binding site and hence increase the percent of binding until the saturation state at (100, 100, and 200 µg.mL-1) homogenate concentration for (benign breast tumors, pre-and post menopausal malignant breast tumors respectively).

The complex precipitate out of solution because of the multivalent nature of both molecules (165). The radioactive antibody has two binding sites, it can cross-link antigenic sites of two different CA15-3 molecules and can produce maximum complex formation and therefore maximum precipitate will occur. When CA15-3 is in greater excess, large complex are again less probable.

In all subsequent experiments the amonts of (100, 100 and 200 µg.mL-1 protein) of tissue homogenate in benign breast tumors and pre-and post menopausal malignant breast tumors were used according to the result obtained in this experiment.

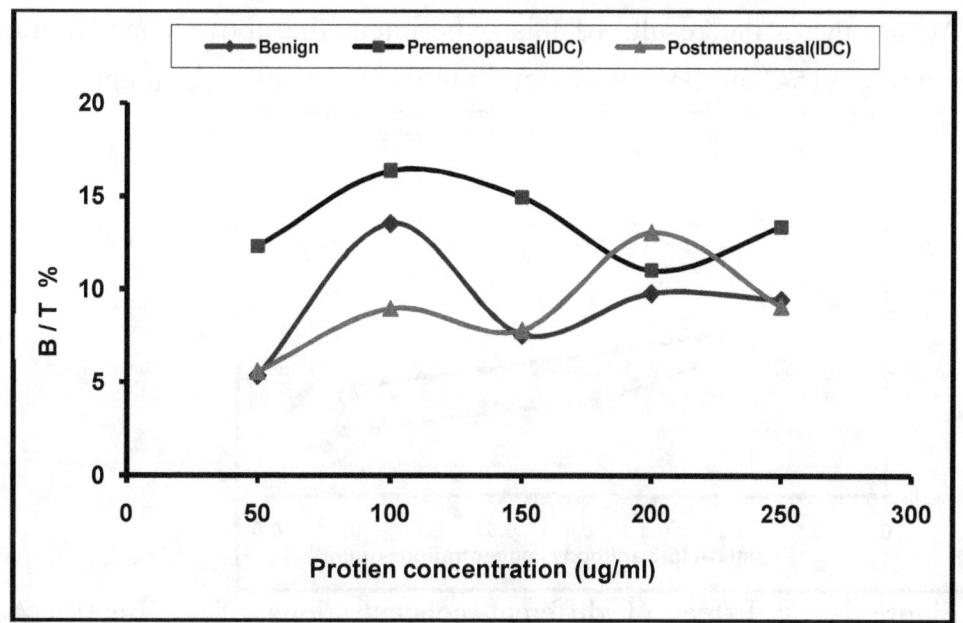

Figure (2.4): Influence of increasing protein concentration on the binding with 125I-anti CA15-3 antibody. (All other details are explained in the text).

The Effect of 125I-Anti CA15-3 Antibody Concentration on the Binding

The experiment was carried out in the presence of fixed amount of protein concentration of the homogenate and increasing concentration of 125I-anti CA15-3 antibody.

The results are illustrated in figure (2.5). Which represent 125I-anti CA15-3 antibody binding curve with supernatant fraction of benign breast tumor, pre-and post-menopausal malignant breast tumors. As shown in figure (2.5) it is obvious that the amount of (125I-anti CA15-3 antibody/CA15-3) complex rises gradually, and then the breast tumor protein was saturated with 125I-anti CA15-3 antibody. When the amount of antibody is in moderate excess, the probability of cross-linking of Ag by Ab in the incubation mixture is more likely, and hence large complex formation is favored. Then the maximum B/T percent was detected. The presence of (0.175, 0.175, 0.14 mg.mL-1) of 125I-anti CA15-3 antibody in benign, pre-and post-menopausal breast tumors homogenates give the optimum concentration of 125I-anti CA15-3 antibody in three groups. Then the binding percent decreased as the amount of 125I-anti CA15-3 antibody increased.

This is because all antigenic sites are covered with antibody and complex formation is inhibited (166). These results indicate that the binding is principally dependent on the amount of the antibody in the reaction mixture (167).

According to the results of this experiment the above concentration of 125I-anti CA15-3 antibody was used in the subsequent experiments.

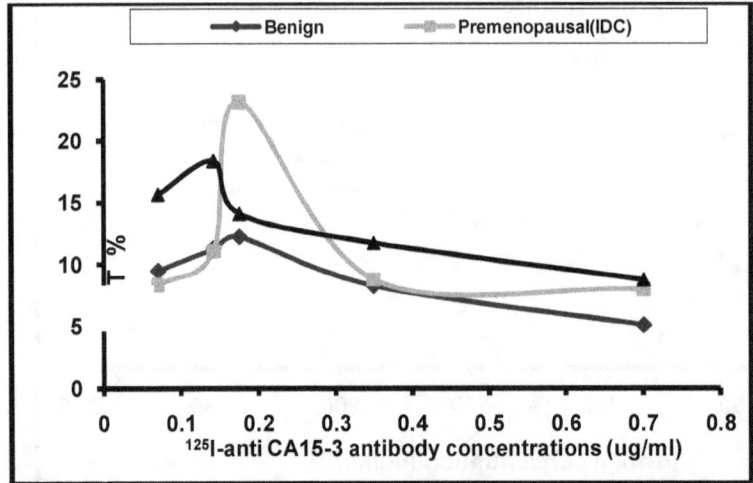

Figure (2.5): Effect of different concentrations of 125I-anti CA15-3 antibody on the binding of with CA15-3. (All other details are explained in the text).

The Effect of pH on the Binding

Figure (2.6) shows the values of the binding of 125I-anti CA 15-3 antibody to CA 15-3 in benign breast tumor, pre- and post-menopausal malignant breast tumors, at different pH values. Maximum value of the binding occurs at (pH 7, pH 7.6, pH 7.8) for benign breast tumor, pre-and post-menopausal malignant breast tumors respectively.

The formation of (125I-anti CA 15-3 antibody/CA 15-3) complex is usually performed at pH between 6.8-8.0; the results indicate that the shift in the pH of the environment may affect the properties of CA 15-13 molecules involved in the binding. This effect may include the protonation deprotonation processes occurring within the possible ionizable groups of the amino acids present in the binding domain of these molecules (168).

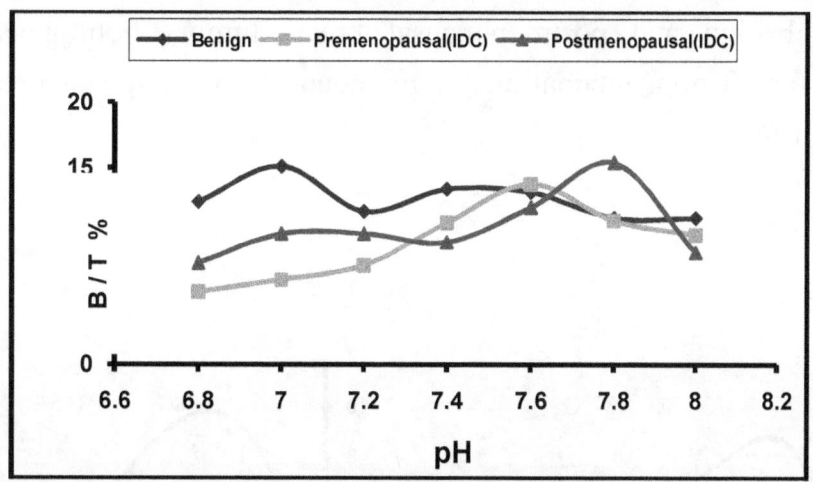

Figure (2.6): Effect of pH on the binding of 125I-anti CA 15-3 antibody with CA 15-3 in breast tumors homogenates. (All other details are explained in the text).

Time Course of the Binding of 125I -Anti CA15-3 Antibody to CA 15-3 in Breast Tumors Homogenates

The results of time course pattern at different temperatures (5, 15, 25, 37, 45oC) indicate the 125I-anti CA 15-3 antibody binding to crude fractions of CA 15-3 is temperature and time dependent process, as shown in figures (2.7), (2.8) and (2.9). The maximum binding was obtained at 45oC after incubation for 90 min. in crude fractions of benign breast tumors and postmenopausal malignant breast tumors respectively, whereas the binding in crude fractions of premenopausal malignant breast tumors occurs at 15oC after incubation for 30 min.

The decrease of the binding activity may be due to reversible dissociation of (125I-anti CA 15-3 antibody/CA 15-3) complex after reaching the equilibrium state.

At 45oC the CA 15-3 molecule preserve the nature of protein structure and gave the maximum binding, but at higher temperature than 45oC denaturation may occur.

In the premenopausal malignant breast tumors the maximum binding occurs at 15oC for 30 min., in this state the energy is enough to overcome the energy barrier and give the maximum binding (169), the decrease in binding after 15oC may be due to proteolytic enzyme.

The difference in incubation time to give the maximum binding may be due to the different source of CA 15-3. According to this results, the binding studies of the subsequent experiments were carried out a 45oC for 90 min incubation for benign and postmenopausal breast tumors homogenate, whereas 15oC for 30 min. incubation for premenopausal malignant breast tumors homogenate.

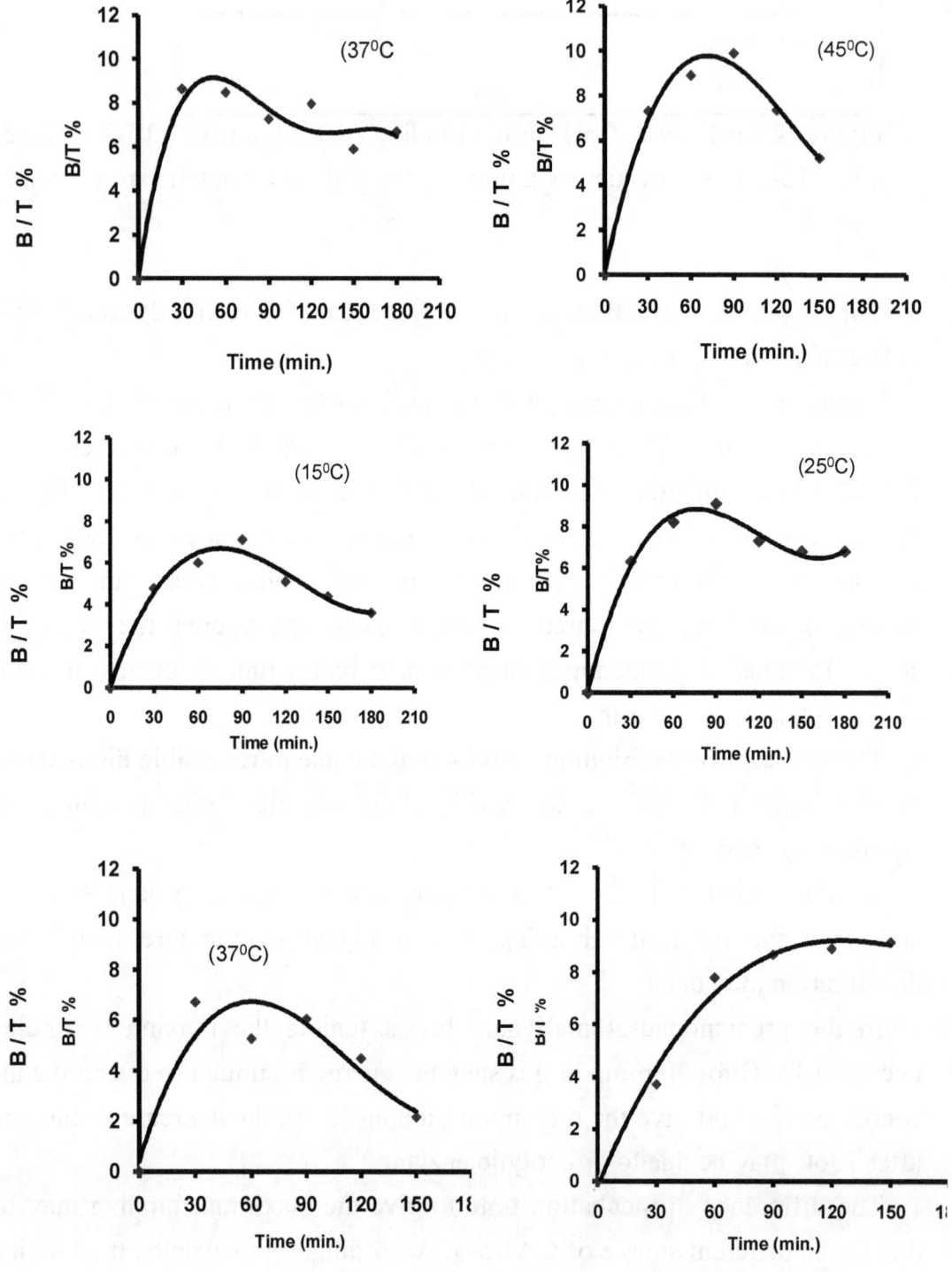

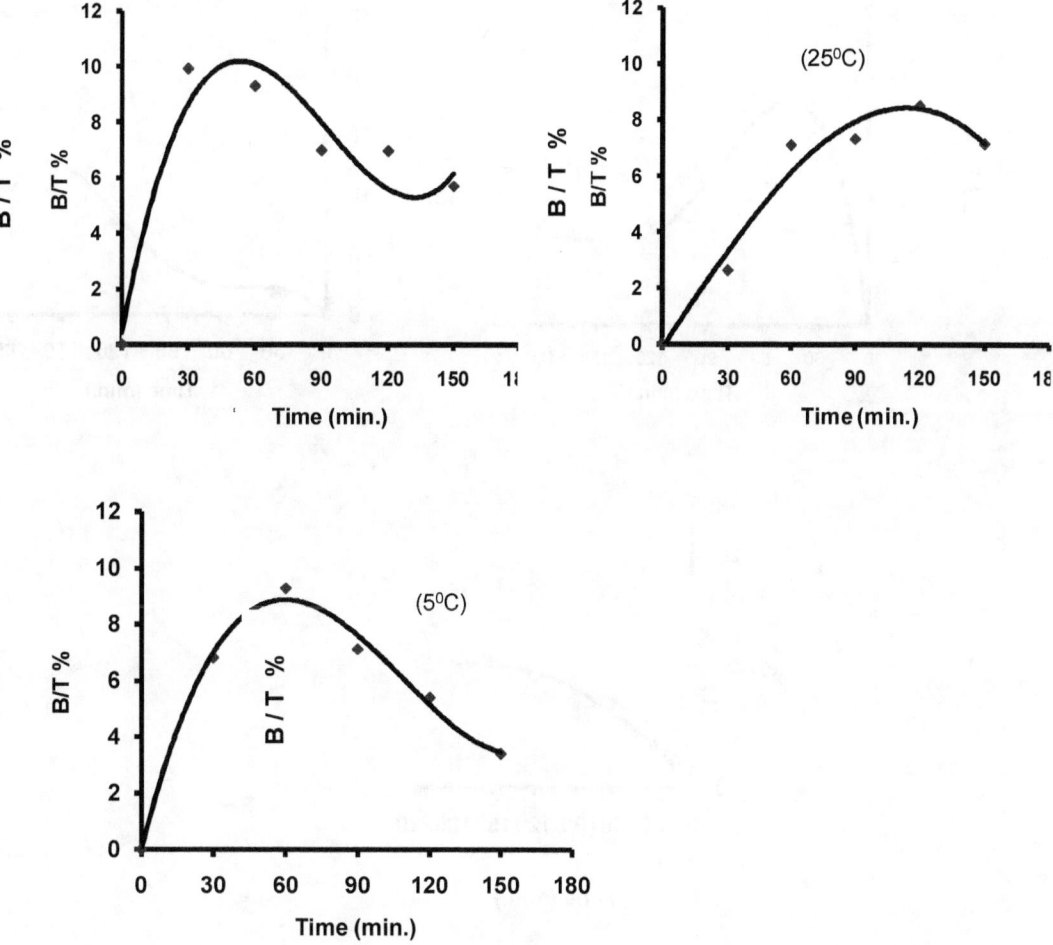

Figure (2.8): Time course of the binding of 125I-antiCA15-3 antibody with CA15-3 in premenopausal malignant breast tumor. (All other details are explained in the text).

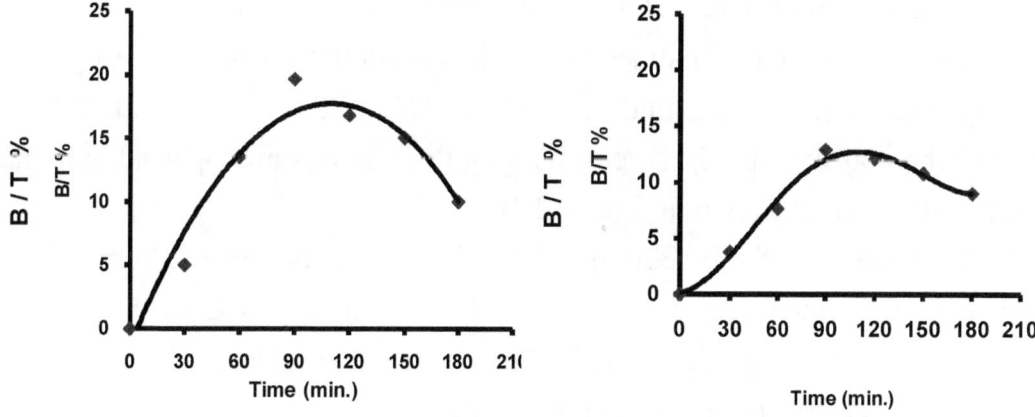

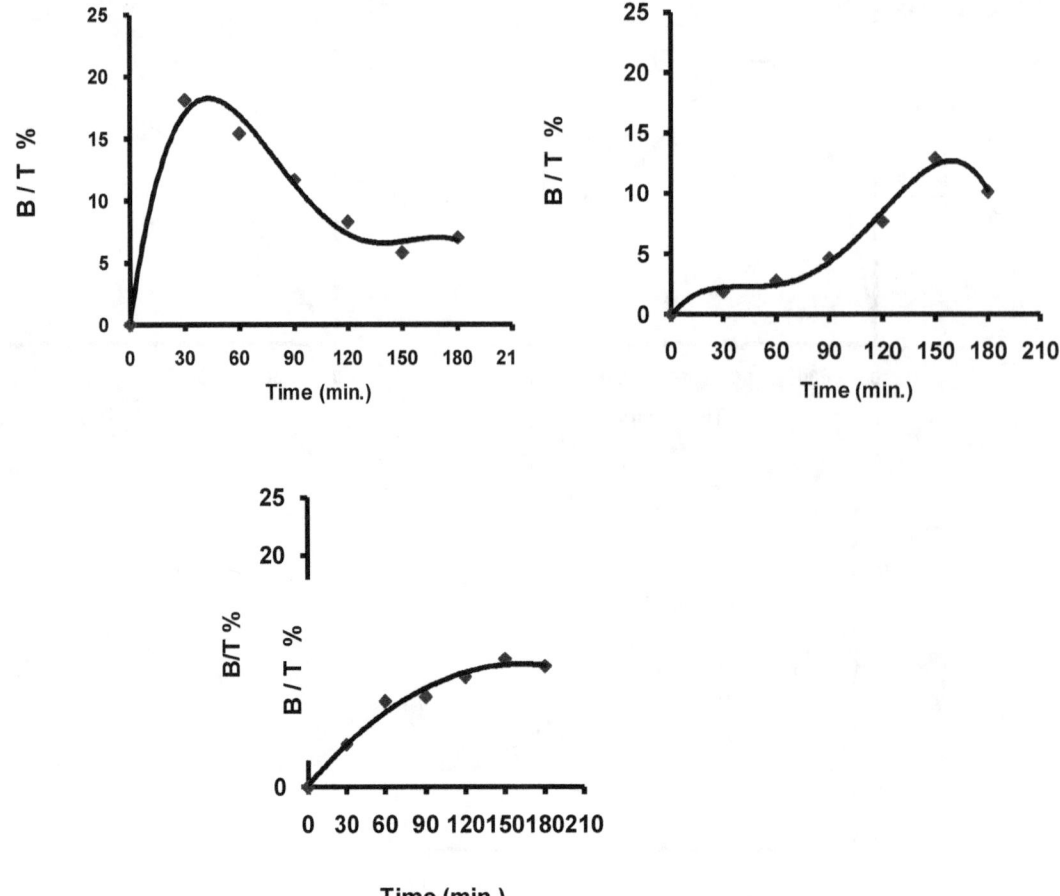

Figure (2.9): Time course of the binding of 125I-antiCA15-3 antibody with CA15-3 in postmenopausal malignant breast tumor. (All other details are explained in the text).

The Effect of Different Halides on the Binding

Different sodium halides at 0.01 M concentration were investigated to study their action on the binding 125I-anti CA 15-3 antibody with CA 15-3 in the three groups (benign breast tumors, Pre-and postmenopausal malignant breast tumors), as shown in figure (2.10).

The presence of the sodium halides in the incubation medium tends to promote the binding of 125I-anti CA 15-3 antibody to CA 15-3 in these groups, the following sequence of effects have occurred.

1. Benign breast tumor tissue homogenate

NaI > NaBr > NaCl > NaF

2. Premenopausal breast cancer tissue homogenate

NaCl > NaI > NaBr > NaF

3.Postostmenopausal breast cancer tissue homogenate

NaCl > NaBr > NaF > NaI

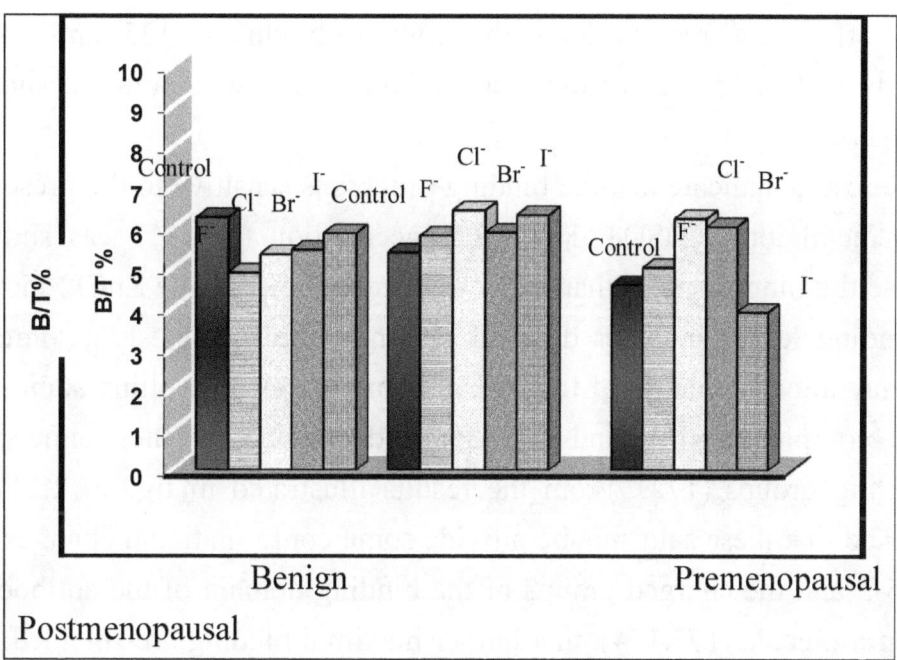

Figure (2.10): Effect of different halides on the binding of 125I-anti CA 15-3 antibody with CA 15-3. (All other details are explained in the test).

As shown in figure (2.10), the sodium halides inhibited the binding in benign breast tumors, according to the decreasing ionic radius and increasing radius of hydration. It seemed that fluoride ion causes lower binding, this could be due to higher electro negativity of fluoride ion that tend to interact with the positive residue in the binding site of the antibody and/or the antigen which lead to decrease the interaction between CA 15-3 and its antibody (170).

Melander and Horvath (1977) reported that the effect of halide salt type on hydrophobic interactions is quantified by its molar surface tension increment (MSTI) that is a measure of the increase in surface tension by the salt (171). On the other hand, figure (2.10) shows the effect of different halides salts at 0.01 M on the extent binding of 125I-anti CA 15-3 antibody to pre-and postmenopausal malignant breast tumors homogenate. It seems that halides salts increased the binding, especially NaCl, this could be due to that NaCl in lower concentration (0.15M) or in physiological concentration, increased the binding between CA 15-3 and its antibody (172).

The Effect of Monovalent and Divalent Cations on the Binding

The effect of different salts on the extent of binding of 125I-anti CA 15-3 antibody to CA 15-3 in benign and malignant breast tumors are shown in figure (2.11).

The results indicate that the binding process is sensitive to the presence of cation metal ions. $CuSO_4.5H_2O$ at concentration (25mM) was shown to increase the binding more than other divalent cations, while $ZnCl_2$ increased the binding less than other divalent cations. One hypothesis assumes that salts may alter the nature of the hydrophobic forces controlling stabilization of the complex formed and these vary depending on the nature of the interacting groups (172). From the results illustrated in figure (2.11), it is suggested that these salts maybe provide some conformational changes in the CA 15-3 and the charged groups of the binding domain of the antibody and antigen molecule (173,174), that hinder maximal binding are shielded. If the interaction is dominated by ionic strength, high salt concentration lowers the affinity.

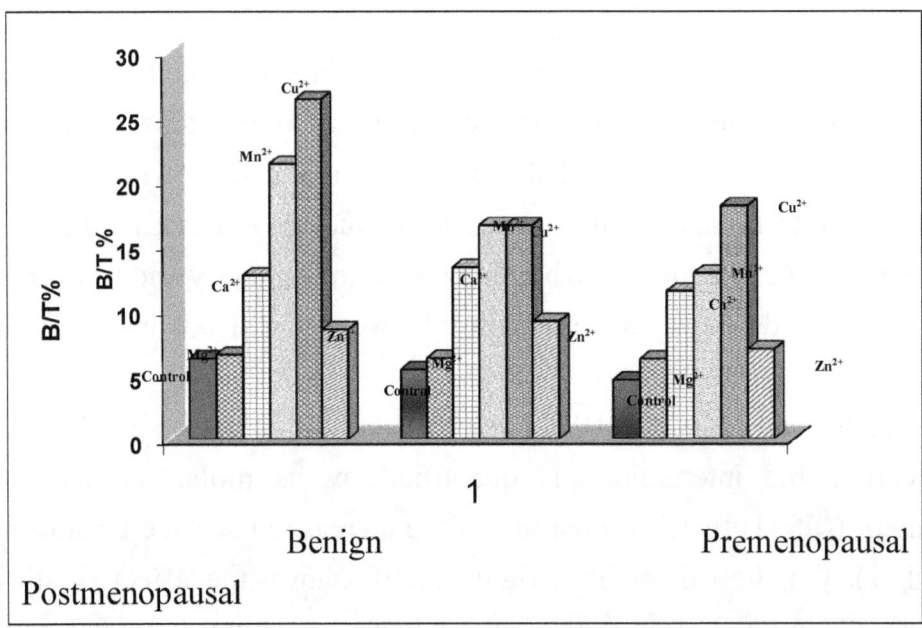

Figure (2.11): Effect of different divalent cations on the binding of 125I-anti CA 15-3 antibody with CA 15-3. (All other details are explained in the text)

Figure (2.12) shows the effect of monovalent cations (KCl and NH4Cl) on the extent of the binding of CA 15-3 to its antibody 125I-anti CA 15-3 in benign and malignant breast tumors. KCl at 25mM was shown to increase the binding in benign and premenopausal malignant breast tumors as compared with the control value, while KCl at the same concentration slightly inhibiting the binding in postmenopausal malignant breast tumors. These results may be due to conformational changes. NH4Cl at 25 mM was shown to inhibit the binding but to a lesser extent.

This result shows that NH4Cl effect on the binding is nearly unremarkable. Presumably, the lesser degree of hydration permits greater interaction of the salt with an anionic group located in the antibody-combining site and then inhibits the complex formation.

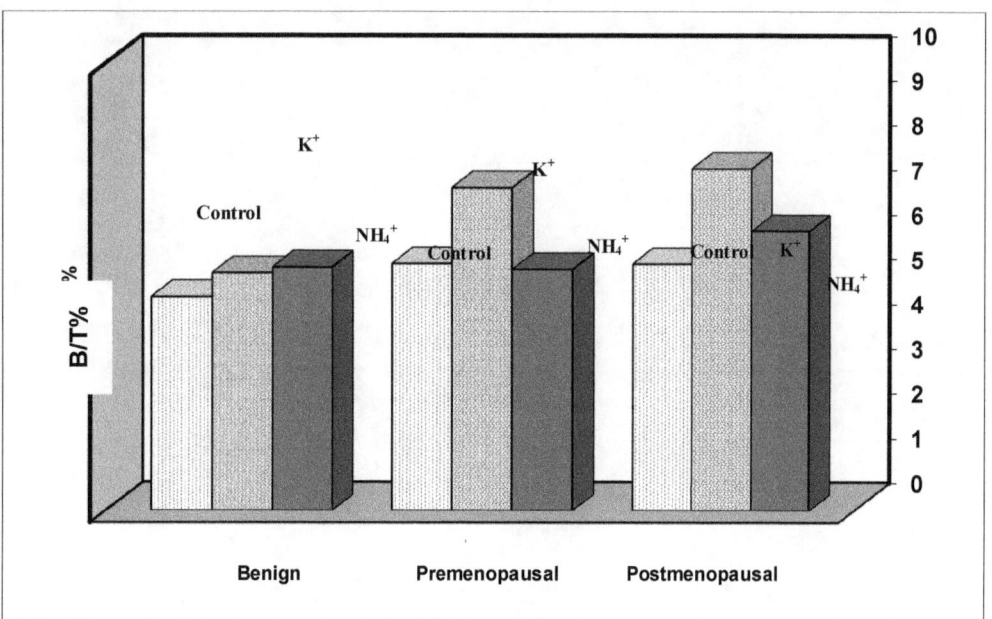

Figure (2.12): Effect of different monovalent cations on the binding of 125I-anti CA 15-3 antibody with CA 15-3. (All details are explained in the text).

Recovery of CA 15-3

This method was used to estimate the percent recovery of CA 15-3 in supernatant fractions of benign and malignant breast tumors homogenates. The results are summarized in table (2.7) and indicate that the CA 15-3 extracted from benign breast tumors, and CA15-3 extracted from malignant breast tissues homogenate were recovered more than CA 15-3 extracted from postmenopausal malignant breast tumors homogenates were recovered more than CA 15-3 extracted from premenopausal malignant breast tumors homogenates. Also the results indicate that total CA 15-3 can be determined through the developed method of immunoradiometric assay, as well as the percent of recovery indicates the precision of the used method.

Table (2.7): Recovery of CA 15-3. (All other details are explained in the text).

Type of CA 15-3	Measured B/T	Expected B/T	Recovery% Measured / Expected
Benign (Fibroadenoma)	16.23	24.84	65.34
Premenopausal (IDC)	20.04	27.64	72.50
Postmenopausal (IDC)	24.20	26.80	90.30

s witAbstract

Gel filtration chromatography technique was used for partial purification of CA15-3 from breast tumor homogenates.

The results revealed the presence of one form of CA15-3 with a high molecular weight (440 KD). This type possesses a high affinity for the binding to its antibody 125I-anti CA15-3 at the same conditions performed in section (2.2.4) of chapter two.

The elution volume (Ve) and the Kav value for elution of CA15-3 from sepharose CL-4B column were calculated. The experiments of optimum conditions of the binding between the partially purified CA15-3 and 125I-anti CA15-3 antibody were determined, in benign breast tumor and premenopausal malignant breast cancer homogenates.

Studies on the stability of both partial purified CA15-3 and crude CA15-3, show that the crude CA15-3 was more stable than the purified CA15-3.

Chapter Three

Purification of CA-15-3

CA15-3 is high molecular weight glycoprotein (>400 KD) identified at the apical side of alevoli and duct of mamary glands (83). Several authors have isolated, purified and characterized CA15-3 from different sources;either by the

isolation of CA15-3 from a breast cancer patient's sera, using affinity chromatography, gel filtration, and then characterized by SDS-PAGE(175,176) ,or by purifing a high molecular weight glycoprotein from human milk and breast carcinoma by using gel filtration, affinity chromatography and then PAGE (177).   In the present study , benign breast tumors and premenopausal malignant breast cancer were used as a source for partial purification of CA15-3 and then determination its yield. The factors effect the binding of partial purified CA15-3 to its antibody 125I-anti CA15-3 antibody were also studied.

Materials and Methods

3.1. Materials
3.1.1. Chemicals
All chemical and reagents mentioned in section (2.1.1) and (2.1.6) were used in the experiments of this chapter.

3.1.2. Instruments
All instruments mentioned in section (2.1.2) were also used in the experiments of this chapter.

3.1.3. Patients
The same patients tissues mentioned in section (2.1.5) were used in the following experiments. Benign breast tumor and premenopausal malignant breast cancer homogenates that showed maximal binding in the preliminary test in section (2.2.3) were used for the purification of CA15-3.

3.2. Methods
3.2.1. Isolation of CA15-3 by Sepharose CL-4B Column
3.2.1.1. Preparation of the Column

The dimensions of the column were chosen according to the following equation (150).

$$\text{Diameter} = \sqrt{\frac{m}{10}}$$

Where:

m= amount of protein in mg.

L = 30 x diameter

Where:

L : length of the column

3.2.1.2. Preparation of Phosphate Buffered Saline

PBS buffer pH 7.0 containing 0.02% sodium azide was prepared as described previously in section (2.1.6).

3.2.1.3. Preparation of the Gel

The gel was prepared by allowing the pre-swollen gel to swell again in PBS buffer (0.05 M) pH 7.0, then left to settle and the excess of buffer was decanted. The step was repeated several times. Suction was then used to degas the gel and slurry was left for 24 hrs to equilibrate with buffer.

The swollen gel was suspended and carefully poured into a vertical glass-column (0.7 x 30 cm) down the wall using a glass rod. After the gel has settled, the column was equilibrated with PBS for 24 hrs.

3.2.1.4. Void Volume Determination

The void volume of the column was determined by using blue dextran 2000 at concentration of 2 mg.mL-1 dissolved in PBS buffer pH 7.0 , then the elution was carried out with the same buffer at a flow rate of 20 mL.hrs-1.

Fractions of 2 mL were collected and their absorbance was measured at 600 nm. Figure (3-1) shows the elution profile of blue dextran 2000. The volume of the buffer required to elute the blue dextran which represents the void volume was (6 mL).

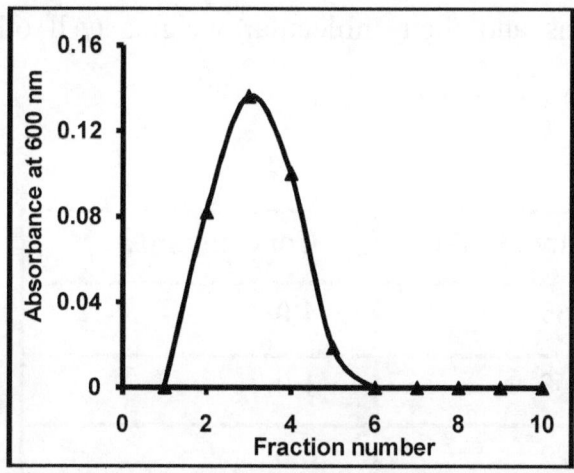

Figure (3.1): The elution profile of blue dextran 2000. (All other details are explained in the text).

3.2.1.5. Column-Calibration

The column was calibrated by gel filtration kit, purchased from pharmacia fine chemicals which contained standard proteins. Standard protein solutions were prepared according to the manufacturers instructions, then applied through two 0.5 mL portions, proteins 1 and 3 in the first portion, protien 2 and 4 in the second portion. Elution was carried out with PBS buffer at a flow rate of 20 ml.hrs-1. the absorbance of the fractions collected was measured at 280 nm to evaluated the elution volume (Ve) of the standard protein.

Standard Proteins

Pharmacia calibration kit for determination of M.wt by gel filtration was used. The kit comprises the highly purified proteins and their high M.wt are detailed in table (3.1).

Table (3.1): Standard proteins and their molecular weights (All other details are explain in text).

Protein	M.wt (KD)	Conc. mg.mL-1
Thyroglobulin	669	4.0
Ferritin	440	1.0
Catalase	322	6.0
Aldolase	158	6.0

Calculations

The Kav values of the proteins eluted were determined using the following equation:

$$K_{av} = \frac{V_e - V_o}{V_t - V_o}$$

Where:

Vo= Void volume

Ve=Elution volume of each protein

Vt=Total gel - bed volume.

The calibration curve of Kav values vs. log M.wt. of the proteins were plotted.

3.2.1.6. Separation Procedure

Reagents

PBS buffer pH (7.0, 7.2 and 7.6) containing 0.02% sodium azide was prepared as described previously in section (2.1.6).

Procedure

The sample of tissue homogenate (0.5 mL) containing approximately 3.43 mg protein was applied to the surface of gel , equilibrated with 0.15 M PBS buffer pH 7.2 for benign and premenopausal malignant breast tumor respectively. The sample was eluted by using the same buffer pH (7.0 and 7.6) for (benign and premenopausal malignant breast tumors respectively) with a flow rate of 20 mL.hrs-1 and fractions volume 2 mL were collected, gel filtration was carried out at 10 oC. The protein content of each fraction was determined using Lowry.et.al method (147).

The fractions contained CA15-3 were identified by the assay method. The binding of each fraction was calculated and plotted against the elution volume. The degree of purification (folds) of CA15-3 was calculated from the following formula.

$$\text{Purification fold of CA15 - 3} = \frac{\text{Specific binding of purified CA15 - 3}}{\text{Specific binding of crude CA15 - 3}}$$

Then yield % was determined as follows:

$$\text{Yield \%} = \frac{\text{Total protein content of purified CA15 - 3}}{\text{Total protein content of crude CA15 - 3}} \times 100$$

3.2.1.7. Dialysis for Concentration

After preparing dialysis tube, the fractions that contained high levels of the binding activity were pooled and concentrated by dialyzing against sucrose at 4 oC for 2hrs to get the required concentration to be used in the next experiments.

3.3. The Choice of the Optimum Conditions for the Binding of the Partially Purified CA15-3 to 125I-Anti CA15-3 Antibody

3.3.1. Optimum Protein Concentration

Reagents

PBS buffer pH 7.0 and 7.6 was prepared as described previously in section (2.1.6).

Procedure

One hundred microliters of increasing amount (50,100,150,200 and 250) μg.mL-1 protein of the dialyzable fractions of the partially purified CA15-3 from benign breast tumor was incubated with 50 μL of 125I-anti CA15-3 antibody (0.35 mg.mL-1) and completed to a final volume of 500 μL with 0.15 M PBS pH 7.0. The assay tubes were incubated for 90 min. at 45 oC. Two additional tubes, containing 50 μL (0.35 mg.mL-1) of 125I-anti CA15-3 antibody only, for total radioactivity computation, were set a side until counting.

Steps 4,5 and 6 of the experiment (2.2.4.1) were repeated. The same experiment was repeated on premenopausal malignant breast tissues homogenates (100 μg.mL-1 protein) with PBS buffer pH 7.6 and incubation time for 90 min at 15 oC.

Calculations

The (B/T) % was calculated as mentioned in experiment (2.2.3) and plotted against increasing amounts of protein concentration.

3.3.2. Influence of 125I-Anti CA15-3 Antibody on the Binding

Reagents

PBS buffer pH 7.0 and 7.6 was prepared as described previously in section (2.1.6).

Procedure

Fifty microliters of increasing concentration (0.070, 0.140, 0.175, 0.210, 0.245, 0.280 mg.mL-1) of 125I-anti CA15-3 antibody were added to 100 μL (150 μg.mL-1 protein) of partially purified CA15-3 from benign breast tumors. The reaction was completed to 500 μL with PBS pH 7.0. The assay tubes were incubated for 90 min at 45 oC. Two additional tubes containing increased concentration of 125I-anti CA15-3 antibody only, for total counts were counted. Steps 4,5 and 6 of the experiment (2.2.4.1) were repeated. The same experiment was repeated on premenopausal malignant breast tissues homogenate (100 μg.mL-1 protein) with PBS pH 7.6 and incubation time for 90 min at 15 oC.

Calculations

The (B/T) % was calculated as mentioned in experiment (2.2.3) and plotted against increasing concentration of 125I-anti CA15-3 antibody.

3.3.3. Optimum pH

Reagents

PBS buffer pH (6.8, 7.0, 7.2, 7.4, 7.6, 7.8, and 8.0) was prepared as described previously in section (2.1.6).

Procedure

To determine the optimum pH, 100 μL of a dialyzable fractions of partially purified CA15-3 from benign breast tumors (150 μg.mL-1 protein) were added to 20 μL of 125I-anti CA15-3 antibody (0.140 mg.mL-1). The volume of each fraction was completed to 500 μL with 0.15 M PBS of different pH (6.8 , 7.0 ,7.2 , 7.4 , 7.6 , 7.8 , 8.0). The assay tubes were incubated for 90 min at 45 oC. Two additional tubes, containing 20 μL (0.140 mg.mL-1) of 125I-anti CA15-3 antibody only , for total count , were set aside until counting. Steps 4,5 and 6 of experiment (2.2.4.1) were repeated. The same experiment was repeated on premenopausal malignant breast tissues homogenates (100 μg,mL-1 protein) and 25 μL (0.175 mg.mL-1) of 125I-anti CA15-3 antibody was incubated for 90 min at 15 oC.

Calculations

The (B/T) % was calculated as mentioned in experiment (2.2.3) and plotted against their corresponding pH values.

3.3.4. Optimum Temperature

PBS buffer pH 7.0 was prepared as described previously in section (2.1.6).

Twenty microliters (0.140 mg.mL-1) of 125I-anti CA15-3 antibody was added to 100 μL dialyzable fractions of partially purified CA15-3 from benign breast tumors (150 μg.mL-1 protein).

The volume of reaction was completed to 500 μL with 0.15 M PBS buffer pH 7.0. The assay tubes were incubated for 90 min at 45 oC. The same steps were repeated at (37, 25, 15, 5oC). Two additional tubes containing 20 μL (0.140 mg.mL-1) of 125I-anti CA15-3 antibody only, for total count, were set aside until counting. Steps 4,5 and 6 of experiment (2.2.4.1) were repeated.

The same experiment was repeated on the premenopausal malignant breast tissues homogenates (100 μg.mL-1 protein) and 25 μL (0.175 mg.mL-1) of 125I-anti CA15-3 antibody in PBS buffer pH 7.0, with incubation time 90 min at 15 oC. The experiment was repeated at different temperatures (45, 37,   25 and 5 oC).

Calculations

The (B/T) % was calculated as mentioned in experiment (2.2.3) and plotted versus temperatures of incubation.

3.3.5. The Effect of Incubation Time

PBS buffer pH 7.0 was prepared as described previously in section (2.1.6).

Twenty microliters (0.140 mg.mL-1) of 125I-anti CA15-3 antibody were added to 100 μL of dialyzable fractions of partially purified CA15-3 from benign breast tumors containing (150 μg.mL-1 protein). The reaction volume was completed to 500 μL with 0.15 M PBS buffer pH 7.0 , then incubated at 37 oC for (30, 60, 90, 120, 150, 180 min). Two additional tubes counting 20 μL (0.140 mg.mL-1) of 125I-anti CA15-3 antibody for total counts , were set aside until counting. Steps 4,5 and 6 of the experiment (2.2.4.1) were repeated. The same experiment was repeated on the premenopausal malignant breast tissues homogenates (100 μg.mL-1 protein) and 25 μL (0.175 mg.mL-1) of 125I-anti CA15-3 antibody with 0.15 M PBS buffer pH 7.0 and incubated at 15 oC for (30, 60, 90, 120, 150 and 180 min).

The (B/T) % was calculated as metioned in experiment (2.2.3) and plotted versus the time of incubation for each group.

3.3.6. Stability of CA15-3 at –20 oC

PBS buffer pH 7.0 was prepared as described previously in section (2.1.6).

Crude and purified CA15-3 were stored at –20 oC for several time intervals. The frozen specimen was thawed at the end of each interval and the binding activity was measured at optimum conditions as described in section (2.2.4) and (3.6). The remaining activity was calculated and plotted against storage periods.

Calculations

The (B/T) % was calculated as mentioned in experiment (2.2.11) and plotted versus time storage for each group.

3.4. Results and Discussion

Partial Purification of CA15-3

Isolation of CA15-3 was performed by gel exclusion chromatography technique. CA15-3 was found to be separated from aggregates and other protein having smaller molecular weight by sepharose CL-4B. Figure (3-2, A & B) shows the elution profile of CA15-3 from benign breast tumors and premenopausal malignant breast cancer homogenates. The homogenate was loaded on the column as described in section (3.2.1). The void volume (Vo) of column was (6 mL) as predicted from the elution profile of the blue dextran. The elution was performed with PBS buffer. The resultant fractions containing the binding activity of CA15-3 were collected, pooled and concentrated, then subjected to protein determination as in section (2.2.1).

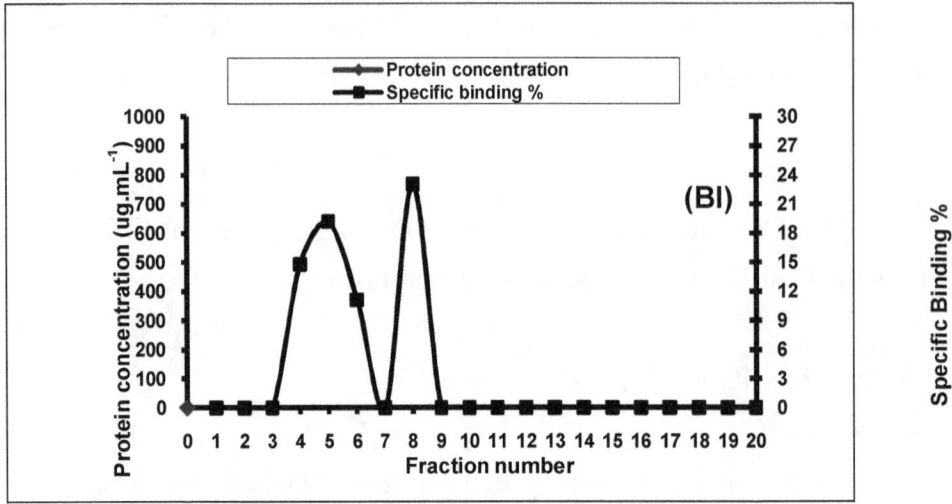

Figure (3.2A): The elution profile of human CA15-3 from benign breast tumors (BI). (All other details are explained in the text).

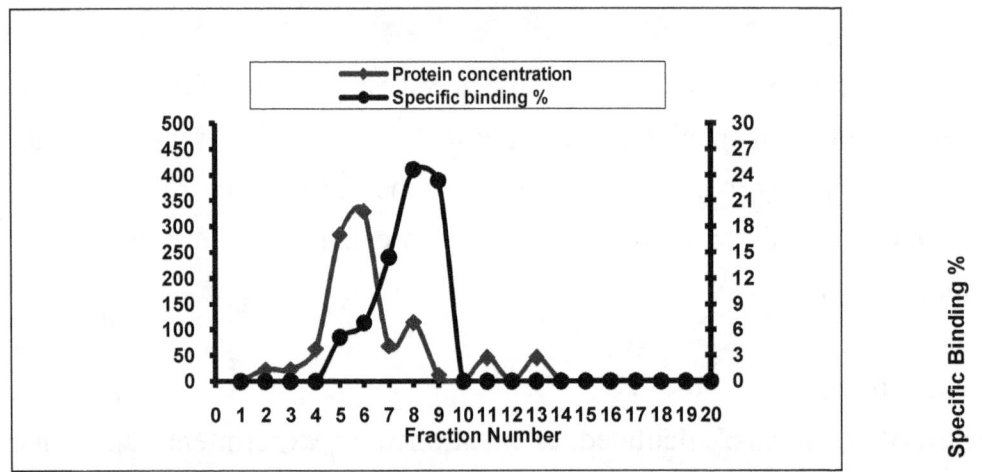

Figure (3.2B): The elution profile of human CA15-3 from premenopausal malignant breast cancer (MI). (All other details are explained in the text).

The elution volume Ve and then Kav values for the two peaks of CA15-3 (BI & MI) from benign breast tumors and malignant breast cancer respectively were calculated. The molecular weight of the partially purified CA15-3 obtained from figure (3-3) was 440 KD for peak (BI) and peak (MI) in two cases.

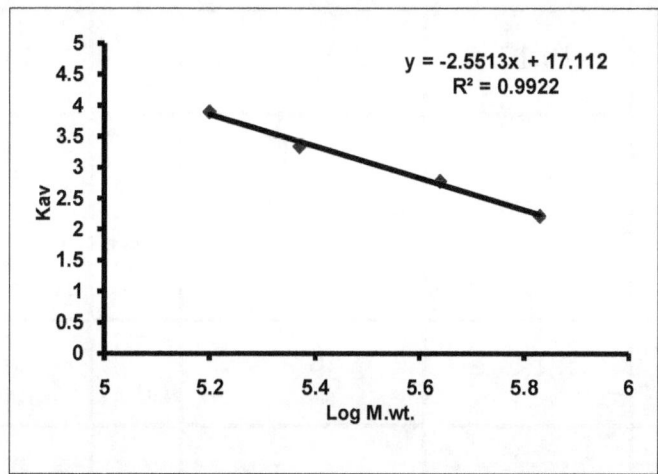

Figure (3.3): Calibration curve for determination of M.wt by gel filtration chromatography. (All other details are explained in the text).

The values ranged from 300-450 KD (178-180). Peaks of partially purified CA15-3 may be heavily aggregated, CA15-3 was obtained near the void volume of the column under separation conditions. From these results it was concluded that these components are capable of binding to the 125I-anti CA15-3 antibody with different affinities and in general CA15-3 type (BI) have lower binding affinities than CA15-3 type (MI), the isolation of CA15-3 from benign breast tumors on gel filtration column showed 3.02 folds of purification for peak (BI), while the isolation of CA15-3 from premenopausal malignant breast cancer showed 5.0 folds of purification. Table (3-2) illustrates the purification parameters for the different purified CA15-3 forms isolated by gel exclusion chromatography technique. The glycosylation of the protein backbone may differ in carcinoma cells from normal epithelial cells causing a wide range of molecular weight for this mucin (181).

Table (3.2): Partial purification of CA15-3 by gel filtration. (All other details are explained in the text).

CA15-3 Source	Total protein mg .mL-1	Specifically bound 125I-anti CA15-3	Specifically binding 125I-anti CA15-3/mg protein	Yield %	Purification fold

Benign	Crude extract	3.43	10.17	2.97	100	1.00
	Gel filtration on sepharose CL-4B	2.91	30.70	10.55	84.84	3.02
Malignant	Crude extract	3.43	8.18	2.39	100	1.00
	Gel filtration on sepharose CL-4B	2.21	40.93	18.52	64.43	5.00

The Choice of Optimum Conditions for the Binding of Partially Purified CA15-3 with 125I-Anti CA15-3 Antibody

Optimum Protein Concentration

Figure (3-4) shows the effect of increasing amounts of partially purified CA15-3 to a fixed amount of 125I-anti CA15-3 antibody to produce (125I-anti CA15-3 antibody/CA15-3) complex, that grow in size until they formed a precipitate. Above this zone an equivalence between CA15-3 and its antibody concentration is obtained, and amount of complex shows no further increases. A further addition of CA15-3 give rise to a solubilization of complex. The results revealed that 150 µg protein was the most appropriate concentration for the binding of (BI) and 100 µg protein for (MI). From these results, it could be concluded that the binding of 125I-anti CA15-3 antibody with its partially purified CA15-3 (BI) needed a higher amount of protein concentration than partially purified CA15-3 (MI). This is may be due to lower concentration of CA15-3 in benign breast tumor as compared with malignant breast tumors. According to these results, in all subsequent experiments, (150 µg.mL-1 protein) in benign breast tumors and (100 µg.mL-1 protein) in malignant breast tumors were used, since they give the highest binding.

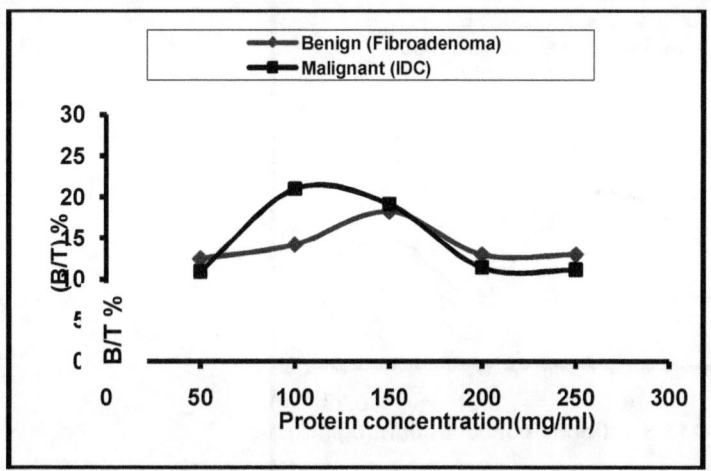

Figure (3.4): Influence of protein concentration on the binding of 125I-anti CA15-3 antibody with partially purified CA15-3 from breast tumors. (All other details are explained in the text).

Influence of 125I-anti CA15-3 Antibody on the Binding

Figure (3.5) illustrate the effect of 125I-anti CA15-3 antibody concentration on the binding with partial purified CA15-3 from benign breast tumors and premenopausal malignant breast cancer.

The maximum binding obtained when 0.140 mg.mL-1 of antibody in benign breast tumors and 0.175 mg.mL-1 of antibody in malignant breast tumors were used. From these results, it was found that (BI) purified fraction was saturated with small concentration of 125I-anti CA15-3 antibody than those required for (MI). This is may be due to the increasement of the epitope (is the part of an antigen molecule that binds to any single antigen-combining site) (182) in partially purified CA15-3 in malignant breast tumors as compared to benign breast tumors.

According to these results, in all subsequent experiments (0.140 mg.mL-1) and (0.175 mg.mL-1) of 125I-anti CA15-3 antibody in benign and malignant breast tumors were used, since they give the highest binding.

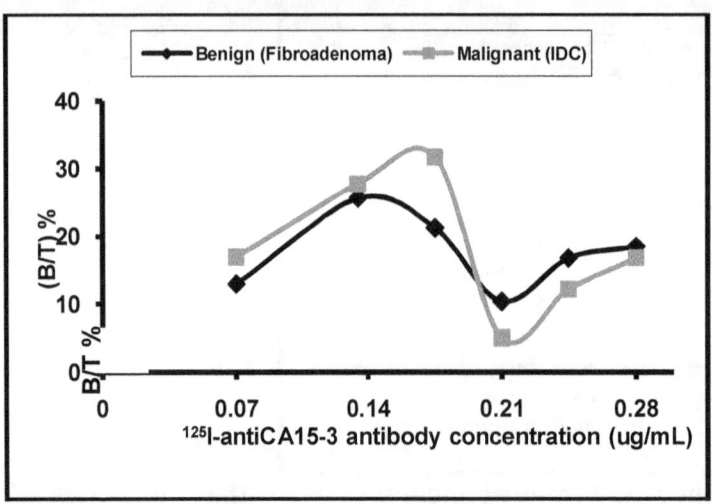

Figure (3.5): Effect of 125I-anti CA15-3 antibody concentration on its binding with partially purified CA15-3 from breast tumors. (All other details are explained in the text).

Optimum pH

Figure (3-6) shows the effect of increasing pH on the binding of 125I-anti CA15-3 antibody to its purified antigen. The results revealed that the optimum pH for (BI) and (MI) purified fractions for the binding with its antibody was 7.0. These results indicate that the binding was pH dependent.

The similarity in pH (7.0) suggests that the CA15-3 isolated from different sources of tissues either benign or malignant breast tissues homogenates possesses the same epitopes in both cases. That means the induction of protonation-deprotonation process (183) occurs within the same changed polar groups on the amino acid residues present in the binding domain. According to the results obtained, the pH of the buffer used in all subsequent experiments was adjusted to pH 7.0.

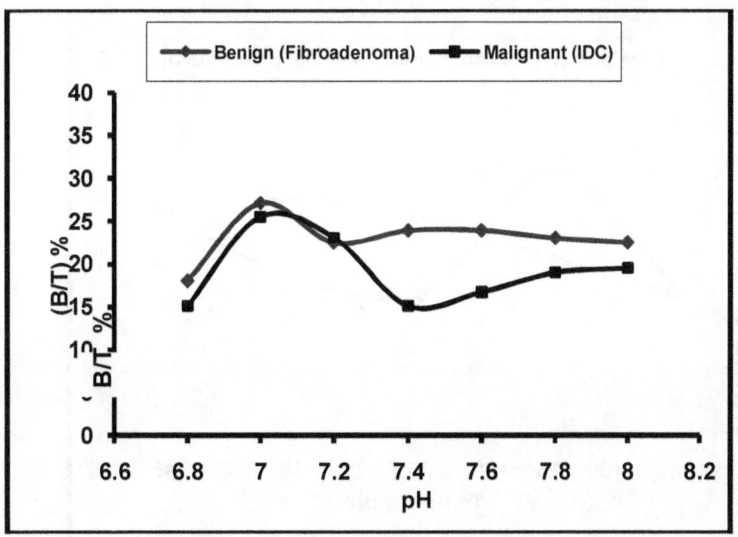

Figure (3.6): pH effect on the binding of 125I-anti CA15-3 antibody with partially purified CA15-3 from breast tumors. (All other details are explained in the text)

Optimum Temperature

The temperature dependency of the isolated CA15-3 binding to its antibody 125I-anti CA15-3 was investigated.

Figure (3.7) show the optimum temperatures on the binding of 125I-anti CA15-3 antibody was 37oC with partially purified CA15-3 (BI) and 15oC with partially purified CA15-3 (MI).

The difference of the temperature between crude and purified CA15-3 occurs in benign breast tumors, i.e. the optimum temperature was 45oC of the binding of 125I-anti CA15-3 antibody to crude CA15-3 while in the purified CA15-3 (BI) was 37oC. On the other hand, the optimum temperature in both crude and partially purified CA15-3 from premenopausal malignant breast tumors was 15oC.

The temperature dependency of the binding suggests that the whole process is controlled by diffusion of the interacting of 125I-anti CA15-3 antibody to CA15-3 in benign and malignant breast tumors (184).

In view of these results, the temperatures (37 & 15 oC) for both benign and malignant breast tumors were used in all subsequent experiments.

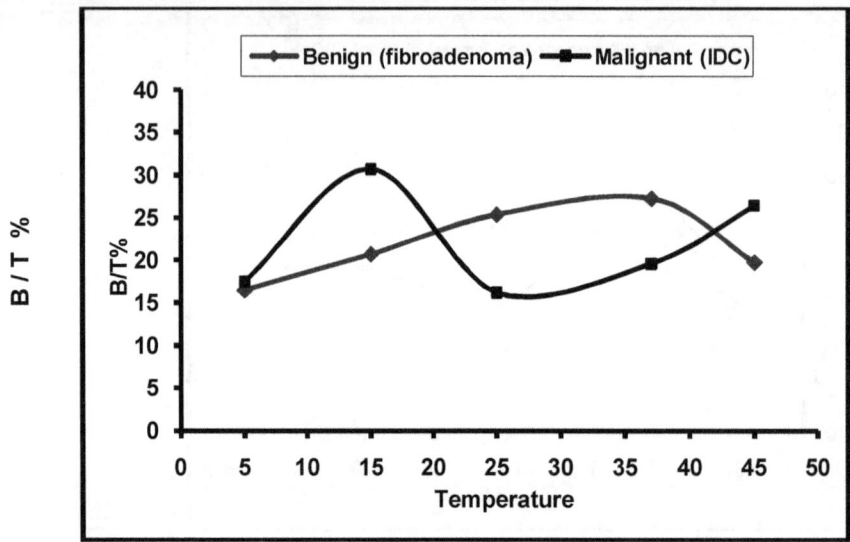

Figure (3.7): Effect of the temperature on the binding of 125I-anti CA15-3 antibody with partially purified CA15-3 from breast tumors. (All other are explained in the text)

The Effect of Incubation Time

Figure (3.8) shows the time required for the highest binding of 125I-anti CA15-3 antibody to partially purified CA15-3 in (BI) and (MI) was 90 min at 37 and 15 oC respectively.

In view of these results, the incubation time used in all subsequent experiments was 90 min.

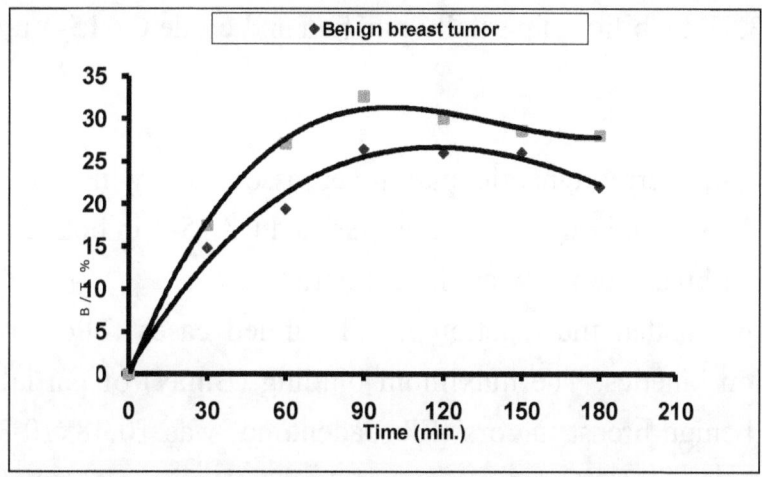

Figure (3.8): Time dependence of 125I-anti CA15-3 antibody binding with partially purified CA15-3 from breast tumors. (All other details are explained in the text)

Stability of CA15-3 at –20 oC

The crude and isolated fractions of CA15-3 from malignant breast tumors were stored at –20 oC during the experiments. It was carried out in order to study the stability of CA15-3 and check their efficiencies of the binding through out the storage period. The results showed that CA15-3 of crude fraction was more stable than the isolated fractions as shows in figure (3-9). This result is in agreement with Al-Atrakchi observations (185).

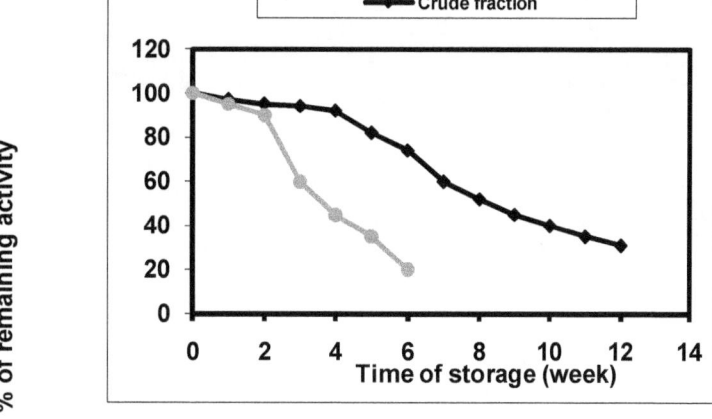

Figure (3.9): Stability of partially purified and crude CA15-3 upon storage at Abstract

Kinetic and thermodynamic parameter associated with the binding of 125I-anti CA15-3 antibody to partially purified CA15-3 in both cases, benign and malignant breast tumors were investigated.

It was shown that the reaction in all studied cases follow pseudo-first order reaction kinetics. The maximum binding (Bmax) of partially purified CA15-3 in benign breast tumors (Fibroadenoma) was 10.48×10^{-3} mg.mL-1 after 90 minutes incubation at 37oC, while the (Bmax) of partially purified CA15-3 in malignant breast tumors (IDC) was 13.38×10^{-3} mg.mL-1. The (Bmax) was decreased with increasing temperature. The values of affinity constant (Ka) were dependent on the temperature, Ka increased from 14.18 mg-1.mL at 5oC to 31.65 mg-1.mL at 45oC in benign breast tumors (Fibroadenoma), while Ka was increased from 13.87 mg-1.mL at 5oC to 23.81 mg-1.mL at 45oC in premenopausal malignant breast tumors (IDC). The association constant K+1 increased with temperature in benign breast tumors (Fibroadenoma). On the other hand, K+1 was independent of temperatures in premenopausal malignant breast tumors (IDC). The Van't Hoff plot demonstrated a linear relationship between Ka and 1/T, using the partially purified CA15-3 in benign and malignant tumor homogenate. Arrhenius plot indicate that there was a linear-relationship between log K+1 and 1/T. The transition state thermodynamic parameters (Ea, ΔH^*, ΔG^*, ΔS^*) for the formation of (125I-antiCA15-3 antibody /CA15-3) were determined.

Chapter Four

Kinetic and thermodynamics of Binding CA-15-3 to its antibody

Introduction

The specific reaction between an antibody (Ab) and an antigen (Ag) is usually driven by electrostatic forces between oppositely charged amino acids, hydrogen bonding, and hydrophobic interactions. The equilibrium reaction, termed "biospecific interaction", is characterized by the affinity of reactants to form Ag-Ab complex (186).

Kinetic studies supplement the information for differences between the initial, final states of each reactant and an intermediate activated complex, (i.e, the pathway taken by the reactants reach the final product) (187). On the other hand, thermodynamics of the binding describes the system in its initial, final states. Using kinetic and equilibrium data also determined thermodynamic formation constant.

Al-Mudhuffar et.al, have many studies on the kinetic and thermodynamic of protein-protein interaction in human breast tissue, like kinetic and thermodynamic of purified steroid receptor of malignant breast tumors with hormone (188), also kinetic and thermodynamic studies on the binding of lectin in human malignant breast to glycoprotein (189).

In this chapter, the basic mathematical analysis was described and used to explain the mechanism through kinetics of binding of CA15-3 from both breast tumor homogenates (fibroadenoma and Infiltrating ductalcarcinoma) to its antibody to form (125I-anti CA15-3 antibody / CA15-3) complex in partially purified fraction.

Materials and Methods

4.1. Materials

4.1.1. Chemicals

All chemical and reagents mentioned in section (2.1.1) in chapter two were used in the experiments of this chapter.

4.1.2. Instruments

All instruments that were described in section (2.1.2) in chapter two were used in the experiments of this chapter.

4.2. Methods

4.2.1. Kinetic Studies

4.2.1.1. The Time-Course of the Binding of 125I-anti CA15-3 Antibody with CA15-3 in Breast Tumor Homogenate

1. One hundred microliters of partially purified CA15-3 from benign breast tumor (fibroadenoma) and premenopausal malignant breast tumor (Infitrating ductal carcinoma, IDC) containing (150 and 100 □g.mL-1 protein) respectively, were added to (20 and 25 μL) of 125I-anti CA15-3 antibody containing (0.140 and 0.175 mg.mL-1) respectively.

2. The volume of reaction were completed to 500 μL with PBS buffer pH 7.0.

3. All tubes were incubated at 37oC at different time intervals (30, 60, 90, 120, 150, 180) min.

4. Steps 3, 4, 5 and 6 of experiment (2-4-2-1) were repeated.

5. To determine the time-course of partially purified CA15-3 binding to 125I-anti CA15-3 antibody at different temperatures, step 1,2,3 and 4 in the same experiment were repeated at different temperatures 5, 15, 25 and 45Co.

Calculation

The values of (B/T)% were calculated as described in section (2.4.1) and plotted against incubation time at each temperature for both types of homogenates.

4.2.1.2. Determination of Kinetic Parameters of 125I-Anti CA 15-3 Antibody Binding with Partially Purified CA 15-3 in Benign and Malignant Breast Tumors

Determination of the affinity constant (Ka) and the maximal binding capacity (Bmax) of:

A. Partially Purified CA15-3 in Benign Breast Tumor Homogenate Binding with 125I-Anti CA15-3 Antibody

1. One hundred microliters of partially purified CA15-3 from benign breast tumor (Fibroadenoma) containing (150 □g.mL-1 protein) were added to increasing volumes (4, 8, 12, 16, 20 and 24 µL) of 125I-anti CA15-3 antibody containing (0.0280, 0.0560, 0.0841, 0.1121, 0.1402 and 0.1684 mg.mL-1) to each assay tube. The final volume of each assay tube was completed to 500 µL with PBS buffer pH 7.0.

2. All tubes were incubated for 90 min at 37oC.

3. Steps 3, 4, 5 and 6 in experiment (2.4.2.1) were repeated at different temperatures (5, 15, 25 and 45oC).

4. The time of incubation required to reach the equilibrium state are reported in table (4-1) according to the following:Table (4.1): The time of incubation for benign and malignant breast tumor homogenate at different temperatures

| Temp. oC | Time (min.) | |
	Benign breast tumor homogenate (Fibroadenoma)	Malignant breast tumor homogenate (IDC)
5	180	180
15	60	90
25	90	150
37	90	90
45	180	90

Calculations

1- The B/F ratio was computed for each tube, where:

B: is the bound radioactivity (mean counts in c.p.m), which represent the formation of (125I-anti CA15-3 /CA15-3) complex.

F: is the free radioactivity (mean counts in c.p.m.), which represents the (unbound or unreacted), 125I-anti CA15-3 antibody.

T: is the total activity (mean counts in c.p.m.)

F = T (total counts) - B (bound radioactivity)

2- The concentration of (125I-anti CA15-3/CA15-3) complex in mg.mL-1 which found after time (t) was calculated from the following equation:

$$B(mg.mL^{-1}) = \frac{B(c.p.m)}{T(c.p.m)} \times Concentration\ of\ ^{125}I-anti\ CA15-3\ antibody\ in$$

the incubation medium in mg.mL^{-1}

3- The affinity constant and maximal binding capacity were determined according to Scatchard equation (190,191).

$$\frac{B}{F} = \frac{1}{K_d} \times (B_{max} - B)$$

$$K_a = \frac{1}{K_d} = \frac{K_{+1}}{K_{-1}}$$

Where: Ka = affinity constant

Kd = dissociation constant

Bmax = maximal binding capacity

The value of affinity constant of the binding Ka at each temperature can be calculated from the slop of the straight line in figure (4.2), while the value of the total concentration of CA15-3 (Bmax) in breast tumor homogenate for each group was calculated from the intercept of the x-axis.

B. Partially Purified CA15-3 in Human Malignant Breast Tumor Homogenate Binding with 125I-Anti CA15-3 Antibody

1. One hundred microliters of partially purified CA15-3 from premenopausal malignant breast tumor (IDC) containing (100 µg.mL-1 protein) were added to increasing volumes (5, 10, 15, 20, 25 and 30 µL) of 125I-anti CA15-3 antibody containing (0.035, 0.070, 0.105, 0.140, 0.175 and 0.210 mg.mL-1) to each assay tube. The final volume of each assay tube was completed to 500 µL with PBS buffer pH 7.0.

2. All tubes were incubated for 90 min at 15oC

3. Steps 3, 4, 5 and 6 in experiment (2.4.2.1) were repeated at different temperatures (5, 25, 37 and 45 oC).

4. The times of incubation required to reach the equilibrium state are reported in table (4.1).

Calculations

The method outlined in experiment (4.3.2.A) was followed exactly to obtain the values of Ka and Bmax at each temperature as shown in figure (4.3).

4.3. The Thermodynamic Studies of 125I-Anti CA15-3 Antibody Binding to Partially Purified CA15-3 in Benign and Malignant Breast Tumors

The same steps mentioned in section (4.2.1.1) and (4.2.1.2) were performed using the dialyzable protein fraction of benign and malignant breast tumor homogenate from fibroadenoma and (IDC) as the partially purified
CA15-3 source.

Calculation

1. The thermodynamic parameters of standard state were obtained from Van't Hoff plot, the values of the natural logarithm of equilibrium constant (affinity constant Ka) obtained at different temperatures were plotted against the reciprocal values of the absolute temperature in Kelvin (1/T), according to the following equation:

$$\ln K_a = \frac{\Delta S^o}{R} - \frac{\Delta H^o}{RT}$$

Where:

ΔH^o = the enthalpy change of the standard state.

ΔS^o = the entropy change of the standard state.

R   = the gas constant (8.314 J.K-1.mol-1).

ΔH^o value obtained from the slop of a linear relationship of the plot.

The change in Gibbs free energy of the standard state ΔG^o was obtained from the following equation:

$\Delta G^o = $ -RT Ln Ka

Where Ka is the affinity constant, while the standard state entropy change was obtained from (192):

$$\Delta S^o = \frac{\Delta H^o - \Delta G^o}{T}$$

2. The thermodynamic parameters of the transition state were obtained from Arrhenius plot of Ln K+1 values against (1/T) values, that given a linear relationship according to the following equation:

$$Ln\ K_{+1} = Ln\ A - \left(\frac{E_a}{RT}\right)$$

Where:

A: Arrhenius constant .

The values of activation energy (Ea) of the binding reaction can be determined from the slop of the straight line.

The enthalpy of transition state ΔH^* was obtained from:

$\Delta H^* = Ea - RT$

Transition state of free energy change ΔG^* is calculated from the following equation:

$$\Delta G^* = -RT\ LnK_{+1} + RT\ Ln\frac{KT}{h}$$

where K and h were Boltzmann and Plank's constant which equal (1.38x10-23 J.K-1), (6.62x10-34 J.sec-1) respectively.

The change in entropy of the transition state AS* is calculated from the following equation:

$$\Delta S^* = \frac{\Delta H^* - \Delta G^*}{T}$$

Results and Discussion

Kinetic Studies

The Time-Course of the Binding of 125I-anti CA15-3 Antibody with CA15-3 in Breast Tumor Homogenate

Figure (4.1.A & B) shows the time – course of the formation of (125I-anti CA15-3 /CA15-3) complex at five different temperatures (5, 15, 25, 37 and 45oC) of partially purified CA15-3 from benign and malignant breast tumors homogenates samples.

The concentration of (125I-anti CA15-3/CA15-3) complex formed after time (t) was calculated from the following equation:

$$[\text{125I-antiCA15-3/CA15-3}] \text{ in mg.mL-1 after time (t)} = \frac{\text{Count (c.p.m.) of 125I-antiCA15-3 specifically bound after time (t)}}{\text{Total counts (c.p.m.) of 125I-anti CA15-3 used in the incubation}} \times \text{Concentration of 125I-antiCA15-3 in the incubation (mg.mL-1)}$$

The results of time-course pattern at different temperatures indicated that the equilibrium binding studies is temperature and time dependent process. In case premenopausal malignant breast tumor (IDC) the maximum binding occurs at 15oC (after incubation for 90 minutes), while in benign breast tumors (fibroadenoma) the maximum binding occurs at 37oC at the same incubation time. This is may be due to the different source of CA15-3. Several authors studied the time – course of purified steroid receptors of malignant breast tumors(188), others studied the time – course on the binding of lectin in human malignant breast to glycoprotein (189), these studies revealed that the time-course must be done to find the maximum binding at different incubation time as a step to prepare the kinetic and thermodynamic studies.

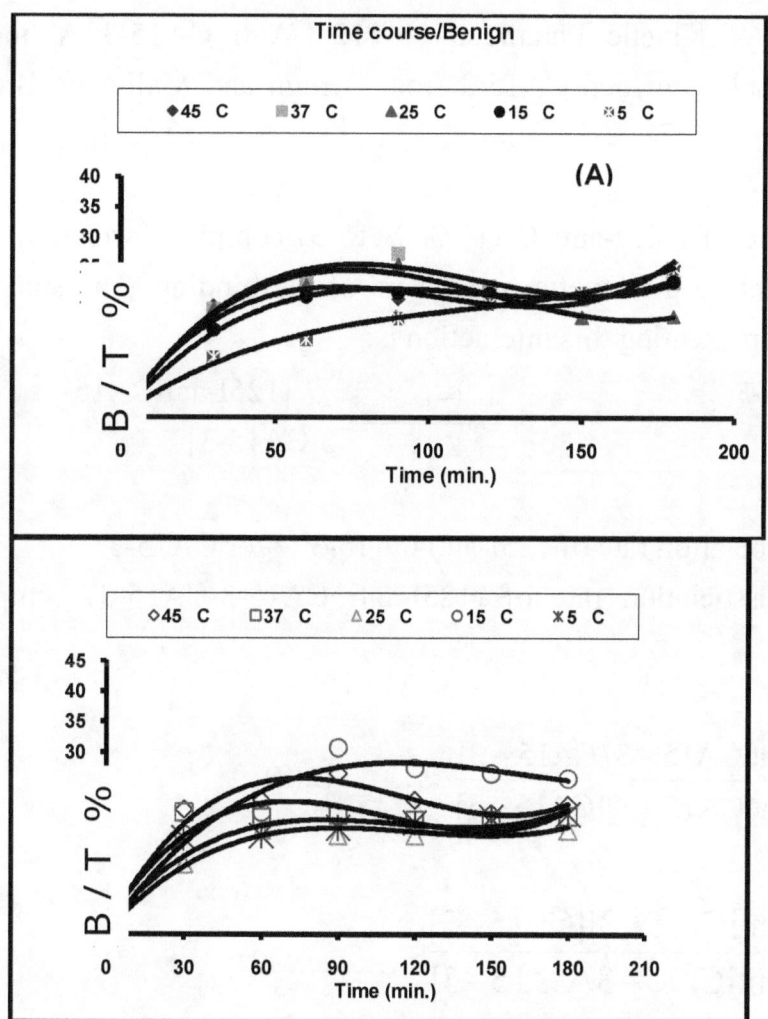

Figure (4.1): Time-Course of 125I-anti CA15-3 binding to partially purified CA15-3 in:

(A)   Benign tumor (Fibroadenoma) tissue homogenate.

(B)   Malignant tumor (IDC) tissue homogenate.

(All other details are explained in the text).

Determination of Kinetic Parameters of 125I-Anti CA15-3 Antibody Binding with Partially Purified CA15-3 from Benign and Malignant Breast Tumors

The time course of (125I-anti CA15-3/CA15-3) complex formation was carried out to describe the kinetic parameters of the binding. The simplest proposed model representing this interaction is:

125I-antiCA15-3   + $\xrightleftharpoons[K_{-1}]{K_{+1}}$ [125I-antiCA15-3/CA15-3]
CA15-3

Where:

K+1: is the association rate of 125I-anti CA15-3 to /or CA15-3.

K-1: is the dissociation rate of (125I-anti CA15-3/CA15-3) complex formed.

At equilibrium:

$$K_a = \frac{[^{125}I - antiCA15 - 3/CA15 - 3]}{[^{125}I - antiCA15 - 3][CA15 - 3]} \ldots\ldots\ldots\ldots(2)$$

$$K_d = \frac{[^{125}I - antiCA15 - 3][CA15 - 3]}{[^{125}I - antiCA15 - 3/CA15 - 3]} \ldots\ldots\ldots\ldots(3)$$

Thus:

$$K_a = \frac{1}{K_d} = \frac{K_{+1}}{K_{-1}} \ldots\ldots\ldots\ldots\ldots\ldots\ldots\ldots\ldots\ldots\ldots\ldots(4)$$

Where:

The value Ka and maximal binding capacity (Bmax). Were calculated from Scatchard plot at five different temperatures at incubation time of 90 minutes, figure (4-2) and (4-3).

It is clear from table (4-2), that the affinity constant (Ka) is depended on the type of the tumor (i.e., benign or malignant) and on the temperature. Ka increased with increased temperature for the same tumor (Fibroadenoma), Ka increased from 14.18 mg-1.mL at 5oC to 31.65 mg-1.mL at 45oC. Whereas the values of dissociation constant (Kd) was calculated by using equation (4), which show that the lowest Kd value of (125I-anti CA15-3/CA15-3) complex occurs at 45oC at time of incubation 180 minutes.

The concentration of CA15-3 in partially purified fractions of (Fibroadenoma) was determined to be 10.48x10-3 mg.mL-1 and the maximum binding (Bmax) occurred after 90 minutes incubation at 37 oC. While in the same table the maximum Ka value for the binding 125I-anti CA15-3 antibody with CA15-3 present in partially purified fraction of (IDC) occurred at 15oC and it was increased with temperature in the following order: 5 >15 >25 >37 > 45 oC.

The lowest Kd value of (125I-anti-CA15-3 /CA15-3) complex occurs at 45 oC at the time of incubation.

Scatchard plot analysis gave straight line as shown in figure (4.2) and (4.3) indicating that the (125I-anti CA15-3/CA15-3) complex is directed against the same epitopes on CA15-3 molecules. On the other hand, the maximum binding occurred at 15oC and was 13.38x10-3 mg.mL-1 also shows that the (Bmax) decreased with increasing temperatures of incubation.

Table (4-2): The Kinetic parameter of 125I-anti CA15-3 antibody binding to partially purified CA15-3 in breast tumor homogenate. (All other details are explained in the text).

Temp oC	Benign breast tumors (Fibroadenoma)			Malignant breast tumors (IDC)		
	Binding Capacity Bmaxx10-3 (mg.mL-1)	Ka (mg-1.mL)	Kdx10-2 (mg.mL-1)	Binding Capacity Bmax x10-3 (mg.mL-1)	Ka (mg-1.mL)	Kdx10-2 (mg.mL-1)
5	9.22	14.18	7.05	10.82	13.87	7.21
15	8.05	16.73	5.98	13.38	20.78	4.81
25	9.02	16.38	6.10	12.57	20.84	4.79
37	10.48	18.66	5.36	9.63	22.22	4.50
45	6.67	31.65	3.16	11.67	23.81	4.20

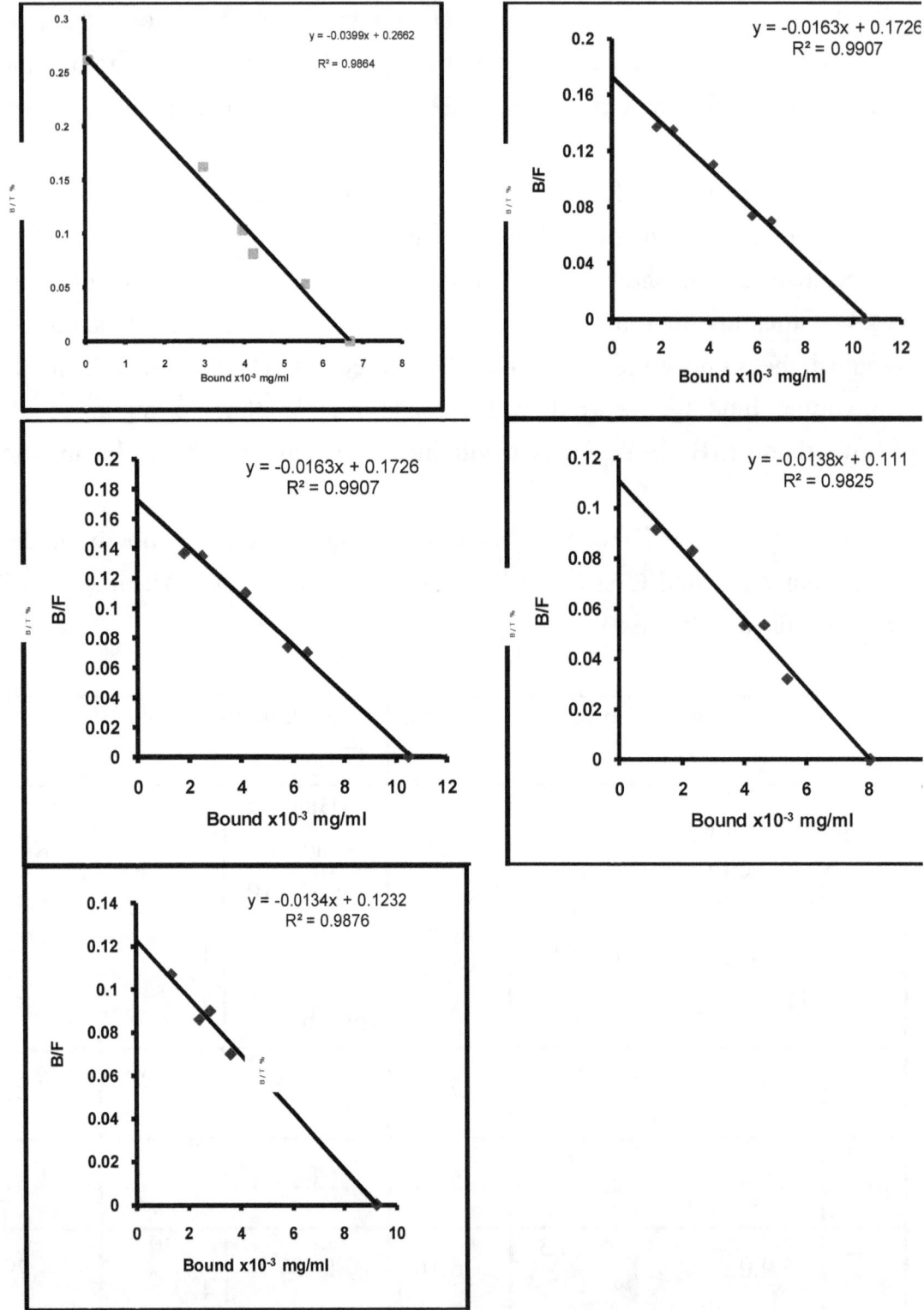

Figure (4-2): Scatchard plot of 125I-anti CA15-3 antibody binding to the partially purified CA15-3 in benign breast tumors (Fibroadenoma) at five different temperatures. All details are explained in the text.

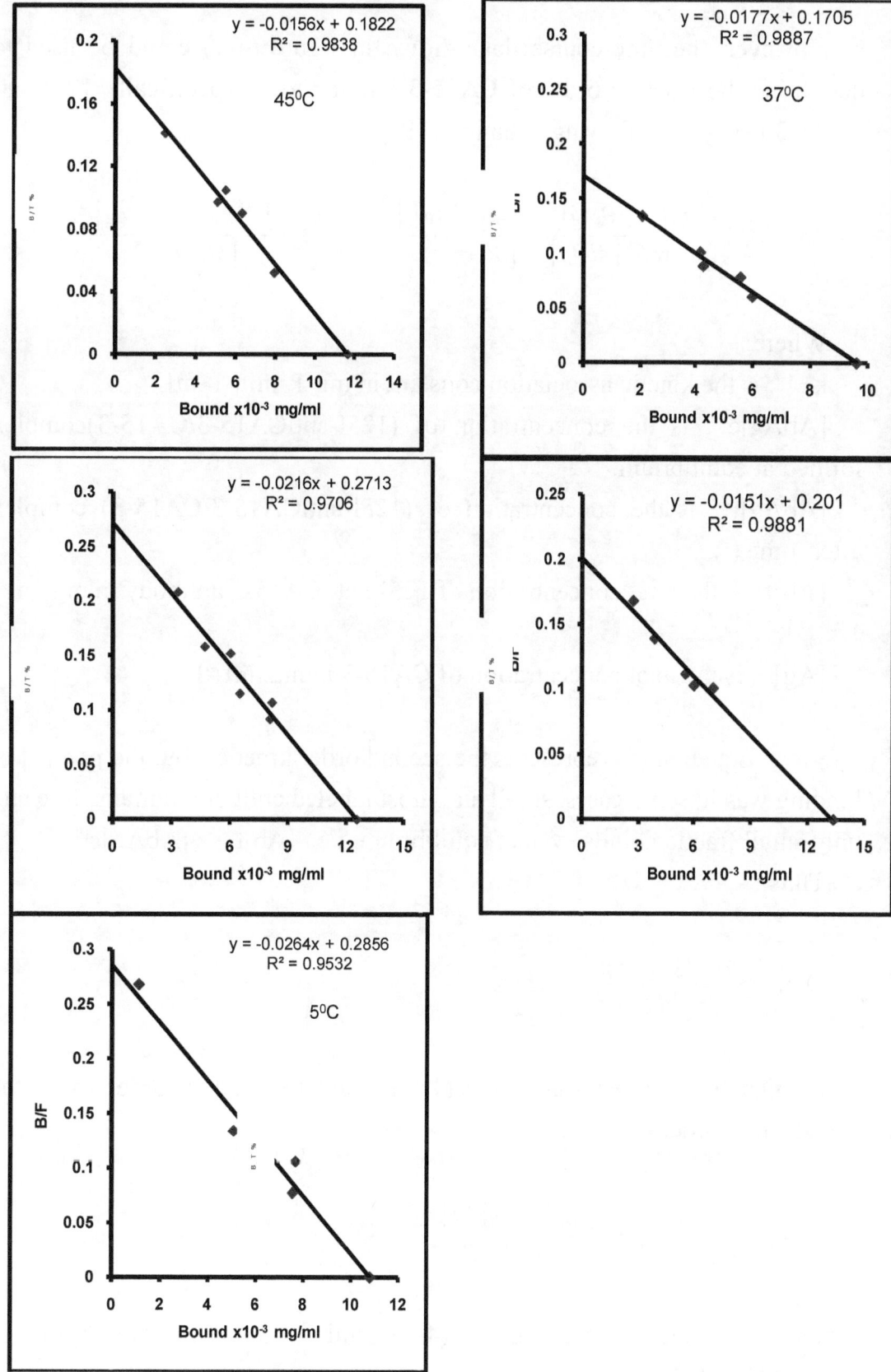

Figure (4.3): Scatchard plot of 125I-anti CA15-3 antibody binding to the partially purified CA15-3 in Malignant breast tumors (IDC) at five different temperatures. All details are explained in the text.

However, the time-course data shown in figure (4-1) could be used to determine the reaction order of CA15-3 binding to its specifically 125I-anti CA15-3 using the following equation (193):

$$Ln[AbAg]_e \left[\frac{[Ab]_t - [AbAg]_t [AbAg]_e / [Ag]_t}{[Ab]_t [AbAg]_e - [AbAg]_e} \right] = K_{+1} t \left[\frac{[Ab]+[Ag]_t - [AbAg]_e}{[AbAg]_e} \right] \quad ......(5)$$

Where:

k+1 : is the kinetic association constant in mg-1. min-1. mL.

[AbAg]e : is the concentration of (125I-antiCA15-3/CA15-3)complex formed at equilibrium.

[AbAg]t : is the concentration of (125I-antiCA15-3/CA15-3) complex after time (t).

[Ab]t : is the total concentration of 125I-anti CA15-3 antibody in mg. mL-1.

[Ag]t : is the total concentration of CA15-3 in mg. mL-1.

Equation (5) represents the second order kinetics, but the percent of binding was in some cases, small and most labeled antibody remains free and only small fraction binds even at equilibrium, i.e , [Ab]t >> [AbAg]e

Thus :

$$[Ab]_t >> \frac{[AbAg]_t [AbAg]_e}{[Ag]_t}$$

So that the following equation (187) could be used in order to fit the pseudo-first order kinetics:

$$Ln \frac{[AbAg]_e}{[AbAg]_e - [AbAg]_t} = K_{+1} t \frac{[Ab]_t [Ag]_t}{[AbAg]_e} \quad ....(6)$$

On the other hand, figure (4-4) and (4-5) show the plot of $\ln \frac{[AbAg]_e}{[AbAg]_e - [AbAg]_t}$ Against time (t) in both benign and malignant breast tumors, which give a straight line with a slope equal to the observed value of first rate constant Kbos in min-1. The rate constant (k+1) in mg-1. mL. min was calculated at five different temperatures by using the following equation (194)

$$K_{obs} = K_{+1} \frac{[^{125}I - antiCA15 - 3]_t [CA15 - 3]_t}{[^{125}I - antiCA15 - 3/CA15 - 3]_e} \dots\dots\dots(7)$$

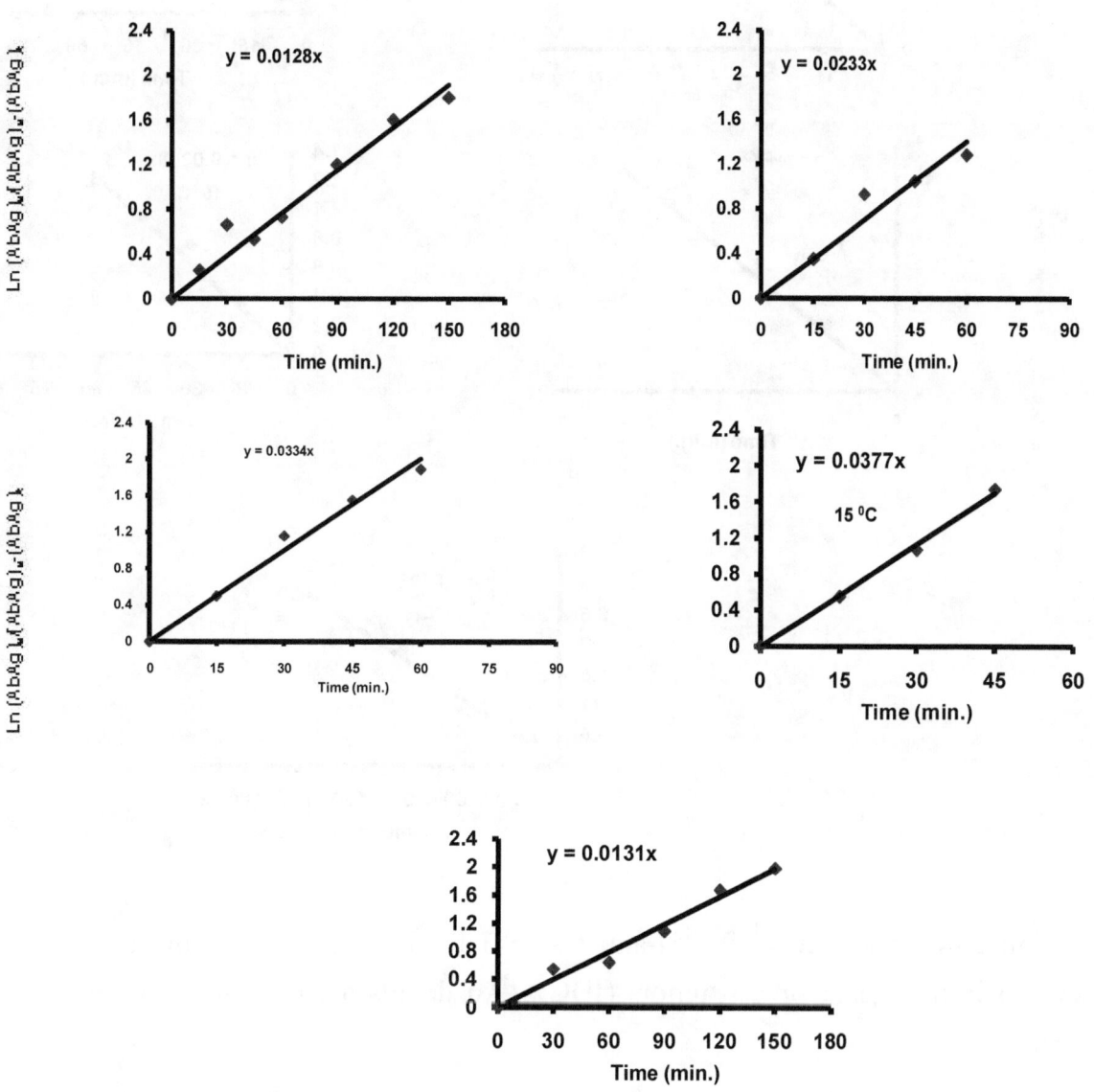

Figure (4.4): Kinetics of 125I-anti CA15-3 antibody binding to partially purified CA15-3 in benign breast tumors (Fibroadenoma). All details are explained in the text.

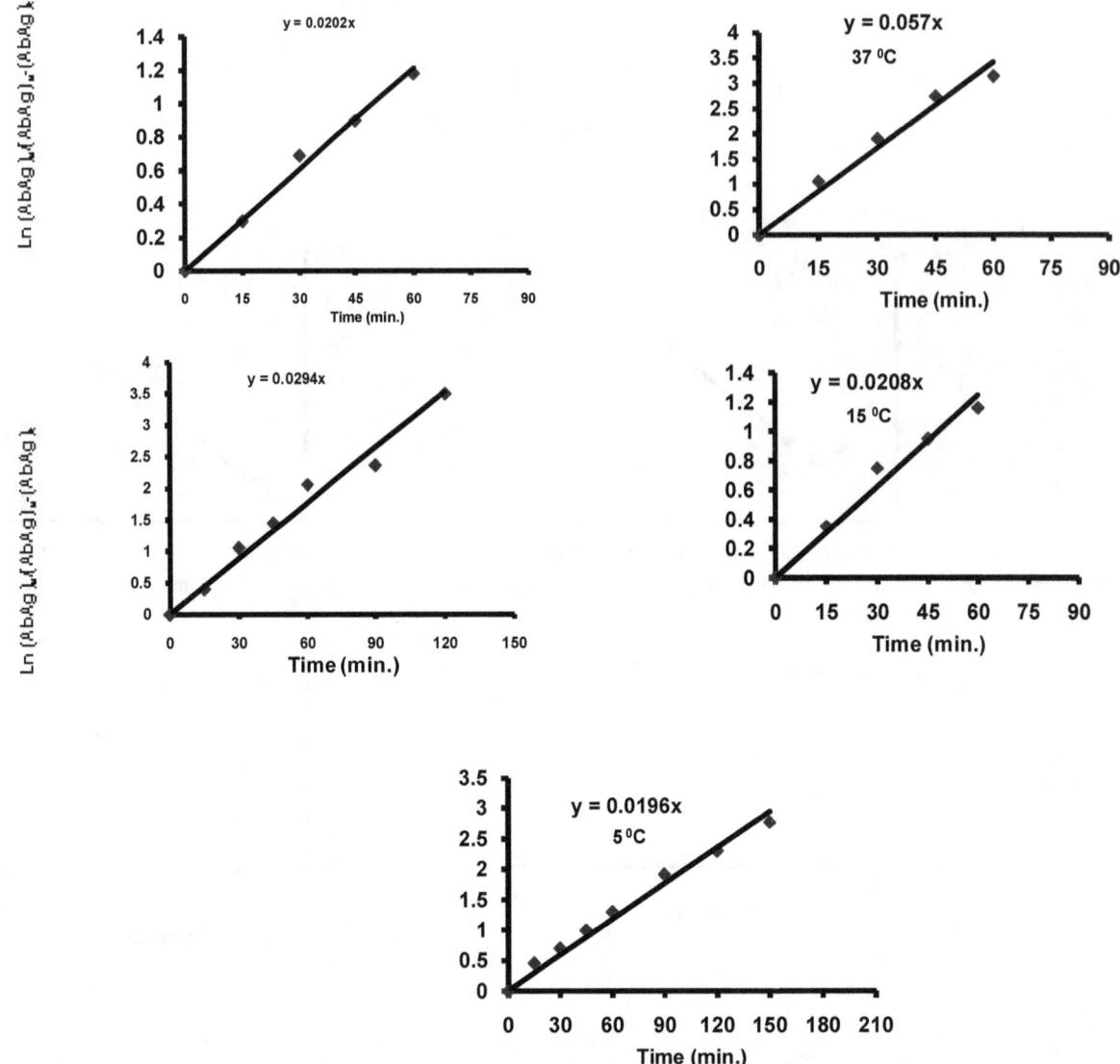

Figure (4.5): Kinetics of 125I-anti CA15-3 binding to partially purified CA15-3 in malignant breast tumors (IDC). (All details are explained in the text).

The value of k-1 at five temperatures was calculated by using equation (4). Whereas, the half-life time of association (t ½)ass. , Which represented the time needed for the formation of half amount of the complex at equilibrium was determined from the concentration of the complex at equilibrium and the time-course curve. The half-life time of dissociation (t ½) diss. , was calculated from the following relation:

$$(t_{1/2})_{diss.} = \frac{\ln 2}{k_{-1}} = \frac{0.693}{k_{-1}}$$

$$(t_{1/2})_{ass.} = \frac{\ln 2}{k_{obs}} = \frac{0.693}{k_{+1}}$$

The value of kobs. , k+1, k-1, (t ½)ass. ,(t ½)diss. at five different temperatures are summarized in table (4.3). Data analysis in this table shows that highest rate for the association reaction k+1 , in benign breast tumors (Fibroadenoma) and malignant breast tumors (IDC) occurs at 37°C and 15°C respectively , while the lowest rate occurs at 45°C. This means the dependence of reaction rate on temperature (Table 4.3) that also shows the values of the rate constant for the reverse reaction k-1 calculated from equation (4). Results show that the rate of dissociation of 125I-anti CA15-3 antibody, from its CA15-3 is temperature independent.

Table (4.3): The effect of temperature on the kinetic parameters of 125I-anti CA15-3 binding to partially purified CA15-3 in benign and malignant breast tumors at five different temperature.

Temp. °C	$k_{obs} \times 10^{-3}$ (min^{-1})		K_{+1} mg^{-1}.ml.min^{-1}		$k_{-1} \times 10^{-1}$ (min^{-1})		$(t_{1/2})_{ass}$ (min)		$(t_{1/2})_{diss}$ (min)	
	Benign (Fibroadenom)	Malignant (IDC)	Benign (Fibroadenoma)	Malignant (IDC)	Benign (Fibroadenoma)	Malignant (IDC)	Benign (Fibroadenoma)	Malignant (IDC)	Benign (Fibroadenoma)	Malignant (IDC)
5	12.8	20.20	48.69	45.81	15.38	34.68	54	34	45	20
15	23.3	57.00	60.65	116.16	32.50	73.75	30	12	21	9
25	33.4	24.9	93.98	35.48	57.37	18.07	21	28	12	38
37	37.7	20.30	103.54	46.61	61.89	22.43	18	34	11	31
45	13.1	19.60	35.40	21.34	24.96	10.58	53	35	28	66

The Thermodynamic Studies of 125I-Anti CA15-3 Antibody to the Partially Purified CA15-3 in Benign and Malignant Tumors

Thermodynamic Parameters of Standard State

Figure (4.6) and (4.7) show Van't Hoff plot of the binding of 125I-anti CA15-3 antibody to the partially purified CA15-3 in benign breast tumors (Fibroadenoma) and malignant breast tumors (IDC) respectively, at different temperatures (5 , 15 , 25 , 37 and 45 °C).

These figures revealed that the equilibrium binding constant (affinity constant) for CA15-3 to its antibody is a temperature dependent. The results indicated that $\Delta H°$, in general, had small values and their positive sign ascertains that the reaction was nearly endothermic. The $\Delta H°$ value in the case of the binding of 125I-anti CA15-3 antibody to partially purified CA15-3 in benign breast tumors 12.71 KJ.mol-1 was higher than that in case of binding in malignant breast tumors (IDC) 6.7 KJ.mol-1, so more energy is needed in case of benign breast tumor for the reaction (binding) to occur. The small positive value of $\Delta H°$ may indicate a favorable interaction between 125I-anti CA15-3 antibody with partially purified CA15-3 in both cases.

These include the non-covalent interaction, which are fundamentally electrostatic in nature such as charge-charge, charge-dipole, dipole-dipole, charge-induced dipole, dipole-induced dipole interactions, and hydrogen bonds. The sum of these types of interactions can yield some stabilization to the folded structure of the complex (195).

The other values of thermodynamic parameters of standard state at five temperatures, such as $\Delta G°$ values and $\Delta S°$ values are summarized in table (4.4) and (4.5).

Table (4.4): Thermodynamic parameters at standard state of 125I-anti CA15-3 to the partially CA15-3 in benign breast tumors (Fibroadenoma). (All other details are explained in the text).

Temp. °C	$\Delta H°$ KJ .moL-1	$\Delta G°$ KJ .moL-1	$\Delta S°$ J .mol-1.K-1
5	12.71	-36.87	137.20
15	12.71	-38.59	138.42
25	12.71	-39.88	138.10

37	12.71	-41.82	139.01
45	12.71	-44.30	143.30

Table (4.5): Thermodynamic parameters at standard state of 125I-anti CA15-3 to the partially purified CA15-3 in malignant breast tumors (IDC). (All other details are explained in the text).

Temp. °C	ΔH° KJ .moL-1	ΔG° KJ .moL-1	ΔS° J .mol-1.K-1
5	6.70	-36.82	156.55
15	6.70	-39.11	159.06
25	6.70	-40.48	158.32
37	6.70	-42.27	157.97
45	6.70	-43.54	157.99

The negative values of ΔG° reflects the stability of the complex hence. The high affinity of the reactants. The high negative values of ΔG° for the binding reaction are controlled by high positive ΔS° values of the complex formed. So, our system is characterized by the sole contribution of ΔS° to the stability of the complex formed, which ΔH° has little or no effect (196). Whereas, the negative values of ΔG° indicates that the reaction is spontaneous at the standard condition. On the other hand, the high positive of ΔS° suggest that the binding was entropically driven. Entropy has a driven force for the occurrence of the binding reaction, this indicates that the hydrophobic interactions played an important role in the stability of complex formation (197).

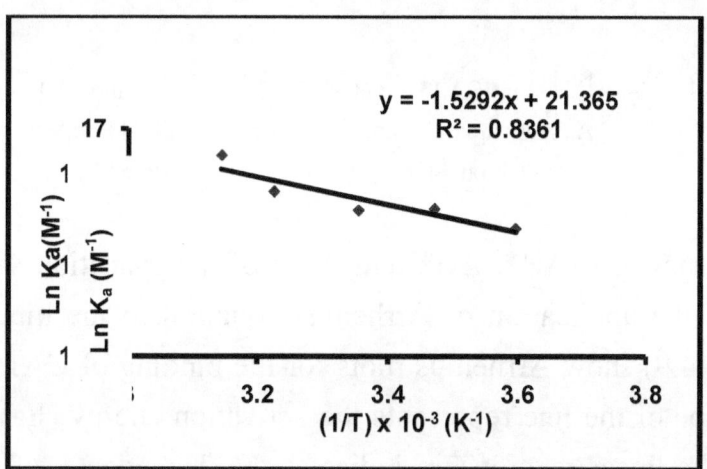

Figure (4.6): Van't Hoff plot for the binding of 125I-anti CA15-3 antibody to the partially purified CA15-3 in benign breast tumors (Fibroadenoma). All details are explained in the text.

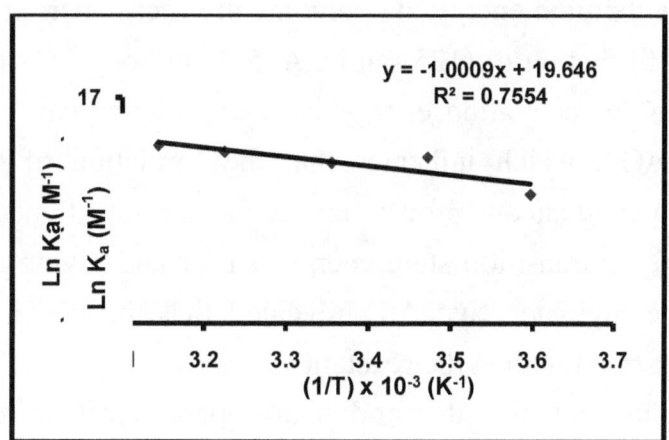

Figure (4.7): Van't Hoff plot for the binding of 125I-anti CA15-3 antibody to the partially purified CA15-3 in malignant breast tumors (IDC). All details are explained in the text.

B. Thermodynamic Parameters of Transition State

Transition state theory postulated that the interaction of two substances to form the final product proceeds through the formation of an activated complex (transition state).

Consequently, the association of 125I-anti CA15-3 antibody with its CA15-3 can be represented as follows:

$$^{125}I - antiCA\,15-3 + CA15-3 \rightarrow \left[^{125}I - antiCA\,15-3/CA15-3\right]^{*} \rightarrow \left[^{125}I - antiCA\,15-3/CA15-3\right]$$

$$\text{State (A)} \qquad\qquad \text{An Activated Complex} \qquad\qquad \text{Final Product}$$

$$\qquad\qquad\qquad\qquad \text{Transition State} \qquad\qquad\qquad \text{State (B)}$$

Thermodynamic parameters (ΔH^*, ΔG^* and ΔS^*) of the transition state were determined from the application of Arrhenius equation to the kinetic data. Figure (4.8) and (4.9) show Arrhenius plots for the binding of CA15-3 to its antibody, the slope of the line represents the activation energy (Ea) of the binding reaction, the linear relationship indicates the dependency of the association rate constant of the binding of CA15-3 to its antibody for benign and malignant breast tumors homogenate on temperature.

Table (4.6) and (4.7) show the values of thermodynamic parameters of the transition state (Ea, ΔH^*, ΔG^* and ΔS^*).

The high values of activation energy 9.96 KJ.mol-1 and 41.76 KJ.mol-1 of CA15-3 partially purified from benign and malignant breast tumors respectively, represents the required energy to overcome the energy barrier of the transition state for the formation of (125I-anti CA15-3 antibody / CA15-3) complex. Also the value of activation energy is in accordance with the high positive values of ΔG^*, which indicates that the formation of the activated complex is a non-spontaneous process and requires a lot of energy (equal to Ea) to overcome the transition state energy barrier and giving the final product, whereas the high negative ΔS^* revealed that the activated complex had a more order structure than the reactants.

From the result obtained of the thermodynamic parameters in the transition state, it can be concluded that the positive values of ΔH^* and high positive values of ΔG^* are favorable to overcome the energy barrier of the transition state, the high negative values of ΔG^* is mainly attributed to the decrease in entropy of the transition state ($\Delta S^* < 0$).

In addition the positive values of ΔH^* show that the heat content of the activated complex is more than that in isolated species (193,198).

It is proposed that the formation of a complex occurs in the two steps. The first is the stabilization of the complex by hydrophobic interactions and second is the stabilization by short range interactions , such as electrostatic interaction, hydrogen bonding and Van der Waals interactions (199).

Hydrophobic interactions contribute to the complex stability via high positive entropy change ($\Delta S^* > 0$), while electrostatic interactions, hydrogen bonding and Van der Waals interactions contribute to the stability of the complex via negative entropy change ($\Delta S^* > 0$) (199,200).

The thermodynamic data indicate that the binding of 125I-anti CA15-3 antibody to partially purified CA15-3 are entropy driven and in agreement with the concept that hydrophobic interaction play an important rote in the formation of (125I-anti CA15-3 antibody / CA15-3) complex.

Table (4.6): Thermodynamic parameters at transition state of 125I-anti CA15-3 antibody to the partially purified CA15-3 in benign breast tumors (Fibroadenoma). (All other details are explained in the text).

Temp. °C	Ea KJ . mol-1	ΔH^* KJ . mol-1	ΔG^* KJ . mol-1	ΔS^* J .mol-1. K-1
5	9.96	7.65	58.94	-184.50
15	9.96	7.57	60.62	-184.20
25	9.96	7.48	61.72	-182.01
37	9.96	7.38	64.06	-182.84
45	9.96	7.32	68.62	-192.77

Table (4.7): Thermodynamic parameters at transition state of 125I-anti CA15-3 antibody to the partially purified CA15-3 in malignant breast tumors (IDC). (All other details are explained in the text).

Temp. °C	Ea KJ . mol-1	ΔH^* KJ . mol-1	ΔG^* KJ . mol-1	ΔS^* J .mol-1. K-1
5	41.76	39.45	59.08	-70.61
15	41.76	39.37	59.09	-68.47
25	41.76	39.28	64.14	-83.42
37	41.76	39.18	66.12	-86.90
45	41.76	39.12	70.00	-97.11

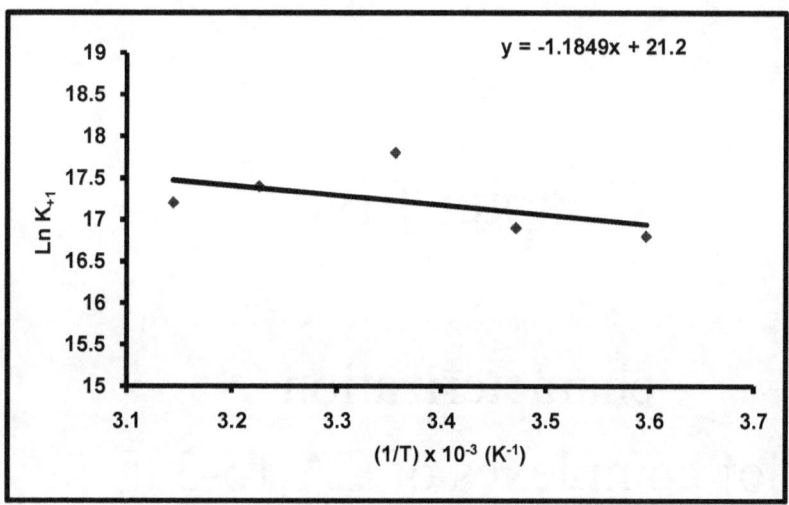

Figure (4-8): Arrhenius plot for the binding of 125I-anti CA15-3 to the partially purified CA15-3 in benign breast tumor (Fibroadnoma). All details are explained in the text.

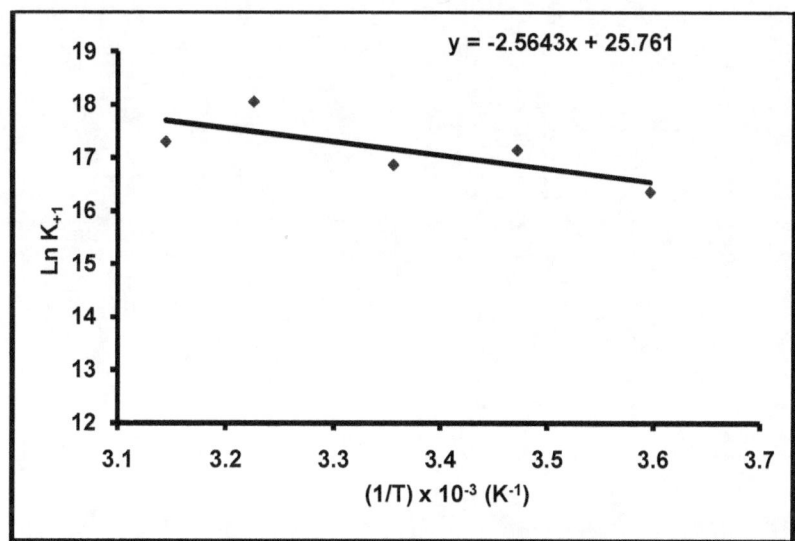

Figure (4.9): Arrhenius plot for the binding of 125I-anti CA15-3 to the partially purified CA15-3 in malignant breast tumor (IDC). All details are explained in the text. Gel filtration technique was used to separate 125I-anti CA 15-3 antibody bound to partially purified CA 15-3 using benign (Fibroadenoma) and malignant (IDC) breast tissue homogenate (as CA 15-3 source) from unbound (Free) 125I-anti CA 15-3 antibody.

Chapter Five

characterization
of complexes of CA 15-3

Introduction

The characterization of the complexes (125I-anti CA 15-3 antibody/ CA15-3) from both benign and malignant breast tumors was carried out through the ultraviolet spectroscopic studies. Factors affecting the absorption properties of the two types of complexes such as pH, solvent polarity (solvent perturbation technique), spectrophotometric pH titration, and thermal stability in the presence of different concentrations of sodium chloride have been studied. pH titration of the two types of the complexes show that about (41.43%) and (44.29%) of histydyl residues are located on the surface of the two types of protein complexes (benign and malignant) respectively, while (40%) and (50%) of tyrosyl residues are buried interiorly in the complexes of (benign and malignant) respectively.

Molecules absorb light; the efficiency of absorption depend on both the structure and environment of the molecule making absorption spectroscopy a useful tool for characterizing both small and large molecule.

The ultraviolet absorption spectra of protein solutions in the region 250 to 310 nm are contributed from phenylalanyl, tyrosyl and tryptophanyl residues. But at the shorter wavelengths the contributions come from other groups such as histidyl residues and the peptide bond (169). Changes in the environment of these chromophores can lead to alteration in the absorption spectrum, and the conformational changes of a protein may also involve environmental changes of its chromophoric groups (1201). A variety of environmental changes (e.g. pH, temperature) can affect the absorption spectrum if the interaction of chromophore and perturbing agent affects the ground and excited states, the altered spectrum of the chromophore can be shifted to longer (red shift) or shorter (blue shift) wavelengths. The shift may or may not be accompanied by a change in intensity of the spectrum (170,202). Saif-Alla, P.H., studied the UV spectra of h-PRL-antibody complex and CA15-3 molecule (203).

Interaction of h-CA 15-3 partially purified from benign (fibroadenoma) and malignant (IDC) tissues homogenate with its antibody is an example of protein-protein association. Although several new immunochemical techniques were developed to study such interactions (204,205), UV spectral remain as one of the most important methods in immunology because it provides a sensitive and quantitative measurements for the study of antibody structure and its specific ligand binding (206,208).

Very limited work concerning the physical properties of CA 15-3 specially those related to UV spectroscopy has been done, also the UV studies on CA 15-3 antibody interaction are not wide spread. Hence, this work is planned to study the association of the partially purified h-CA 15-3 and its antibody at different conditions.

Materials and Methods

5.1. Materials

5.1.1. Chemicals

All chemicals and reagents used in the experiments of this chapter were mentioned in section (2.1.1).

5.1.2. Instruments

The instruments used in this chapter are Shimadzu double beam UV-Visible spectrophotometer type 160, and instruments listed in section (2.1.2).

5.1.3 Buffers and Reagents

Buffers and reagents mentioned in section (2.1.6) are used in this chapter. Other additional solutions are indicators in each experiment.

5.2. Methods

5.2.1. Gel Filtration Technique for Separation of Free and Bound125I - Anti CA 15-3 Antibody

5.2.1.1. Preparation of the Column

The dimensions of the column were (1x30 cm) chosen according to the equation in section (3.2.1.1).

5.2.1.2. Preparation of the Gel and Determination of Void Volume

The sepharose CL-4B was used to separate free and bound 125I - anti CA 15-3 antibody, and was prepared as mentioned in section (3.2.1.3) and (3.2.1.4), the void volume was determined and found to be 10 mL.

5.2.1.3 Separation Procedure of (125I-Anti CA 15-3 Antibody/CA15-3) Complex

A) Partially Purified CA15-3 from Benign Breast Tumor (Fibroadenoma) and its Antibody 125I -Anti CA 15-3

Reagents

Buffer PBS 0.15M, pH 7.0 containing 0.02% sodium azide was prepared as described previously in section (2.1.1.3).

Procedure

1-   Partially purified CA 15-3 (475μL) containing (0.665 mg. mL-1) was incubated with 120 μL of 125I-anti CA 15-3 antibody (0.8412mg. mL-1) and complete the reaction to a final volume of 700 μL with PBS buffer 0.15 M pH 7.0. The tubes were incubated for 90 min. at 37oC.

2-   At the end of incubation, the mixture was applied to the surface of a sepharose CL-4B (1x30 cm) with a bed volume (23.5 cm3) equilibrated with PBS buffer 0.15M, pH 7.0. Elution was carried out using the same buffer to separate CA 15-3 bound to 125I-anti CA 15-3 antibody from unbound (Free) CA 15-3 and 125I-anti CA 15-3 antibody with a flow rate (1 mL per 7 min), and fraction volumes of 1 mL were collected.

3-   The radioactivity of each fraction was counted by gamma counter for one minute.

4-   Protein concentration was measured at 280 nm.

5-   One hundred and twenty microliters of 125I-anti CA 15-3 antibody (0.84 mg. μL-1) was completed to 700 μL with PBS buffer (0.15M, pH7.0), then this volume was injected to the column as mentioned in step2, then steps 2,3 and 4 were repeated.

Calculations

1. Radioactivity (c.p.m) of each eluted fraction was plotted against the fraction number.

2. The absorbance of each eluted fractions was measured at 280nm, and the absorbance was plotted against the fraction number.

3. The percent radioactivity was calculated by dividing the sum of the radioactivity of the fractions under each peak by the sum of radioactivity of all peaks appeared in the profile:

$$\text{Percent radioactivity of each peak} = \frac{\text{Radioactivity per peak (c.p.m)}}{\text{Sum of radioactivity of all peaks (c.p.m.)}} \times 100$$

B) Partially Purified CA15-3 from Premenopausal Malignant Breast Tumors (IDC) and Its Antibody 125I-anti CA 15-3

Reagents

Buffer PBS 0.15 M, pH 7.0 containing 0.02% sodium azid was prepared as described previously in section (2.1.1.3).

Procedure

1.   Four hundred and twenty four microliters of partially purified CA 15-3 (0.147 mg. mL-1 protein) and incubated with 106 μL of 125I-anti CA 15-3 antibody (0.743 mg.mL-1) in a final volume 700 mL with PBS buffer 0.15M pH 7.0. The tubes were then incubated for 150 min at 15oC.

2.   Steps 2,3,4 and 5 in section (5.2.1.3 A) were repeated.

Calculation

The same calculation that mentioned in section (5.2.1.3 A) was used to calculate the radioactivity; protein was measured at 280nm and the percent of radioactivity of each peak was determined.

5.2.2. The UV Spectrum of (125I-Anti CA 15-3 Antibody/CA15-3) Complex from Benign and Malignant Breast Tumors

The gel filtration profile in section (5.2.1.3 A&B) gave two peaks. The fractions under each peak were pooled and the absorption spectrum was scanned in UV Region against the appropriate blank in the reference beam.

5.2.3. The UV. Spectrum of 125I-Anti CA 15-3 Antibody

Half milliliter of 125I-anti CA 15-3 antibody was placed in a 0.25 cm cuvette in the sample beam and the absorption spectrum was measured immediately against an appropriate blank in the reference beam.

5.2.4. The UV Spectrum of Partially Purified CA 15-3

Half milliliter of partially purified CA 15-3 from benign (Fibroadenoma) and malignant (IDC) breast tumors was placed in a 0.25 cm curette in the sample beam and the absorption spectrum was measured immediately against an appropriate blank in the reference beam.

5.2.5.Factors Affecting the Absorption Properties of (125I-Anti CA 15-3 Antibody/CA 15-3) Complex from Benign and Malignant Breast Tumors

5.2.5.1. The pH Effect on the Complex

Reagents

1. KCl-HCl buffer (pH 2) was prepared as follows:

Solution A: Potassium chloride (0.15M), 1.11825 gm was dissolved in a final volume of 100mL deionized distilled water.

Solution B: Hydrochloric acid (0.15M).

The required pH (2.0) was prepared by mixing a volume of solution A with an appropriate amount of solution B to obtain the required pH.

1. Citrate-phosphate buffer at different pH was prepared as follows:

Solution A: Citric acid (0.15M); 2.8815 gm citric acid dissolved in 100mL deionized distilled water.

Solution B: Dibasic sodium phosphate (0.15M); 2.1294 gm of Na_2HPO_4 was dissolved in a final volume of 100 mL deionized distilled water.

Working buffer pH (4 and 6) was prepared by mixing a volume of solution A with an appropriate amount of solution B to obtain the required pH.

2. Phosphate buffer at different pH values was prepared as follows:

Solution A: Dibasic sodium phosphate (0.15M), 2.1294 gm Na_2HPO_4 was dissolved in a final volume of 100 mL deionized distilled water.

Solution B: Monobasic sodium phosphate (0.15M), 1.7997 gm NaH_2PO_4 was dissolved in a final volume of 100 ml deionized distilled water.

Phosphate buffers at different pH rang (7-8) were prepared by mixing a volume of solution A with an appropriate amount of solution B to obtain the required pH.

3. Glycine - NaOH buffer was prepared as follows:

Solution A: Glycin (0.15M); 1.12575gm C2H5NO2 was dissolved in a final volume of 100 mL deionized distilled water.

Solution B: Sodium hydroxide (0.15M); 0.6gm NaOH was dissolved in a final volume of 100 mL deionized distilled water.

Working buffer pH (9-11) was prepared by mixing a volume of solution A with an appropriate a mount of solution B to obtain the required pH.

Procedure

Two hundred and fifty microliters of pooled fractions under the first peak that represent (125I-anti CA 15-3 antibody/CA 15-3) complex, was completed to 500µl with different buffers at different pH values (4 to 11), then each sample beam and the buffer at the adjusted pH in the reference beam. The absorption spectrum was scanned.

Calculations

The molar absorption coefficient ($\square$) for (125I-anti CA 15-3 antibody/CA 15-3) complex at 278 nm was calculated from Lambert-Beer's law.

5.2.5.2. Effect of Solvent Polarity on UV Spectra of the Complex

The effect of 20% ethanol, and the same amount for ethylene glycol, glycerol, sucrose, urea, dimethyl sulphoxide, dioxane, and polyethylene glycol; on the complex. Two hundred and fifty microliters of complex from benign and malignant breast tumors of pooled fractions under the first peak were completed to 500 µL with phosphate buffer containing any of the following solvent at pH 7.4 in the test cell and the 20% ethanol, ethylene glycol, glycerol, sucrose, urea, dimethyl sulphoxide, dioxane, and polyethylene glycol was adjusted and placed in the reference cell using 0.25 cm cuvette (i.e., the experiment was repeated by using solvents individually).

Calculations

The absorption spectrum of each sample was scanned immediately in the area of (200-350 nm).

5.2.5.3. Spectrophotometric pH Titration on the Complex

A series of complex from benign (Fibroadenoma) and Malignant (IDC) breast tumors (250 μL) were completed to 500 μL with buffer at pH ranging from 8 to 11. The maximum absorbance of each sample was measured at 295 nm; the absorbance of λ max at each pH value was plotted versus the corresponding pH. Other series of complexes isolated from benign (Fibroadenoma) and malignant (IDC) breast tumors (250 μL) were completed to 500 μL with buffer at pH ranging 4 to 8. The maximum absorbance of each sample was measured at 211nm. The absorbance of λmax at each pH value was plotted against the corresponding pH.

5.2.5.4. The Effect of NaCl Concentration on the Thermal Stability of the Complex by UV Spectral Studies

Reagents

Twenty percent ethylene glycol buffur was prepared by dissolving 20mL of ethylene glycol in 80mL of phosphate buffer. NaCl (0.01M) in 20% ethylene glycol was prepared by dissolving 0.05844 gm of NaCl in 100mL of 20% ethylene glycol buffur, while NaCl (0.1M) in 20% ethylene glycol was prepared by dissolving 0.5844 gm of NaCl in 100mL of 20% ethylene glycol buffer.

Procedure

Two hundred and fifty microliters of complex from benign (Fibroadenoma) or malignant (IDC) breast tumors were completed to a final volume 500 μL with 20% ethylene glycol buffer pH7.4 containing 0.01 M NaCl Each mixture was placed in 0.25 cm cuvette in the sample beam and the buffer at the adjusted pH in the reference beam.The absorbtion was measured at the wavelength of (292 and 295 nm) at different temperatures 20, 30, 40, 50, 60, 70oC. The experiment was repeated for each complex with another solution (20% ethylene glycol 0.1 M NaCl), at 295 nm.

Calculations

The absorbance of each complex was plotted against the different temperatures at two wavelengths (292 and 295 nm).

5.2.5.5. Effect of Urea, KCl and (Urea, KCl) Mixture on the Spectrum of the Complex

Reagent

1. Eight molar of urea was prepared by dissolving 24.02gm of Urea in a final volume of 50 mL of PBS buffer at pH 7.4.

2. KCl (0.03 M) was prepared by dissolving 0.2737gm of the salt in a final volume of 50mL of corresponding buffer.

3. PB buffer solution was prepared as described in section (5.2.5.1).

Procedure

Two hundred and fifty microliters of complex isolated from benign (fibroadenoma) and malignant (IDC) were pipetted in a set of three tubes. The volume was completed to 500 μL with PBS buffer at pH 7.4 contains (0.03 KCl, 8 M urea and mixture 1:1 of both 0.03 KCl and 8M Urea) respectively, then each sample was placed in 0.25cm cuvette in the sample beam and the buffer at the same pH in the presence of the same salt in the reference beam.

Calculations

The absorption spectrum of each sample was scanned immediately in the area of (200-350 nm).

5.3. Results and Discussion

Protein UV light maximum absorption is at approximately 280nm, caused by tryptophan, tyrosine and (to a lesser extent) phenylalanine residues, and at lower wavelength (215-230 nm) due to polypeptide chain backbone. Absorbance at 280 nm varies for each protein. The absorbance at lower wavelengths is directly related to the amount of polypeptide material and is usually considerably more sensitive than at 280nm.however,many buffers and other molecules also absorb at these lower wavelengths (phosphate and tris buffers are acceptable but the preservative sodium azide absorbs strongly).

Absorbance at 215-230 nm is useful for monitoring peptides that may not contain tryptophan or tyrosine (205).

Gel Filtration Technique for Separation of Free and Bound 125I-Anti CA15-3 Antibody

Figure (5-1) and (5-2) show the results of gel filtration technique to separate 125I-anti CA 15-3 antibody bound to partially purified CA 15-3 from benign (Fibroadenoma) and malignant (IDC) breast tumors respectively. The profile of separation revealed two peaks. The first peak represents (125I-anti CA 15-3 antibody/CA 15-3) complex, the second peak represents the unbound (Free) 125I-anti CA 15-3 antibody. Figure (5-3) show the gel filtration profile of 125I-anti CA 15-3 antibody, the results revealed only one peak in the same position of the second peak of figures (5-1) and (5-2), which represent the unbound 125I-anti CA 15-3 antibody. The percent of 125I-anti CA 15-3 antibody/ CA 15-3) complex was 49.74% in benign (Fibroadenoma) breast tumors patients, while the percent of complex was 56.20% in malignant breast tumors patients (IDC). On the other hand the percent of 125I-anti CA 15-3 antibody was 34.40% in benign breast tumors (Fibroadenoma) and 31.42% in malignant breast tumors (IDC). This is because the epitope of CA 15-3 in malignant breast tumors was higher than in benign breast tumors.

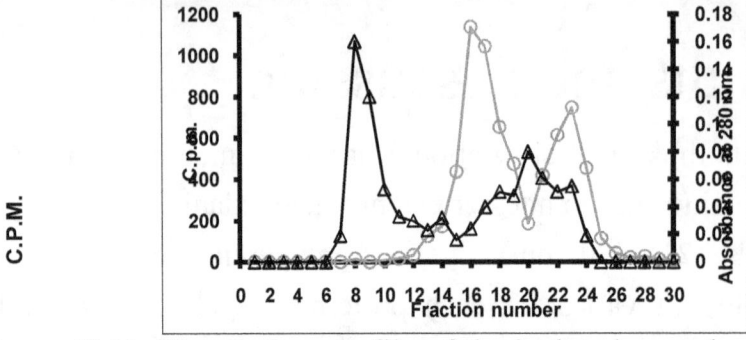

Figure (5.1): The elution profile of the isolated complex (125I-antiCA15-3 antibody/CA15-3) and free antibody in benign breast tumors on Sepharose CL-4B. (○) radioactivity, (△) protein. (All other details are explained in the text).

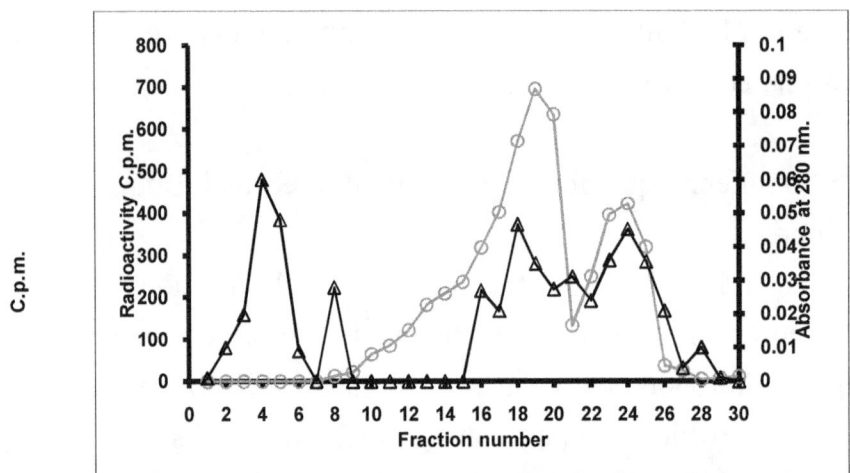

Figure (5.2): The elution profile of the isolated complex (125I-antiCA15-3 antibody/CA15-3) and free antibody in malignant breast tumors (IDC) on Sepharose CL-4B, (○) radioactivity, (△) protein. (All other details are explained in the text).

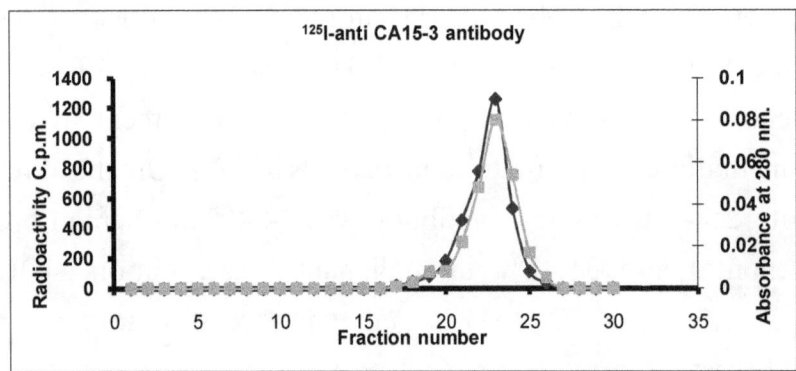

Figure (5.3): The elution profile of the 125I-antiCA15-3 antibody on Sepharose CL-4B, (■) radioactivity, (◆) protein. (All other details are explained in the text).

The UV Spectra of Partially Purified CA 15-3, Anti CA 15-3 Antibody and (125I-Anti CA 15-3 Antibody/CA 15-3) Complex Molecules

The UV spectra of partially purified h-CA 15-3, 125I-anti CA 15-3 antibody and (125I-anti CA 15-3 antibody/CA 15-3) complex were scanned from 200-350 nm to determine the absorption spectra, and the alternation in the UV spectra as a results of their interaction.

The UV Spectrum of Partially Purified CA 15-3

The UV spectra of partially purified h-CA15-3 in benign tumors (Fibroadenoma) and malignant tumors (IDC) at neutral pH shows that the λmax for purified CA15-3 from benign (Fibroadenoma) consisted of two peaks; a large one at 208nm and smaller one at 270nm, while the UV spectra of purified CA 15-3 from malignant tumors (IDC) shows two peaks at 205 and 270nm as shown in table (5.1). Therefore it seemed that each human CA 15-3 has a characteristic spectrum and can be identified by its peaks, the first peak (at 208nm or 205nm) such results could be due to the amide group in polypeptide bond of h-CA 15-3 molecule with contribution of the histidyl residues (207), while the second peak (at 270) is assigned to the side chain chromophore of phenylalanine or tryptophyl residues (208).

The UV spectrum of 125I-Anti CA 15-3 Antibody

The UV spectrum of 125I-anti CA 15-3 antibody at neutral pH shows that the λ max consisted one peak at 203.6nm, which is assigned to the amide groups in the polypeptide bond (207), with contribution of hisidyl residues (209) as shown in table (5.1) .

The UV spectrum of (125I-Anti CA 15-3 Antibody/CA 15-3) Complex

The UV spectra of partially purified CA 15-3 extracted from benign (Fibroadenoma) and malignant (IDC) bound to 125I-anti CA 15-3 antibody at neutral pH show that the λ max is consisted of two peaks at (203.4nm and 274nm) in benign complex, while the λ max is consisted of two peaks at (204.2 nm and 278nm) in malignant complex as shown in table (5-1). The first peak at (274nm or 278nm) is assigned to tyrosyl residues(208), it is very weak band and it seems that the tyrosyl residues in the benign or malignant complexes is located on the surface of protein complex.

The strong absorption of the second peaks (at 203.4 or 204.2nm) arises form electronic transition in the peptide backbone itself and is therefore sensitive to backbone conformation (207).

Table (5-1): The λ max valves of (125I-anti CA 15-3 antibody/CA 15-3) complex, partially purified CA 15-3 and unbound (Free) 125I-anti CA 15-3 antibody in both cases benign and malignant breast tumors. (All other details are explained in the test).

No.	Fractions	Benign λmax (nm)	Malignant λmax (nm)
1	CA 15-3 partially purified	208, 270	205, 270
2	125I-anti CA 15-3 antibody	203.6	203.6
3	125I-anti CA15-3 antibody/ CA15-3) complex	203.4, 274	204.2, 278

Factors Affecting the Absorption Properties of (125I-Anti CA15-3 Antibody/ CA15-3) Complex from Benign and Malignant Breast Tumors

The Effect of pH on the Complex

The pH of the solvent determines the ionization state of ionizable chromophores in the protein molecule (208). The UV spectrum of isolated (125I-anti CA 15-3 antibody/CA15-3) complex from benign (Fibroadenoma) and malignant (IDC) breast tumors was determined at different pH (2, 4, 6, 7, 7.4, 8, 9, 10, and 11). Table (5-2) shows the effect of different pH on both complexes. At an acidic pH 2 and neutral pH (7,7.4) the both complexes benign (Fibroadenoma) and malignant (IDC) have one maximum wavelength near 200 nm as compare to UV spectrum of h-CA 15-3 and the 125I anti CA15-3 antibody.

The λ max of CA 15-3 (270 and 208 nm) in benign (Fibroadenoma) and its antibody λ max (203.6) disappeared. The λ max of CA 15-3 (270 and 205 nm) in malignant (IDC) and its antibody λmax (203.6) also disappeared. The absorption near 200 nm is characteristic of the amide group in the polypeptide bond of the complex (209). The blue shift is due to the increasing of hydrogen bond formed in the presence of highly positively charged state (210). The disappearance of λmax 280 nm of tyrosine and phenylalanine due to conformational changes and chromophore in native complex were buried in the interior of their complexes(211,212). Protein shows a strong absorption in range (180-225 nm), absorption at such wavelength arises from electronic transition in the polypeptide backbone itself and is therefore sensitive to back bone conformation(207).

At pH (4, 6, 9, 10, and 11) no band was observed and all peaks disappeared. The disappearance of the λ max at these pH's may be due to conformational changes of the protein complex.

Table (5-2): The effect of different pH on λ max values of (125I-anti CA 15-3 antibody/CA 15-3) complex. (All other details are explained in the text).

pH	λ max (nm)	
	(125I-anti CA 15-3 antibody/CA15-3) benign complex	(125I-anti CA 15-3 antibody/CA 15-3) malignant complex
2	200	200
4	-	-
6	-	-
7	200	200
7.4	200	200
8	200	200
9	-	-
10	-	-
11	-	-

Effect of Solvent Polarity on UV Spectra of the Complex

The immediate environment of a chromophore affects its absorption. The determination of whether an amino acid is internal or external by measuring the spectra of protein in a polar and non-polar solvent is called the solvent perturbation method (208). In fact, proteins are rarely studied in completely non-polar solvents because most proteins are either insoluble or denatured in these solvents. However, significant solvent effects can be induced by use of a mixture of water and substance of a reduced polarity such as ethanol, ethylene glycol, polyethelyne glycol, sucrose, dioxane and dimethyl sulfoxide (DMSO)(208). Several spectra changes were obtained in the precence of these perturbants, like the alteration of λmax positions and intensities of protein spectrum and the appearance of new chromophores on the surface of the complex. These chromophores on the region of the protein disappeared in the absence of the solvent. One of the main assumptions of the solvent perturbation technique is that solvent alters the peak positions and intensities by altering the energy and probably of electronic transitions. Other considerations include the following (213,214):

a. Polarization effect

b. Change in permanent dipole moment during excitation, which will tend to produce either a short wave or a long wave shift depending on the nature of the electronic transition and wheather the solute is a hydrogen donor or hydrogen acceptor (215).

The effects of different solvents on the (125I-anti CA 15-3 antibody /CA 15-3) complex from benign (Fibroadenoma) and malignant (IDC) breast tumors at pH 7.4 were investigated. The data obtained are illustrated in table (5-3). It was found that one λ max specific for the amide groups of polypeptide bond at pH 7.4, this shift toward the shorter wavelength is due to the n-π* transitions in the presence of 20% ethanol, ethylene glycol and glycerol. In the presence of polyethylene glycol there was a significant red shift in the λ max (204 nm) in benign (Fibroadenoma) complex and λ max (205nm) in malignant (IDC) complex. When 20% Dioxane was used there were a significant red shift in the λ max (220nm) of the amide bond at pH 7.4, which assigned to tyrosyl residue. The value of λ max is for n-π* transitions which occur at longer wavelength because the nonbonded electrons in the anion are available for interaction with the π electron system of the ring (215), while in the presence of 20% sucrose the complex has a slight blue shift and show λ max at 202 nm and 201nm in both benign and malignant complexes. Finally the effect of 20% DMSO on the complex, show that the amide bands at pH 7.4 were disappeared, this may be due to the denaturation of protein complex in presence of 20% DMSO.

The application of spectrophotometric solvent perturbation on the complex is to determine the location of tyrosyl residues, whether they are buried and inaccessible or exposed and accessible to the solvent approach (216). Laskowski (201) has listed the major assumptions of solvent perturbation experiments. There are: (1) buried chromophors are unperturbed, that is only the groups located on the surface or near the surface of the protein should experience the perturbing effects of the solvent; groups buried in the interior of the protein, not accessible to the solvent; which should not be affected and consequently could not contribute to the overall spectral shift observed. (2) No conformational changes take place upon addition of perturbant, and (3) the solvation layer around the chromophore contains the same concentration of perturbation experiments when employed at convenient concentrations (often 20%), do not appear to produce conformational changes in most protein studied under reasonable conditions of pH, ionic strength, and temperature. This concentration is large enough to cause measurable shifts in the spectra of chromophoric residues. Conformational changes can be expected if perturbation is carried out under conditions in which the protein structure has marginal stability (low-or high pH for many protein)(201,216). Chromophore may not completely bury. It has been, distinguished between chromophores in crevices and chromophores that are partially buried (201). The former are observed to be fully perturbed by perturbant solvent smaller than a certain critical size (e.g ethanol), but not by larger perturbants (e.g polyethylene glycol). The degree of exposure is thus determined only by the size of perturbant molecule (solvent) or by the size of the crevice in which the chromophore is located (216). Partially buried chromophores on the other hand, show a degree of exposure that depends on the nature of the perturbant, rather than on its size. The observed degree of exposure decrease in the order:

Sucrose ≥ Glycerol ≥ Ethyleneglycol ≥ Methanol, Ethanol > Polyethylene glycol ≥ Dimethyl sulfoxide.

The first perturbant in this series modify the solvent nonspecifically, while the later ones in the series may specifically interact with chromophore(216).

When comparing the effects of the six solvents used, ethanol, ethleneglycol, glycerol, dioxane, polyethylene glycol and dimethylsulfoxide at pH 7.4 on the UV spectrum, especially on the shift of λ max, which is due to tyrosyl residues. It seems that the maximum effect was observed in the presence of 20% dioxane as perturbant solvent, where there was a shift in the λ max about 16nm, while minimum effect was observed in the presence of 20% polyethylene glycol where the λ max remained unchanged. Since the change in the λ max of tyrosyl residues does not depend on the size of the perturbant solvent, the tyrosyl residues showing the changes in λ max ; absorbance must be partially buried.

Table (5-3): The effect of 20% of ethanol, ethyleneglycol, glycerol, polyethylene glycol, sucrose, dioxane, DMSO and on the λ max of (125I-Anti CA 15-3 Antibody/ CA15-3) complex at pH 7.4. (All other details are explained in the text).

Solvent of 20% of	λ max (nm)	
	(125I-anti CA 15-3 antibody/ CA15-3) benign complex	(125I-anti CA 15-3 antibody/ CA 15-3) malignant complex
Ethanol	Near 200	200
Ethylene glycol	Near 200	Near 200
Glycerol	Near 200	Near 200
Polyethylene glycol	204	205
Sucrose	202	201
Dioxane	220	220
DMSO	-	-

Spectrophotometric pH Titration of the Complex from Benign and Malignant Breast Tumors

To study (125I- anti CA 15-3 antibody/ CA15-3) complex structure, this requires the determination of pka values for proton dissiociation from ionizable amino acid side chains, because these values give an indication of the location of amino acid in the protein. This can often be done spectrophotmetrically because dissociation often changes the spectrum of one of the chromopores (tyrosyl)(208). For proteins this usually amounts to the titration of the phenolic groups of tyrosine residues. By the measurement of the absorption at 295 nm (λ max for the ionized form of tyrosine), or observation of histidine dissociation by measurment at 211nm.

The titration curves of (125I- anti CA 15-3 antibody/ CA15-3) complex from benign (Fibroadenoma) and malignant (IDC) for both histidyl and tyrosyl residues are illustrated in figure (5-4 A&B) respectively. Figure (5-4) shows that the pka for histidine is (6.69) for (125I- anti CA 15-3 antibody/ CA15-3) complex from benign breast tumors, while the pka for histidine is (6.65) for (125I- Anti CA 15-3 Antibody/ CA15-3) complex from malignant (IDC) breast tumors. From the same curve it could be concluded that about (41.43%) histidyl residues are located on the surface of the protein complex (217) of benign (Fibroadenoma), while about (44.29%) histidyl residues are located on the surface of the protein complex from malignant (IDC). The other residues are buried interior the benign and malignant complex. Figure (5-4 B) shows that the pka value of the benign complex of tyrosyl residues is (8.9) and it's about (40%) at tyrosine residues are internal and a large arise in the absorbance at very high pH was observed. While in the malignant (IDC) complex the pka value of tyrosyl is (8.4) and it's about (50%) this indicates that the internal tyrosines have become exposed to the solvent, which is the protein complexes in folded (become denatured)(217).

The two curves also illustrated the low content of histidine compared to the high content of tyrosine in the benign and malignant complex.

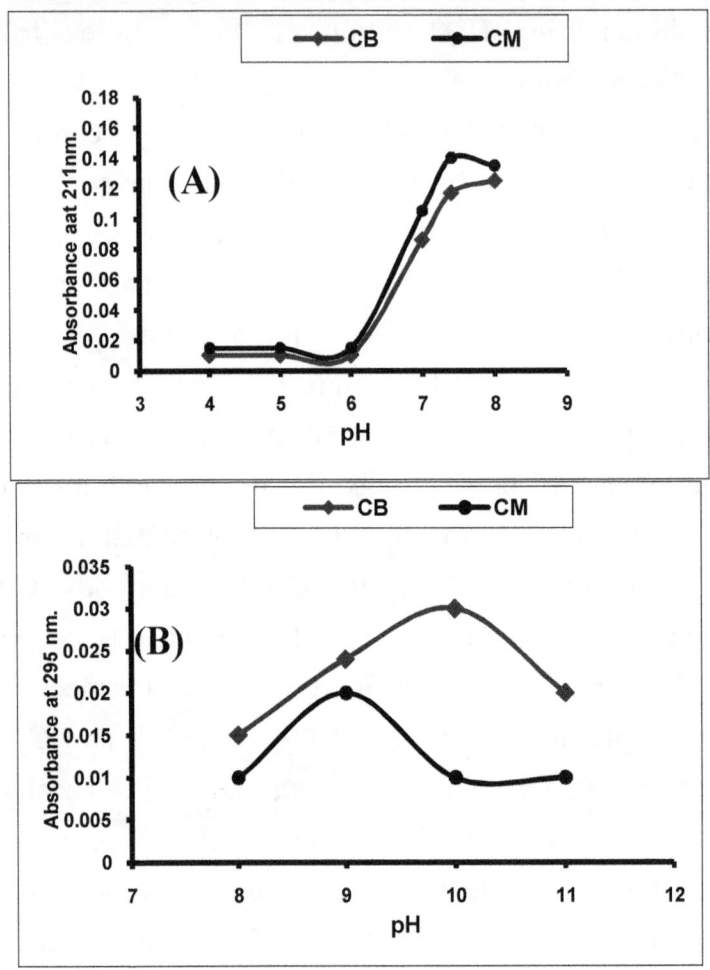

Figure (5.4): Spectrophotometric pH titration of 125I-anti CA15-3 antibody/CA15-3 complex from benign and malignant breast tumors:

(A)   for histidine, (B) for tyrosine.

(CB): Complex of benign breast tumors, (CM): Complex of malignant breast tumors. (All other details are explained in the text).

The Effect of NaCl Concentration on the Thermal Stability of the Complex by UV Spectral Studies

The effect of different concentrations of NaCl on the thermal stability of the protein complex isolated from benign and malignant breast tumors was examined in this experiment. The values of absorbance at λ max (292, 295nm) for tryptophyl and tyrosyl residues respectively, in two different concentrations of NaCl 0.01 M and 0.1 M in 20% ethylene glycol buffer are shown in figure (5.5 A&B) and (5.6 A&B). The λ max was used to examine if the protein contains internal tryptophans and tyrosines .

As shown in figure (5.5 A&B), the absorbance of both tryptophane and tyrosine reach higher absorbance at 60oC, in the presence of 0.01 M NaCl in benign and malignant complex. The increment in the absorbance of both tryptophyl and tyrosyl residues with increasing temperature could be due to that buried chromophores becomes exposed to the solvent during thermal denaturation (209).

Figure (5.6 A) shown the absorbance of tyrosin reach higher absorbance at 70oC in the presence of 0.1 M NaCl in benign and malignant complex. On the other hand figure (5.6 B) shown the absorbance of tryptophane reach higher absorbance at 60oC and 30oC in benign and malignant breast tumors complexes in presence of 0.1 M NaCl respectively. Which means that the complexes were very stable at 70oC in presence of higher concentration of NaCl, 70oC was needed for unfolding benign and malignant complex at λ max 292 nm and benign complex was more stable at 60oC in presence of 0.1 M NaCl,while the temperature is decreased to 30 oC in the presence of 0.1M NaCl at λ max 295. This is due to conformational changes required more energy 70oC in presence of 0.1 M NaCl than in 0.01 M NaCl.

The decreased absorbance in presence of 0.1 M NaCl as compared with that in 0.01 M NaCl could be due to salt concentration. Each protein in solution containing salts will collect around it a counter ion atmosphere enriched in oppositely charged small ion (chloride ion, sodium ion) and such a cloud of ions will tend to screen the protein, the more effective electrostatic screening will be, and decrement in the absorption intensity will be observed (207).

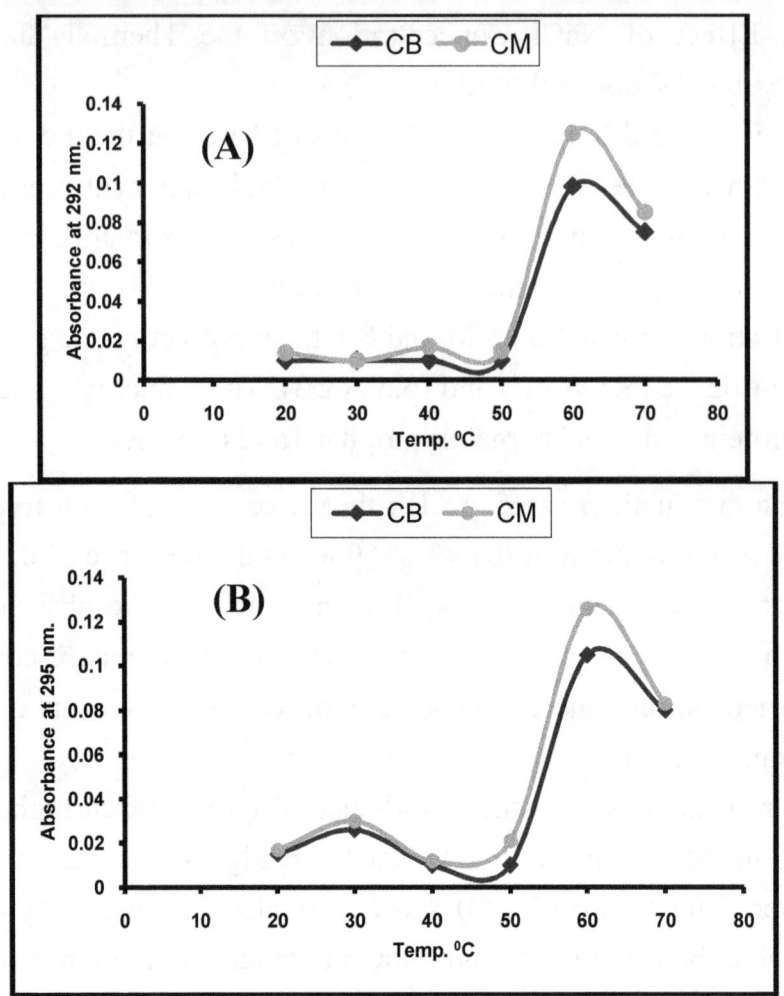

Figure (5.5): Thermal stability curve for benign and malignant: (A) at □max 292 in the presence of 0.01 M NaCl, (B) at □max 295 in the presence of 0.01 M NaCl. (CB): Complex of benign breast tumors, (CM): Complex of malignant breast tumors. (All other details are explained in the text).

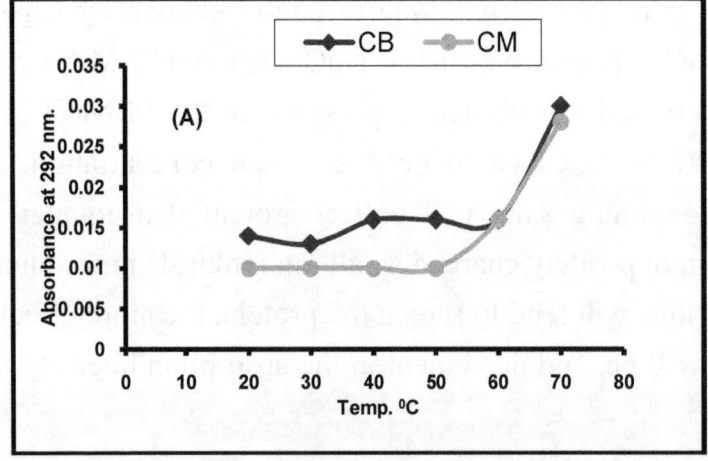

140

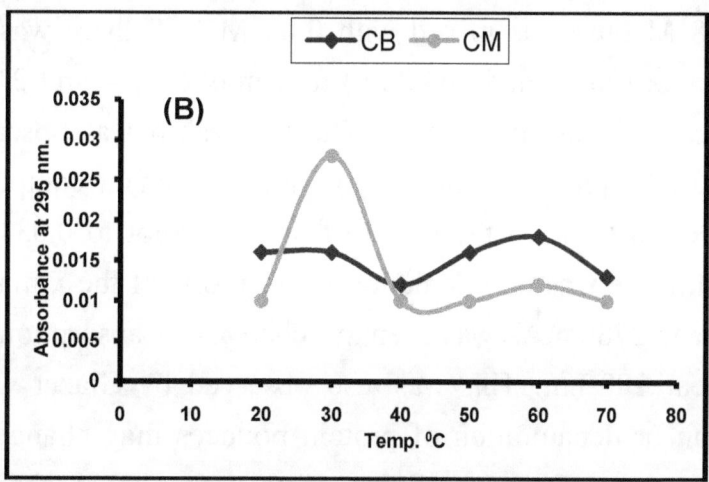

Figure (5.6): Thermal stability curve for benign and malignant: (A) at □max 292 in the presence of 0. 1 M NaCl, (B) at □max 295 in the presence of 0.1 M NaCl. (CB): Complex of benign breast tumors, (CM): Complex of malignant breast tumors. (All other details are explained in the text).

Effect of Urea, KCl and (Urea, KCl) Mixture on the Spectrum of the Complex

The effect of 8 M urea, 0.03 M KCl and a mix of 1:1 of 8 M urea and 0.03 M KCl on the λ max of the benign (fibroadenoma) and malignant (IDC) complexes, were examined. The values of λ max are illustrated in table (5-4). When table (5-4) is compared with table (5-1), it seems that the presence of 8 M urea at pH 7.4, there was a red shift of the λmax1 of polypeptide bond from 200 to 227.4 nm in benign complex and a red shift of λmax1 from 200 to 226 nm in malignant complex respectively. While λmax2 of aromatic amino acid i.e., tyrosine residues in both complexes was disappeared. The red shift is due to intramolecular hydrogen bonding between the oxygen of the amide group and the solvent (218).

When 0.03 M KCl was used, there was no alternation in the position of the λ max2 of the tyrosyl at pH 7.4 in both benign and malignant complexes. There was a slight blue shift (3-4nm) in the λ max1 of the polypeptide bond in the benign and malignant complex spectra respectively. On the other hand the λ max of the aromatic ring of tyrosyl residues at (274 or 278nm) disappeared. Such blue shift can arise by introducing positive (K+) or negative (Cl-) charges near the chromophore (the amid group), which might interact with □-electron system of the amide group (201).

When 8 M urea was mixed with 0.03 M KCl there was significant red shift in λ max (203.4 and 204.2nm) to λ max (221.4 and 219.4nm) in both benign and malignant complexes. The same shift was observed when 8 M urea was used alone with each benign and malignant complexes, this mean that the red shift due to the effect of urea, but not to 0.03 M KCl. On the other hand, there was no alternation in positions of the λ max of the tyrosyl residues near 278nm.As was seen,the changes in absorption were near 230 nm and near 280 nm. This was also observed by Glazer who that solvent perturbation or denaturation of protein poduces may changes in absorption near 230 nm and 280 nm. Some of this change in absorption may be produced by change in the n-□□□absorption of poly peptide bond in protein either because of a change in their geometrical arrangement, or because of an environment changes (219).

Table (5-4): The effect of 8M urea, 0.03M KCl and mixture (urea+KCl) on the λ max of the complex UV spectrum at pH 7.4. (All other details are explained in the text).

Solvent	λ max (nm)	
	(125I-anti CA 15-3 antibody/ CA 15-3) Benign Complex	(125I-anti CA 15-3 antibody/ CA 15-3) Malignant Complex
Urea 8M	227.4	226
KCl 0.03M	200	200
Urea+ KCl mixture 1:1	221.4 278.6	219.4 278

Chapter six

Immunoradiometric assay

Abstract

Asolid-phase Immunoradiomertric Assay sandwich technique (IRMA) was used for the determination of the carbohydrate antigen 19-9 (CA19-9) defined by a monoclonal antibody 125I-anti CA19-9. The antibody 125I-anti CA19-9 reacts with CA19-9 found at low concentrations in sera of healthy women but increased slightly in sera of patients with breast cancer.

The factors affecting the binding of 125I-anti CA19-9 antibody with CA19-9 in the breast tumor homogenate (benign and pre-and post-menopausal malignant) were determined. The results revealed that 100, 75 and 75 µg protein was the most appropriate amount of protein used in each incubation at pH 7.8, 8.0 and 7.0 respectively, with 0.0565 mg. mL-1 of 125I-anti CA19-9 antibody for 4,1 and 6 h incubation time at optimum temperatures 25, 37 and 45 oC respectively. The use of 0.01 M sodium halides and 0.025 M of divalent salts were shown to cause different effects on the binding in the three groups.

The recovery of the method was calculated and found to be 99% , 98% and 95% for binding CA19-9 present in (benign and pre-and post-menopausal malignant) breast tumor homogenates respectively.

Introduction

The Carbohydrate antigen 19-9 (CA19-9) (Koprowski etal.,1979) (118), is specific carbohydrate fraction of a circulating antigen found in sera of normal adults (Koprowski etal.,1981) (220), has sialyl Lewisa structure and is present in individually expressing the Lewisa and /or Lewisb blood group antigen (114). CA19-9 is identified as a glycolipid- that is , sialylated lacto-N-fucopentose II ganglioside (221). In serum, it exists as a mucin , a high molecular mass (200-1000 KD) glycoprotein complex (54). In Normal tissues, sialyl Lewisa antigen is present in ductal epithelium of breast, kidney, salivary gland, and sweatglands(115-117).

CA19-9 is measured with a double monoclonal immuno-radiometric assay (178). Another techniques used for the detection of CA19-9 in tissues and sera were performed by an immunoperoxidase assay (126) and by radioimmunoassay (125) of samples from patients, and enzyme immunoassay (124) for quantitative determination of CA19-9 in human serum. The upper limit of normal value 37.0 U.mL-1 (121,222). The abnormal expression of the sialyl Lewis a is closely correlated with various forms of cancer including pancreatic cancer (223-225), gall bladder (226) and bile duct (227) cancer.

A monoclonal antibody CA19-9 against sialyl Lewis a is a popular diagnostic agent for these tumors. The antibody is useless for cancer diagnosis when a patient is lacking the enzyme for the synthesis of sialyl Lewis a. In Japan, about 5-10% of the population lacks this enzyme leading to false negative results (228). CA19-9 represents the most important and basic carbohydrate tumor marker. The immunohistologic distribution of CA19-9 in tissues is consistent with the quantitative determination of higher CA19-9 concentrations in cancer than in normal of tissues (126,229). Recently reports indicates that serum CA19-9 level is frequently elevated in the serum subjects with pancreatic (80%), hepatobiliary (67%), gastric (40-50%), hepatocellular (30-50%), colorectal (30%) and breast (15%) cancer (51).

Research studies demonstrate that serum CA19-9 values may have utility in monitoring subjects with the above-mentioned diagnosed malignancies(230-232). A declining CA19-9 value may be indicative of a favorable prognosis and good response to treatment (233). Therefore, the development of immunoradiometric assay was planned to carry out the determination of the optimum conditions of 125I-anti CA19-9 antibody.

Materials and Methods

6.1. Materials

6.1.1. Chemicals

All chemical and reagents mentioned in the section (2.1.1) were used in the experiments of this chapter; other reagents used were indicated in each experiment.

6.1.2 Instruments

All instruments described in section (2.1.2) all were used in the experiments of this chapter.

6.1.3 Patients and Blood Samples

Thirty breast patients and specimens mentioned in section (2.1.3) were used in this chapter, classified to three group of patients, one group with benign and two groups with malignant breast tumors. The fourth group is a healthy women used as control.

• Group I: Consisted of 10 patients with benign (Fibroadenoma) breast tumors.

• Group II: Consisted of 10 premenopausal patients with breast cancer (IDC).

• Group III: Consisted of 10 postmenpausal patients with breast cancer (IDC).

• Group IV: Consisted of 10 normal healthy subjects.

Blood samples were prepared as described in section (2.1.4). PBS buffer was prepared as described in section (2.1.6), while homogenization of breast tumor tissues was carried out as described in section (2.1.7). Statistical analysis was determined by student's t-test as mentioned in section (2.1.8).

6.2. Methods

6.2.1. Determination of CA19-9 Levels in Sera of Patients with Benign and Malignant Breast Tumors

Reagents

The reagents IRMA-ELSA CA19-9 Kit was provided from CIS-bio international ORIS Group/France.

1. Anti CA19-9 monoclonal antibody coated on the ELSA fixed in the bottom of the tube.

2. Anti 125I-CA19-9 monoclonal antibody, radioactivity content < 10 µCi (<370 KBq)

3. Six standard ready for use, Human serum, Human CA19-9 in sodium azide (0,14,30,66,130 and 255 U.mL-1).

4. Diluent (0.0 U.mL-1), human serum in sodium azide.

5. Control (35 U.mL-1), human serum, human CA19-9 in sodium azide. Patients sera and control were used without dilution in this assay.

Procedure

The assay protocol is described in table (6-1).Table (6.1): IRMA protocol of serum CA19-9 (U.mL-1).

	CA19-9 (U.mL-1)						Control		Unknown Samples	
	0	14	30	66	130	255	Level I	Level II	1	2 etc.
Coated tube no.	1,2	3,4	5,6	7,8	9,10	11,12	13,14	15,16	17,18	19,20
Standards (µL)	←						100 µL			→
Control serum or samples (µL)	←						100 µL			→
Buffer (µL)	←						200 µL			→
	Incubation for 3 h. at 37 oC in water bath									
	The solution was aspirated, and washed the tubes 3 times with 3 mL distilled water									
125I-anti CA19-9 (µL)	←						300 µL			→
	All tubes were mixed gently with vortex-type mixer and									
	Incubated for 3 hrs. at room temperature (18-25 oC)									
	The solution was aspirated, the tubes were washed 3 times with 3 mL distilled water									
	The remaining bound radioactivity was measured with gamma counter.									

Calculations

1. The mean net count for each group of tubes was counted in gamma counter for 1 min, represents the bound c.p.m.

2. The standard curve was constructed by plotting counts per min. (Y-axis) versus concentration of CA19-9 standard (X-axis) figure (6.1). Then the points were connected with straight-line segments.

6.2.2. Preliminary Test of the Binding of CA19-9 in Breast Tumor Tissues with 125I-Anti CA19-9 Antibody in Breast tumors Homogenates

Reagents

Phosphate buffered saline pH 7.2 was prepared as described in section (2.1.6).

Procedure

The pellet and the cytosol fractions were obtained from the supernatant of breast homogenate were centrifuged at 4000 r.p.m. In order to detect CA19-9, 20 μL of crude cytosol fraction having 1100 μg protein were incubated with 60 μL (0.1356 mg.mL-1) of 125I-anti CA19-9 antibody. The volume of mixture was completed to 500 μL with PBS buffer pH 7.2, and then incubated at 37 oC for 3 hrs. The assay tubes were centrifuged at 4000 r.p.m. for 45 min. at 45 oC. The supernatant was discarded, the rims at tube were swabbed with cotton piece, then the complex formed was counted in gamma counter for 1 min. Pellet CA19-9 were determined by dissolving the sediment in PBS buffer pH 7.2 with ratio 1:5 (weight: volume), then 20 μL of supernatant fraction of pellet breast homogenate having 800 μg protein, was added to 60 μL (0.1356 mg.mL-1) of 125I-anti CA19-9 antibody. The same steps mentioned above were followed to determine the radioactivity of the complex formed. For total radioactivity two additional tubes with 60-μL of 125I-anti CA19-9 antibody were counted in gamma counter.

Calculations

1. The counted radioactivity in each tube (expressed in c.p.m.) represents the bound fraction (B); (i.e., 125I-anti CA19-9 antibody/CA19-9 complex).

2.   The counted radioactivity in the tubes counting 125I-anti CA19-9 antibody only represents the total radioactivity (T).

3.   The (B/T) % ratio for each tube was calculated as follows:

$$(B/T)\% = \frac{\text{Sample counts (B)}}{\text{Total counts(T)}} \times 100$$

6.2.3.Factors Effecting of 125I-Anti CA19-9 Antibody Binding to CA19-9 in Breast Tumors Homogenates

6.2.3.1. Effect of Protein Concentration on the Binding
Reagents
All reagents prepared is described in section (2.1.6) and (2.2.3.1).

Procedure
Sixty microliters (0.1356 mg.mL-1 protein) of 125I-anti CA19-9 antibody were added to 20 µL of cytosolic fraction of benign (Fibroadenoma) and malignant (premenopausal IDC and postmenopausal IDC) breast tumors respectively, containing increasing amounts of protein (50, 75, 100, 150, 200 and 250 µg.mL-1) and were completed to a final volume of 500 µL with 0.15 M PBS pH 7.2. The assay tubes were incubated for 3 hrs. at 37 oC. At the end of incubation, the assay tubes were centrifuged at 4000 r.p.m. for 45 min. at 4 oC. The supernatant was decanted; the rims at the tube were swabbed with cotton piece. The radioactivity of the complex formation was counted using gamma counter.

Calculations
1. The (B/T) % values were determined as in section (6.2.2).
2. Values of (B/T) % were plotted against their corresponding amount of protein of the breast tumor homogenate.

6.2.3.2. Effect of 125I-Anti CA19-9 Antibody Concentration on the Binding
Reagents
All reagents prepared is described in section (2.1.6) and (2.2.3.1).

Procedure

Sixty microliters of increasing amounts (0.0226, 0.0452, 0.0565, 0.113, 0.1356, 0.226 mg.mL-1) of 125I-anti CA19-9 antibody were added to 20 μL of crude cytosolic fraction (100, 75 and 75 μg protein) for benign (fibroadenoma) and malignant (premenopausal IDC and postmenopausal IDC) respectively, completed to a final volume 500 μL with 0.15 M PBS pH 7.2. After incubation for 3 hrs at 37 oC the bound CA19-9 was determined as mentioned in section (6.2.2).

Calculations

1. The (B/T) % values were determined as in section (6.2.2).
2. Values of (B/T) % were plotted versus the concentrations of 125I-anti CA19-9 included.

6.2.3.3. Effect of pH on the Binding

Reagents

All reagents prepared is described in section (2.1.6) and (2.2.3.1).

Procedure

Twenty microlites (100, 75 and 75 μg protein) of cytosolic fraction (fibroadenoma, premenopausal IDC and postmenopausal IDC respectively) were added to 25 μL (0.0565 mg.mL-1) of 125I-anti CA19-9 antibody respectively.The volume of the mixture was completed with PBS buffer of different pH (6.8, 7.0, 7.2, 7.4, 7.6, 7.8, 8 and 8.2) to a final volume 500 μL. After incubation for 3hrs at 37 oC, the bound CA19-9 was determined as mentioned in section (6.2.2).

Calculations

1. The (B/T) % values were determined as in section (6.2.2).
2. Values of (B/T) % were plotted versus the corresponding pH.

6.2.3.4. Effect of Temperature on the Binding

Reagents

All reagents prepared is described in section (2.1.6) and (2.2.3.1).

Procedure

Twenty microliters (100, 75 and 75 µg protein) of cytosolic fraction (Fibroadenoma , premenopausal IDC and postmenopausal IDC) were added to 25 µL (0.0565 mg.mL-1) of 125I-anti CA19-9 antibody respectively. The volume of mixture was completed to a final volume 500 µL with PBS buffer at pH 7.8 for fibroadenoma , pH 8.0 for premenopausal (IDC) and pH 7.0 for postmenopausal (IDC). The experiment was carried out at (5, 15, 25, 37 and 45oC) for 3hrs. After incubation the bound CA19-9 was determined as mentioned in section (6.2.2).

Calculations

1. The (B/T) % values were determined as in section (6.2.2).
2. Values of (B/T) % were plotted versus the temperature.

6.2.3.5 Effect of Incubation Time on the Binding

Reagents

All reagents prepared is described in section (2.1.6) and (2.2.3.1).

Procedure

Twenty microliters (100, 75 and 75 μg protein) of cytosolic fraction (fibroadenoma , premenopausal IDC and postmenopausal IDC) were added to 25 μL (0.0565 mg.mL-1) of 125I-anti CA19-9 antibody respectively. The reaction mixture was completed to a final volume 500 μL with PBS buffer pH (7.8 , 8.0 and 7.0) respectively. The experiment was carried out at 25 oC , 37 oC and 45 oC for fibroadenoma , premenopausal (IDC) and postmenopausal (IDC) respectively. The incubation was carried out at different time intervals (1, 2, 3, 4, 5 and 6 hrs). The bound CA19-9 was estimated as mentioned in section (6.2.2).

Calculations

1. The (B/T) % values were determined as in section (6.2.2).
2. Values of (B/T) % were plotted versus incubation time.

6.2.3.6.Effects of Different Halides on the Binding

Reagents

3. Phosphate buffer (PB) were prepared as described in section (2.1.6) without addition of NaCl .

4. Halid reagents were prepared in concentration of 0.01M PB at pH (7.8, 8.0 and 7.0) individually, by dissolving each of 0.021gm of NaF, 0.0292gm of NaCl, 0.0515gm of NaBr, and 0.075gm of NaI in a final volume 50mL of PB and the pH was adjusted.

5. The breast tumors homogenates (fibroadenoma , premenopausal IDC and postmenopausal IDC) were prepared as described in section (2.1.7), except using PB-buffer instead of PBS at the same pH and same concentration was carried out the homogenization.

Procedure

The experiment was carried out at optimum conditions as mentioned in section (6.2.3) using three groups of human breast homogenate (i.e., fibroadenoma, premenopausal IDC and postmenopausal IDC), by incubating 20 µL of the homogenate from each group containing (100, 75 and 75 µg protein) respectively with 25 µL (0.0565 mg.mL-1) of 125I-anti CA19-9 antibody. The reaction mixture was completed to a final volume 500 µL with PBS buffer pH (7.8, 8.0 and 7.0) containing 0.01 M of each of the following salts: NaF, NaCl, NaBr and NaI in each assay tube (A sample without the addition of any salt was used as a control). The assay tubes were incubated for (4,1 and 6 h) at 25 ,37 and 45oC for three group individually. The bound CA19-9 was estimated as mentioned in section (6.2.2).

Calculations

1.The (B/T) % values were determined as in section (6.2.2).

2.Values of (B/T) % were plotted versus 0.01 M of NaX.

6.2.3.7.Effects of Monovalent and Divalent Cations on the Binding

Reagents

1. Phosphate buffer (PB) were prepared as described in section (2.1.6) without addition of NaCl .

2. Monovalent and divalent cations (0.025 M) were prepared in PB buffer, and then the pH was adjusted to 7.8, 8.0 and 7.0 individually by dissolving each of 0.0931 gm of KCl, 0.0668 gm of NH4Cl, 0.2541 gm of MgCl2.6H2O, 0.1388 gm of CaCl2.2H2O, 0.2474gm of MnCl2.4H2O, 0.3150 gm of CuSO4.5H2O, 0.1703 gm of ZnCl2 , in a final volume 50 ml of PB and the pH was adjusted.

Procedure

The experiment was carried out at optimum conditions using three groups of human breast homogenate (i.e., fibroadenoma, premenopausal IDC and postmenopausal IDC) respectively.

The same steps mentioned on section (6.2.3.6) were followed to determine the effect of monovalent and divalent cations on the binding , except ; the buffer solution was PB (0.15 M) containing 0.025 M of the following salts: KCl , NH4Cl , MgCl2.6H2O, CaCl2.2H2O, MnCl2.4H2O, CuSO4.5H2O and ZnCl2.

Calculations

1.The (B/T) % values were determined as in section (6.2.2).

2.Values of (B/T) % were plotted versus the 0.025 M of monovalent and divalent cations.

6.2.3.8 Recovery of CA19-9

Reagents

All reagents prepared is described in section (2.1.6) and (2.2.3.1). Standared concentration of CA19-9 255 U.mL-1 was used.

Procedure

The experiment was carried out at optimum conditions. Known concentration of CA19-9 (255 U.mL-1) was added to the three group of benign (fibroadenoma) and malignant (premenopausal IDC and postmenopausal IDC) breast tissues homogenates. The experiment was carried ou at optimum conditions that was obtained in the experiment of section (6.2.3).

Calculations

1. The bound (c.p.m.) of the reaction mixture added to tissue homogenate with 125I-anti CA19-9 antibody, represent the measured value.

2. The bound (c.p.m.) of CA19-9 in tissue homogenate with 125I-anti CA19-9 antibody only , represent the expected value.

3. The recovery % (yield) calculated as follows:

$$Recovery\% = \frac{Measured\ values\,(c.p.m)}{Expected\ values\,(c.p.m)} x100$$

Results and Discussions

Determination of CA19-9 levels in Sera of Patients with Benign and Malignant Breast Tumors

Serum CA19-9 levels were measured by a solid-phase "sandwich" Immunoradiometric Assay (IRMA), which is specifically recognized by the anti CA19-9 monoclonal antibody.The monoclonal antibody is coated on the solid phase, or radiolabeled with the iodine 125 and used as a tracer. The radioactivity of the bound is directly proportional to the amount of CA19-9 presents at the beginning of the assay.

CA19-9 levels in sera of patients with benign breast tumors (group I) and (pre-and post-menopausal) malignant breast tumors (group II and group III) were measured by immunoradiometric assay. Three groups were matched with one group of control subjects. Table (6.2) shows the results obtained from this study. CA19-9 concentration of specimens and control were determined directly from standared curve in figure (6.1) .The level of serum CA19-9 in benign breast tumor patients was found to be 31.0 U.mL-1 ($p < 0.05$), where that of (pre-and post-menopausal) malignant breast tumor patients were found to be 33.1 U.mL-1 ($p < 0.05$) and 32.1 U.mL-1 ($p < 0.0005$) respectively. While in control, the level was found to be 28.8 U.mL-1 .Matching case and control subject proved to be important for controlling undesired variability. The mean CA19-9 was significantly high in postmenopausal patients ($p < 0.0005$) while in premenopausal and benign breast tumors the mean of CA19-9 was significantly low ($p < 0.05$ Student's t-test).

Table (6-2): Sera CA19-9 levels (U.mL-1) in patients with benign and malignant breast tumors. (All other details are explained in the text).

Group	Patients	No. of Cases	Age (year)	Serum CA19-9 U.mL-1 (mean ± SD)	P values
I	Benign breast tumors	10	18-35	31.0 ± 1.52	P<0.05
II	Premenopausal malignant breast tumors	10	35-43	33.1 ± 2.79	P<0.05
III	Postmenopausal malignant breast tumors	10	53-65	32.1 ± 0.13	P<0.005
Control	Control	10	25-35	28.8 ± 0.631	

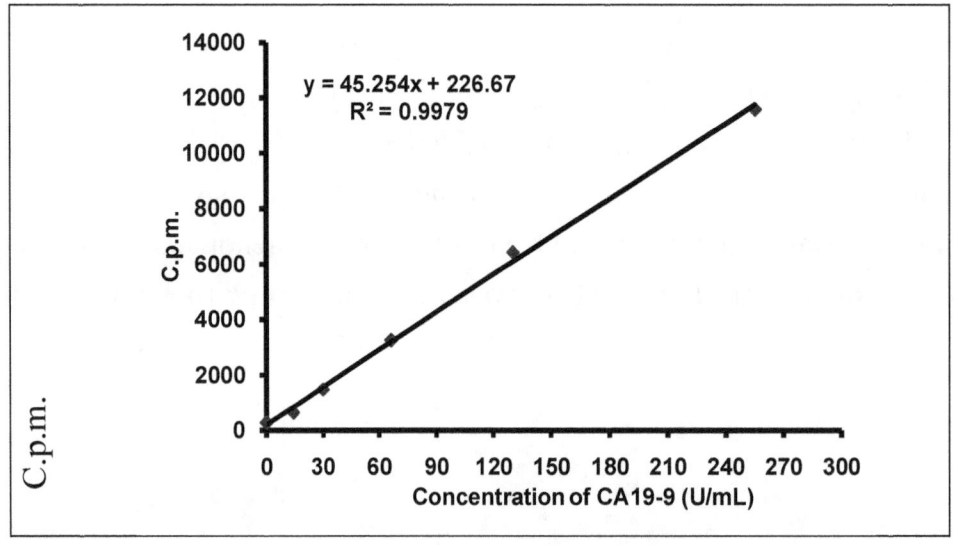

Figure (6.1): Standard curve of CA19-9. (All other details are explained in the text).

CA19-9 was at low concentration in sera of healthy individuals, these results are in agreement with several authors previously (120).

There were few studies to evaluate CA19-9 in breast tumors patients. Several investigators (222) detected CA19-9 in bone metastasis in breast cancer patients and in patients without documented metastases and reported that

CA19-9 level elevated in patients with metastases breast cancer.

When patients were analyzed with respect to the menopausal status, significant differences between the monastic and non monastic patients was detected (222).

Several studies proved the possibility of the role of carbohydrate antigen 19-9 as a tumor marker in colorectal cancer (132), pancreas (234), gastric (235), liver disease (236) and esophageal cancer (125). Recently, European group proved that CA19-9 monitored in patients with tumors of gastrointestinal tract and endometrial cancer could be used as a tumor marker and can be helpful (237) in monitoring patients with breast cancer. They observed significant increase of CA19-9 and CA15-3 levels (237) in all patients.

Preliminary Test of the Binding of CA19-9 with 125I-Anti CA19-9 Antibody

Supernatant and pellet obtained at speed (4000 r.p.m) were investigated in the three groups of human breast tumor homogenate (fibroadenoma, premenopausal IDC and postmenopausal IDC). In each fraction, CA19-9 was detected through the incubation of 125I-anti CA19-9 antibody with crude fraction supernatant and pellet individually for 3 h at 37oC in PBS buffer pH 7.2 as a medium to complete the reaction.

The separation of the bound antibody from unbound was carried out at 4000 r.p.m for 45 min. to precipitate the 125I-anti CA19-9 antibody/CA19-9 complex formed.

Table (6.3): Incidence of CA19-9 in supernatant and pellet fractions in three different breast homogenate. (All other details are explain in the text) .

| Groups | Age(year) | B/T % | |
		Supernatant fraction	Pellet fraction
Benign	34	5.32	1.43
Premenopausal (IDC)	43	5.48	2.03
Postmenopausal (IDC)	63	5.86	2.47

Table (6-3) shows the amount of binding B/T % values of pellet and supernatant fractions. The data revealed that CA19-9 in cytosolic fraction obtained from supernatant was higher in incidence than in pellet fraction, according to these results cytosolic fraction was collected. CA19-9 collected and the pellet was then discarded.

Factors Effecting of 125I-Anti CA19-9 Antibody Binding to CA19-9 in Breast Tumors Homogenates

Effect of Protein Concentration on the Binding

To obtain the optimum protein concentration of cytosolic fraction for the binding of CA19-9 with 125I-anti CA19-9 antibody, cytosolic fraction containing increasing amount of soluble CA19-9 in the presence of fixed amount of 125I-anti CA19-9 antibody was carried out as it was mentioned in section (6.2.3.1). Figure (6-2) represent the formation of (125I-anti CA19-9 antibody/CA19-9) complex in three cases (fibroadenoma, premenopausal IDC and postmenopausal IDC) and shows that (100, 75 and 75 μg protein) were the most appropriate concentration to give the maximum values of binding in crude fraction of three cases respectively. The decrease of the binding at high concentration of cytosolic fraction (in three cases) in the reaction mixture may be due to a conformational change in CA19-9 and 125I-anti CA19-9 antibody rather than the formation of reversible inactive

(125I-anti CA19-9 antibody/CA19-9) complex (238) and may be due to splitting antigen into large fragments with proteolytic enzymes (239).

In all subsequent experiments an amount of (100, 75 and 75 µg protein in three cases respectively), were used in the incubation mixture.

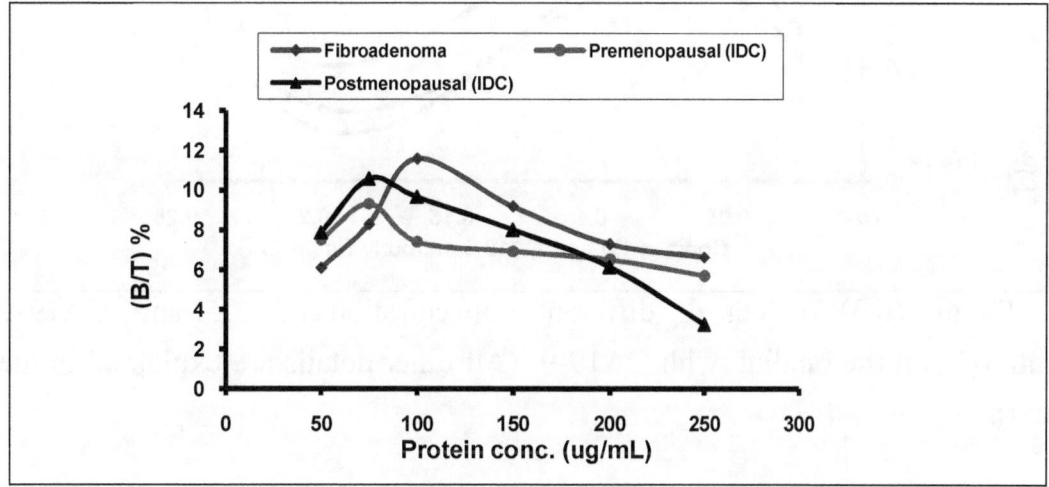

Figure (6.2): Influence of increasing protein concentrations on the binding of CA19-9 with 125I-anti CA19-9 antibody. (All other details are explained in the text).

Effect of 125I-Anti CA19-9 Antibody concentration on the Binding

One of the most important factors that effect binding is the concentration of 125I-anti CA19-9 antibody. To determine the suitable concentration of 125I-anti CA19-9 antibody, cytosolic sample (100, 75 and 75 µg protein) in the three cases (fibroadenoma, premenopausal IDC and postmenopausal IDC) respectively were incubated with increasing concentration of 125I-anti CA19-9 antibody, the incubation was carried out for 3 h at 37 oC. The results revealed that the optimum concentration of the 125I-anti CA19-9 antibody to give the maximum binding in all three cases was (0.0565 mg.mL-1). The results showed that an increase in the conc. of 125I-anti CA19-9 antibody caused a decrease in the binding %. This is because the soluble complexes, and the excess of antibody cover all antigentic sites, which leads to complex formation inhibition. Accordingly in all subsequent experiments, 0.0565 mg.mL-1 of 125I-anti CA19-9 was used as the optimum conc., which gives the highest binding %.

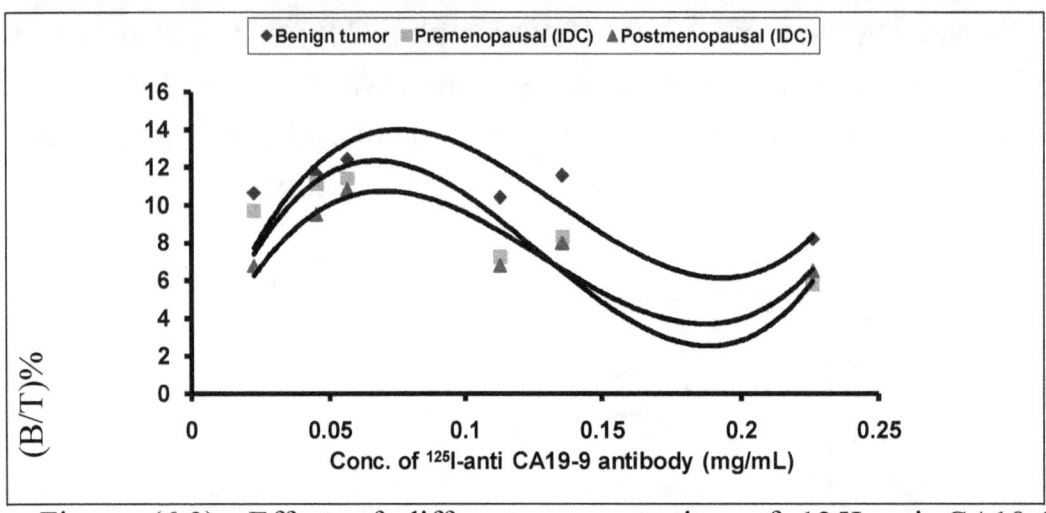

Figure (6.3): Effect of different concentration of 125I-anti CA19-9 antibody on the binding with CA19-9. (All other details are explained in the text).

Effect of pH on the Binding

The effect of pH on the binding of radioactivity CA19-9 to its antigen CA19-9 was investigated. Figure (6-4) shows that the maximum binding of 125I-anti CA19-9 antibody to its antigen CA19-9 was found to be (7.8, 8.0 and 7.0) in the three cases used (fibroadenoma , premenopausal IDC and postmenopausal IDC) respectively. The shift in pH of the environment may involve a protonation-deprotonation process occuring within the change of polar groups of the amino acids residues present in the binding domain (240) .According to these results, the pH of the buffer used in all subsequent experiments were (7.8, 8.0 and 7.0) for the three cases respectively.

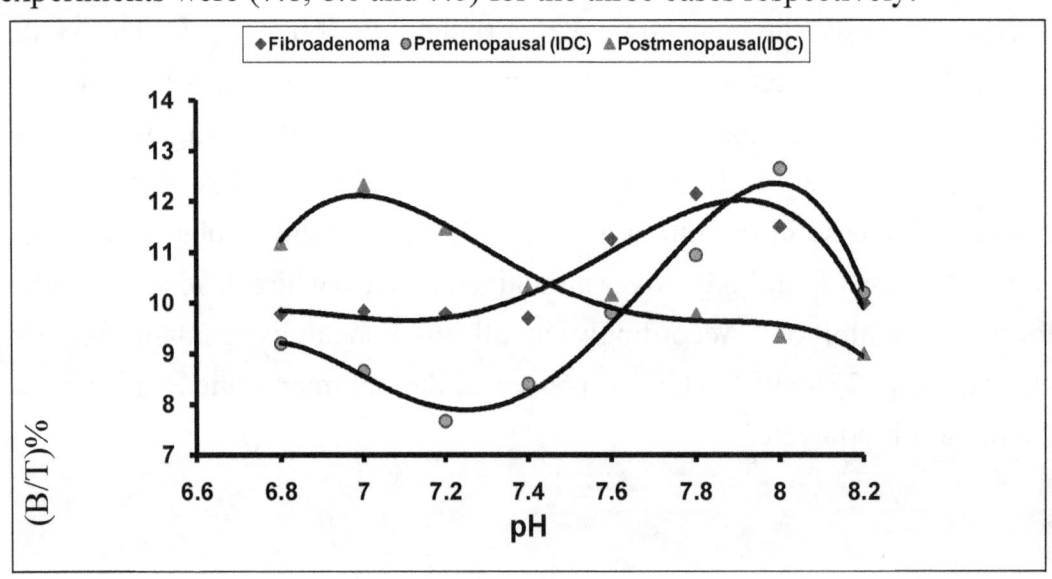

Figure (6-4): The effect of pH on the binding of CA19-9 with its antibody 125I-anti CA19-9 antibody with CA19-9. (All other details are explained in the text).

Effect of Temperature on the Binding

Temperature dependency of the association of 125I-anti CA19-9 antibody to its cytosolic fraction CA19-9 was investigated. Cytosol fraction of benign and malignant breast tumors was incubated for 3 hrs at different temperatures (5, 15, 25, 37 and 45 oC). Figure (6-5) reveals that the binding of 125I-anti CA19-9 antibody to its cytosol fraction CA19-9 was increased when the temperature was raised from 5 to 25 oC in fibroadenoma and the maximal binding was obtained at 25 oC and from 5 to 37 oC in premenopausal (IDC) and the maximal binding was obtained at 37 oC. Finally from 5 to 45 oC in postmenopausal (IDC) and the maximal binding was obtained at 45 oC. The decrease in the binding at temperature higher than the optimum temperature is probably due to denaturation of CA19-9 molecules (241) or due to proteolytic degradation of enzyme (150). According to these results (25 oC , 37 oC and 45 oC) respectively they will be used in all the subsequent experiments for the three cases used.

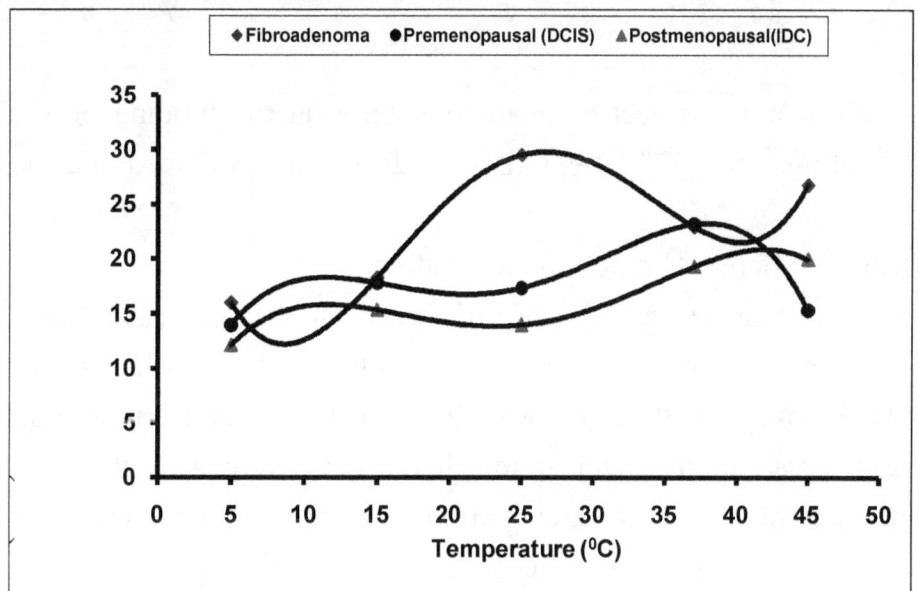

Figure (6-5): Effect of temperature on the binding of 125I-anti CA19-9 antibody with CA19-9. (All other details are explained in the text).

The Effect of Incubation Time on the Binding

To choose the most appropriate incubation time at (25, 37 and 45 oC) for the three cases used in this study (fibroadenoma, premenopausal IDC and postmenopausal IDC) respectively , the experiments were carried out at different time intervals. Figure (6-6) shows the results of this analysis. It seemed that the specific binding of 125I-anti CA19-9 antibody to cytosolic fraction homogenate for the three cases were maximal at (4,1 and 6 hrs) respectively. In view of these results, the incubation time used in all subsequent experiments were (4,1 and 6 hrs) respectively.

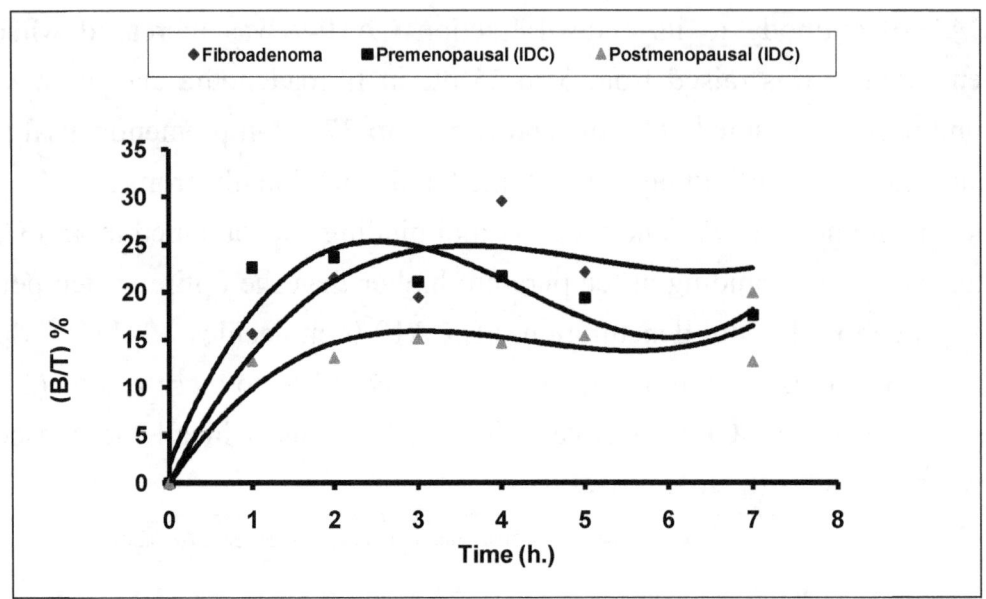

Figure (6.6): The effect of incubation time on the binding of 125I-anti CA19-9 antibody with CA19-9. (All other details are explained in the text).

Effect of Different Halides on the Binding

Figure (6.7) shows the effect of different halides salts (i.e., NaF, NaCl, NaBr and NaI) at 0.01 M concentration on the extent of 125I-anti CA19-9 antibody binding to their cytosol fraction homogenate in benign and malignant breast tumors. The sodium halides (ion radius) in the incubation mixture of benign and postmenopausal malignant breast tumors induced inhibition of the percent of binding according to the following sequence:

NaI>NaF>NaCl>NaBr

While the sodium halides in the incubation mixture of premenopausal malignant breast tumor (IDC) induced activation of the percent of the binding in the order:

NaF<NaCl<NaI<NaBr

164

Melander and Horvath (1977) reported that the effect of halide salt type on hydrophabic interactions is quantified by its molar surface tension increment (MSTI) which is a measure of the increasing in a surface tension by the salt (171) , also they found that parameter increases as the following sequence:

NaF>NaCl>NaI

The same researches found that halides with higher MSTI values will strengthen the hydrophabic interactions while halides with lower MSTI values reverse this effect. Thus the dependence of the extent of the binding in benign and malignant (pre-and post-menopausal) breast tumors on MSTI values of the corresponding halide further implicates the low involvement of hydrphobic forces in maintaining the stability of (125I-anti CA19-9 antibody /CA19-9) complex formed.

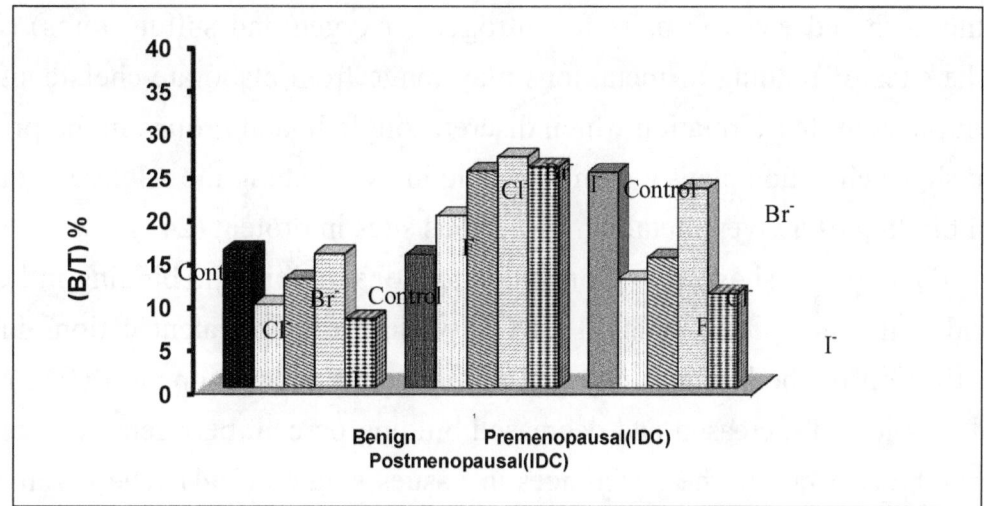

Figure (6-7): Effect of different halides on the binding of of 125I-anti CA19-9 antibody with CA19-9. (All other details are explained in the text).

Effect of Monovalent and Divalent Cations on the binding

Figure (6.8) and (6.9) show the effect of different divalent and monovalent cations respectively on the binding value in benign and malignant breast tumors. The results indicate that the binding process is sensitive to the presence of cation metal ions. CuSO4.5H2O at concentration 25 mM was showed to increase the binding two folds than the control as compared with other divalent cations.

CaCl2.2H2O induced activation in the binding in benign (fibroadenoma) and malignant (premenopausal IDC), while induced inhibition in the binding in malignant (postmenopausal IDC). ZnCl2 decreased the binding in two groups (fibroadenoma and premenopausal IDC) , while ZnCl2 increased the binding in malignant (postmenopausal IDC).

The frequency of the stimualtion of the binding of 125I-anti CA19-9 antibody to its cytosolic fraction CA19-9 homogenate of the three groups by divalent cations is according to the following:

Postmenopausal breast cancer tissue homogenate (IDC)

$Cu+2>Zn+2>Mn+2>Mg+2>Ca+2$

Premenopausal breast cancer tissue homogenate (IDC)

$Cu+2>Ca+2>Mn+2>Mg+2>Zn+2$

Benign breast tumor tissue homogenate (Fibroadenoma)

$Cu+2>Ca+2>Mg+2>Mn+2>Zn+2$

The binding of metal ions to proteins is a function of pH among the different classes of groups, such as carboxyl, amino, imidozol and tyrosyl (the unshared electron pairs for nitrogen , oxygen and sulfur atoms) (242). The sites of binding of metal ions may range from elaborate chelate sites to simple complex formation which discrete single ligand groups in the protein. In short, chelation plays a dominant role in establishing the relative strengths of binding of a given metal ion by various sites in protein (243).

Figure (6-9) shows that monovalent cations inhibit the binding in benign and malignant premenopausal (IDC), while the monovalent cations induce activation of the binding in-group of malignant postmenopausal (IDC). The alternation of increased and decreased binding percent between these cations may be ascribed to the differences in tissues studied (244). The variation of results obtained between these divalent cations may be ascribed to the difference in tissue studied (245) .

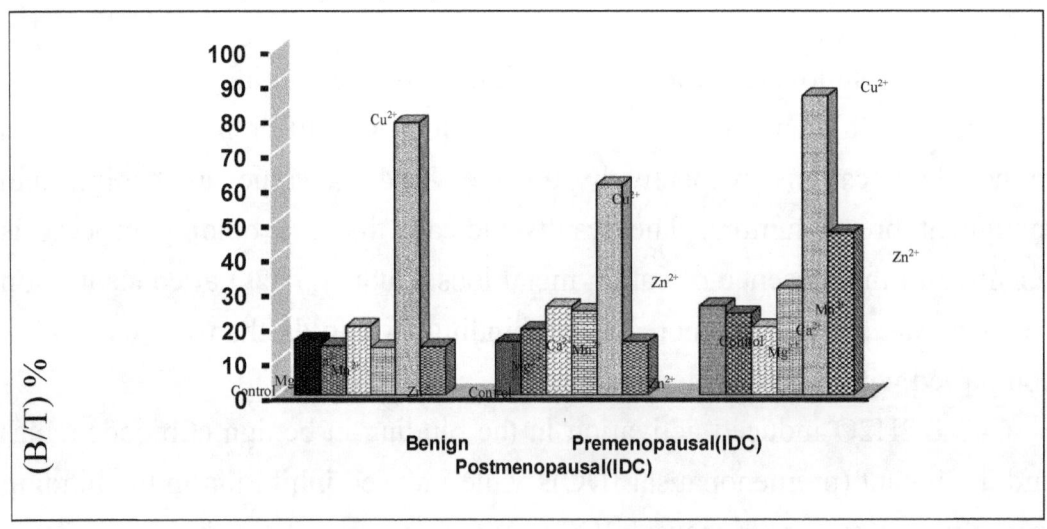

Figure (6.8): Effect of different cations on the binding of 125I-anti CA19-9 antibody with CA19-9 in different human breast tumor homogenate. (All other details are explained in the text).

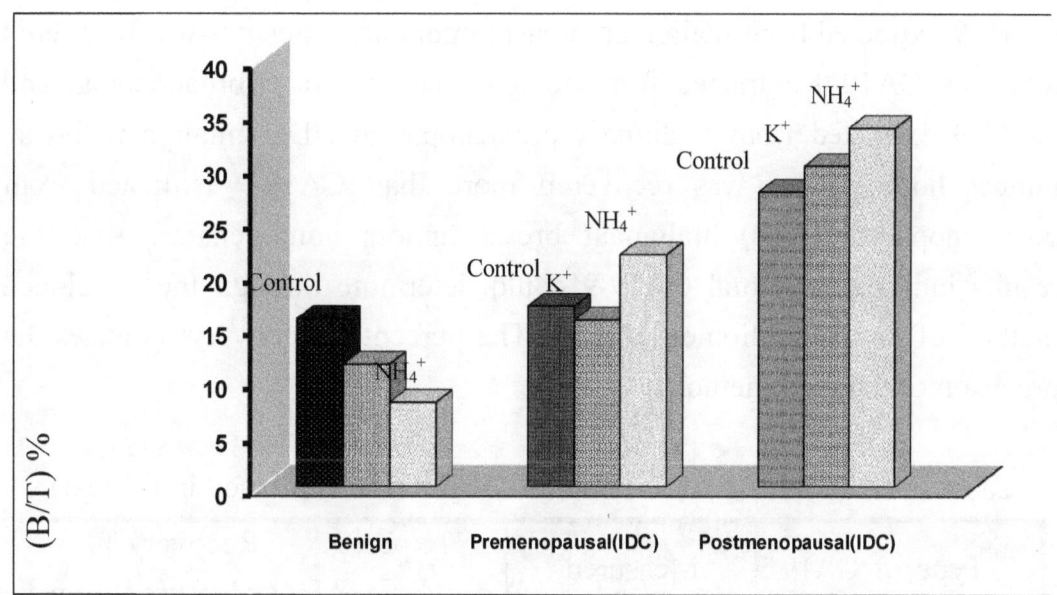

Figure (6.9): Effect of different monovaleat cations on the binding of 125I-anti CA19-9 antibody with CA19-9 in different human breast tumor homogenate. (All other details are explained in the text).

Recovery of CA19-9

The method used to estimate the percent recovery of cytosolic fractions of benign (Fibroadenoma) and malignant (pre-and post-menopausal IDC) breast tumors homogenates. The results summarized in table (6.4) indicate that CA19-9 extracted from malignant breast tumors homogenates was recovered less than CA19-9 extracted from benign breast tumor (fibroadenoma) and CA19-9 extracted from malignant premenopausal (IDC) malignant breast tumors homogenates was recovered more than CA19-9 extracted from postmenopausal (IDC) malignant breast tumors homogenates. Also the results indicate that total CA19-9 could determine through the developed method of immunoradiometric assay. The percent of recovery indicates the precision of the used method.

Table (6.4): Recovery of CA19-9 (All details are explained in the text).

Type of CA19-9	Measured B/T %	Expected B/T %	Recovery % Measured/ Expected %
Benign	103	104	99
Premenopausal	192	195	98
Postmenopausal	166	175	95

Conclusion

1. CA15-3) complex in the two cases benign and malignant breast tissues have a characteristics spectrum.

2. The developed protocol for the assay of CA15-3 or CA19-9 is suitable for the assessment of CA15-3 or CA19-9 in tissues.

3. The magnitude of elevation in CA15-3 is more than CA19-9 in the same sera of patients with breast tumors. This indicates that CA15-3 as a tumor marker is more specific than CA19-9.

4. Partially purified CA15-3 from benign and malignant breast tumors homogenates shows high affinity to 125I-anti CA15-3 antibody than crude CA15-3.

5. Kinetic studies of 125I-anti CA15-3 antibody with partially purified CA15-3 in benign and malignant breast tissues homogenates show that the reaction is temperature and time dependent. Pseudo first order kinetics at (5, 15, 25, 37, and 45 oC) was observed, in all cases.

6. The results obtained from the thermodynamic studies on the association of 125I-anti CA15-3 antibody with partially purified CA15-3 in benign and malignant breast tissues homogenates indicate that the binding reaction occurs spontaneously $\Delta G° < 0$, and entropically driven since $\Delta S° > 0$.

References

1. Porth, C.M.; (1994). "Path physiology", 4th ed. Philadelphia. J.B. Lippincott.

2. Berkow, R.; Beers M.H; Fletcher A.J.; Bogin R.M.; (2001). "The Merck manual of medical information". Home ed. ht, Whitehouse Station. Merck & Co., Inc.; Chapter 238, Section 22.

3. World Health Organization: Hostological typing of breast tumors. In: International Histological Classification of Tumors; (1981). 2nd ed. Geneva, World Health Organization P19.

4. Cotran, R.S.; Kumar V.; Collins T.; (2000). "Robbins pathologic basic of disease", 6th ed. Philadelphia. W.B. Saunders Company. Chapter 25, pp 1102-1107.

5. Dixon, J. M. ; Mansel R.E.; (1995). "Congential proplems and aberrations of normal breast development and involution", In: Dixon J. M Jed) ABC of Breast Diseases. BMJ Publishing Group, London, Chapter1, pp6-11.

6. Flectcher, J.A; Pinkus G.S; Weidner N., Morton C.C.; (1991). Am. J. Pathaol., 138: 1199-1207.

7. Dupont, W.d., Page D.L., Parl F.F. (1994). N. Engl. J. Med., 311: 10-15.

8. Burnet, K.L.; (2001). "Holistic breast care", 1st ed. Harcourt Publishers Limited. Chapter 2, p23.

9. Belieu, R.M.; (1994). Obstet. Gynecol. Clin. North Am., 21:461.

10. Rosai, J.; (1996). "Ackerman's surgical pathology", 8th ed. Philadelphia. Mosby Yer Book, St. Louis, Vol 2, pp: 1565-1568.

11.Casciato, D.A; Lowitz B.B.; (2000). "Manual of clinical oncology" 4th ed. Philadelphia. Awolters Kluwer Company. Chapter 10, pp218-237.

12.Rubin, P.; Williams J.P; (2001). "Clinical oncology, a multidisciplinary approach for physical and students", 8th ed. Philadelphia. W.B.Saunders Company. Chapter 17, pp 267-299.

13.Iraqi cancer Registry (ICR) Results; (1993). Ministry of Health, (1989-1991). Iraqi Cancer Borad.

14.Iraqi cancer Registry (ICR) Results; (1995). Ministry of Health, (1992-1994). Iraqi Cancer Borad.

15. Iraqi cancer Registry (ICR) Results;(1998). Ministry of Health, (1995-1997). Iraqi Cancer Borad.

16. Iraqi cancer Registry (ICR) Results;(2000). Ministry of Health, Iraqi Cancer Borad.Unpublished.

17. Pazdur, R.; Coia L.R.; Hoskins W.J.; Wagman L.D.; (1996). "Cancer management: a multidisciplinary approach, medical, suergical & radiation oncology", 1st ed. Princeton. Bristol-Myers Squibb Company, Chapter2.p 22.

18. Osborne, C.K.; (1994). "Internal medicine", 4th ed. Philadelphia. Mosby, St. Louis, pp 924-926.

19. Miller, A.; Howe G.; Sherman G.; (1989). N. Eng. J. Med., 321: 328.

20. Lata C.; (2000) Cancer. http://www.vhihealthe.com

21. Kohlmeier, L. ; Mendez M.; (1997). Proc. Nutr. Soc., 56: 369.

22. Sala, E.; Warren R.; Duffy S.; (2000). Br. J. Cancer, 83(1): 121-6.

23. Fiedenreich, G.; Howe G.; Miller A.; (1993). Am. J. Epidemiol., 137:512.

24. Williams, E.L.; (1994). Am. J. Epidemiol., 140: 956-958.

25. Newcomb, P.; Storer B.; Longnecker M.; (1994). N. Eng. J. Med., 330:81.

26. Landis, A.; Murray D.; Bolden M.; (1999). Cancer Statistis, 49:1.

27. Frykery, E.R.; Masood S.; Copeland E.M.; (1993). Surg. Gynecol. Obstet, 177: 425-440.

28. Wood, W.C.; (1996). Semin. Oncol., 23:446-452.

29. Goldschmidt, R.A, Victor T.A.; (1996). Semin. Surg. Oncol., 12: 314-320.

30. Garne, J. P.; (1994). Cancer, 73:1438.

31. Di Costanzo,D.; Rosen P.P.; Gareen I.; (1990). Am. J. Surg. Pathol., 14:12-23.

32. Cavalli, F.; Hansen H.H.; Kaye S.B.; (1997). "Text book of medical oncology", 1st ed., London, Martin Dunitz Ltd, Chapter 4, p58.

33. Mann, C.V.; Russel R.C.G.; William N.S.; (1995). "Baily & Love's short practice of surgery", 22nd ed. London, Chapmann & Hall Medicine, Chapter 39, p543.

34. Giuliano, A.E.; (1995). Ann. Surg., 222: 394.

35. Tiernery, L.M.; Mc Phee S. J.; Papadakis M.A.; (1999). "A large medical book, current medical diagnosis & treatment", 38th ed. New Yourk. Appleton & Lange, Chapter 16, pp678-703.

36. Hellman, S.; (1994). J. Clin. Oncol., 12: 2229-2234.

37. Fisher, B.; Redmond C.; (1992). J. NCI., 11:7-13.

38. Veronesi, U et al; (1995), 222:612.

39. Devita, J.R.; Vincent T.; Sanmel H.; Hellman S.; Rosenberg S.A.; (1997). "Cancer principle and proactice of oncology", 5th ed. Philadelphia, J.B. Lippincott-Raven publishers, p1562.

40. Cooke, A.L.; (1995). Int. J. Radiat. Oncol. Bio. Phys., 31:777.

41. Guenther, J.M.; Tokita D.M.; Guiliano A.K.; (1994). Cancer, 73:2613

42. Haagensen, CD.; (1997).Int. Radiat Oncol. Biol. Phys., 2: 975-980.

43. Valero, V.; (1997). Oncology, 11:34.

44. Cameron, D.A.; Gabra H.; Leonard R.C.; (1994). Br. J. Cancer, 70: 120-124.

45. Christman, K., Muss H.B., Stanley V.; (1992), JAMA, 268: 57-62.

46. Muss, H.B., (1995). Semin. Oncol., 22:14-16.

47. Bondaontra, G., Zambetti M., Valagussa P., (1995), JAMA, 542-547.

48. Powels, T.J.; (1997), Semi Oncol; 24 (suppl): 48-54.

49. Sundeland, M.C., Osborne C.K.; (1991). J. Clin. Oncol.,9:1283-1297.

50. Russel, R.C.G.; Williams N.S; Bulstored C.T.K; (2000). "Bailey & Love's short practice of surgery" 23rd. arnold, a member of the holder healine Group. Chapter 46, PP 750-759.

51. Burtis, C.A.; Edward R.; Ashwood E.R.; (1999). "Tietz text book of clinical chemistry", 3rd ed. Philadelphia, W.B. Saunders Company. Chapter 23, pp 722-748.

52. Anderson, S.C.; Cockayne S.; (1993). "Clinicla chemistry, concepts and applications", An HBJ☐int.ed. Philadelphia, W.B. Saunders company. Chapter 16, pp 322-330.

53. Kalstan, M. B.; Onyekwere O.; Sidransky D.; Vogelstein B.; Craig R.W.; (1991). Cancer Res., 51: 6304.

54. Burtis, C.A.; Ashwood E.R.; (1994). "Tietz textbook of clinical chemistry", 2nd ed. Philadelphia, W.B. Saunders company. Chapter 21, pp 899-920.

55. Eurepean Group of Tumors Markers (EGTM). http://www.med.uni.muenchen.de/egtm/detail/4.htm.

56.Stearns, V.; Yamauchi H.; Hayes D.F.; (1998). Breast Cancer Res. Treat., 52: 239-259.

57.Schwartz, M. k.; (1994). Adv. Exp. Med. biol., 353: 47-53.

58.Hayes, D.F.; (1994). "Tumor markers for breast cancer: Current utilities and future prospects", In: Hayes DF (ed) Hematology/ oncology clinics of North Amirica: philadelphia, W.B. Sounders Company, pp 485506.

59.Safi F.; Kohler I.; Rottinger E.; Boger H.G.; (1990). Cancer, 68 (3): 574-582.

60.Ordonez, N.G.; (1989). Cancer Bull, 41: 142-151.

61.Sell,S.; (1990). Human Pathol., 21: 1003-19.

62.Soletormos, G.; Nielsen D., Schioler V.; (1996). Clin. Chem., 42: 564-575.

63.Bjorklond, B.; Bjorklund V.; (1957). Arch. Allergy, 10: 153-184.

64.Karaloglu, D.V.; Yasusever N., Dalay E.N; (1995). Eur. J. □□Gynaec. Oncol., 5:363-367.

65.Blijlevens, N.M.A.; Oosterhuis W.P.; Oosten H.R.; Mulder N.H.; (1995). Anticancer Res., 15: 2711-2716.

66.Schuurman, J.J.; Bong S.B.; Einarsson R.; (1996). Anticancer Res., 16: 2169-2172.

67.Locker, G. J.; Mader R.M.; Braun J.; Sieder N.E.; Marosi C.; Rainer H.; Jakesz R.; Steger G.G.; (1995). Oncology, 52:140-144.

68.Gion, M.; Mione R.; Leon A.E.; Dittadi R.; (1999). Clin. Chem., 45 (5): 630-637.

69.Correale, M.; Abbate I.; Gargano G.; (1992). In . J. Biol. Markers, 7: 43-46.

70.Jcobs, I.; Bast R.C.; (1989). Hum. Reprod., 4: 1-12.

71.Helzlsouer, K. D.; Bush T.L.; Albrg A. J.; Bass K.M.; Zacur H.; Comstock G.W.; (1993). J. Am. Med. Assn., 269: 1123-1126.

72.Kaneko, J.J.; harvey J.W.; Bruss M.J.; (1997). "Clinical biochemistry of domestic animals", 5th ed. New York, Academic Press, Chapter 26, p764.

73.Ward, B.G.; Mc Guckin M.A.; Rarnm L.E.; Coglan M.; (1993). Cancer, 71: 430-438.

74.Chatterjea, B.M.N.; Shinde R.; (1995). "Textbook of medical biochemistry" 2nd ed. India, Medical Publishers (P) LTD. Chapter 41, part III, pp1088-1098.

75.Yasasever, V.; karaloglu D.; Erturk N.; Dalay N.; (1994). Eur. J. Gynaec Oncol., 1: 33-36.

76.Hilkens, J., Kroezen V.; Bonfrer J.M.G.; Bakker M. D.; Bruning P.F.; (1986). Cancer Res., 46: 2582-2587.

77.Hilkens, J.; Buijs, F; (1988). J. Biol. Chem., 263(9): 4215-4222.

78.Galectine-4. http://www.albany.edu/chemistry/sarma/cwabstiactsmar98.htm.

79.The American Society of Clinical Oncology; (1996). J. Clin Oncol, 14(10): 2843-2877.

80.Tandon, A.K.; Clark G.M.; Chamness G.C.; (1990). N. Engl. J. Med., 322: 297-302.

81."http://www.asco.org/prof/pp/html/guide/tumor/m-tumor 15. htm"

82.Hilkens, J.; Buijs F.; Hilgers J.; Hayeman P.; Calofat J.; Sonnenberg A; (1984). Int .J. Cancer, 34: 197-206.

83.Thomas, C.M.G.; (1995). Ned. Tijdschr. Klin. Chem; 20 (6): 298-300.

84.SaFi, F.; Kohler I.; Rottinger E.; Beger H.G.; (1991). Cancer, 68(3): 574-582.

85.Sekine, H.; Ohno T.; Kufe D.W.; (1985). J. Immunol., 135: 3610-3615.

86.Shimizu, M.; Yamauchi K.; (1982). J. Biochem., 91: 515-524.

87.Gendler, S.; Papadimitrion J.T.; Duhig T.,; Rothbard J.; Burchell J.; (1988). J. Biol. Chem., 263: 1280-12823.

88.Cordell, J.; Richardson T.C.; Pulford K.A.; Ghosh A.K.; Gatter K.C.; Heyderman E.; Mason D.Y.; (1985). Br. J. Cancer, 52: 347-354.

89.Wesseling, J.; (1997). "The Carcinoma- Associated Mucin Episialin (MUC1) in Cell Adhesion and Tumor Progression" Ph. D. Thesis, Department of Tumor Biology, The Nether lands Cancer Institute.

90.Hou, M.F.; Huang T.J.; Hsieh J.S.; Huang Y.S.; Huang C.J.; Chan H.M.; Wang J.Y.; Chen Y.L.; Jong S.B.; Yang C.C.; (1995). Kaohsiung J. Med. Sci.; 11: 660-666.

91.Wojtacki, J.; Bokiniec A.D.; Kowalski D.M.; Zoltowska A.; Cresielski D.; Suszko M.; (1996). Neoplasma, 43 (4): 225-229.

92.Kufe, D.; Inghirami G.; Abe M.; Hayes D.; Justiwheeler H.; Scholm J.; (1984). Hybridoma, 3: 223-232.

93.Ligtenberg, M. J. L.; Vos H.L.; Genissen A.M.C.; Hilkens J.; (1990). J. Biol. Chem., 265: 5573-5578.

94. Swallow, D.M.; Gendler S.; Griffiths B.; Corney G.; Taylor P.J.; Bramwell M.E.; (1987). Nature, 328: 82-84.

95. Jentoft, N.; (1990). Trends. Biochem. Sci., 15:291-294.

96. Hilkens, J.; Wesseling J.; Vos H.L.; Storm J.; Van der Valk S.W.; Maas M.C.E.; (1995). Ned. Tijdschr. Klin. Chem., 20 (6): 293-298.

97. Hilkens, J.; Ligtenberg M.J.L; Vos H.L; Litvinov S.V.; (1992). Trends. Biochem. Sci., 17:359-363.

98. Tsubura, a.; Morii S.; Vdea S.; Sasaki M.; Zother S.; Watzing V.; Mooi W.; Hageman P.C.; Hilkens J.; Tweel J.V.; (1987). Arch. Dermatol. Res., 279:550-557.

99. Zoher, S.; Lossnitzer A.; Hageman P.C.; Delemarre J.G.; Hilkens J.; Hilgers J.; (1987). Lab. Invest., 57: 193-199.

100. Zotter, S.; Hageman P.C.; Lossnitzer A.; Mooi W.; Hilgers J.; (1988). Cancer Rev., 11-12: 55-101.

101. Zaretsky, J.Z.; Weiss M.; Tsarfaty I.; Hareuveni M.; Wreschner D.H.; Keydar I.; (1990). FEBS Lett; 265: 46-50.

102. Hilkens, J.; Buys F.; (1988). J. Biol. Chem., 263: 4215-4222.

103. Linsley, P.S.; Kallestadt J.C.; Horn D.; (1988). J.Biol.Chem., 263: 8390-8397.

104. Ligtenberg, M.J.L.; Buijs F.; Vos H.L.; Hilkens J.; (1992). Cancer Res., 52: 2318-2324.

105. Special, Article by the American Society of Clinical Oncology; (1996). J. Clin. Oncol., 14(10): 2843-2877.

106. Hilkens, J.; Ligtenberg M.J.L.; Vos H.L.; Litvinov S.V.; (1992). Trends. Biochem. Sci., 17: 359-363.

107. Braga, V.M.; Pew berton L.F.; Duhig T.; Gendler S.J; (1992). Development; 115: 427-437.

108. Vande Wiel-van Kemenade, E.; Ligtenberg M.J.L.; de Boer A.J; Buijs F.; Vos H.L.; Melief C.J.M; Hilkens J.; Figdor C.G.; (1993). J. Immunol., 151: 767-776.

109. Jerome, K.R.; Barnd D.L.; Bendt K.M.; Boyer C.M.; Taylor Papadimitriou J.; Mckenzie I.F.C; Bast R.C.; Finn O.J.; (1991). Cancer Res., 51: 2908-2916.

110. Jerome, K.R.; Domenech N.; Finn O.J.; (1993). J. Immunol., 151: 1654-1662.

111. Ioannides, C.G.; Risk B.; Jerome K.R.; Irimura T.; Warton J.T.; Finn O.J.; (1993). J. Immunol., 151: 3693-3703.

112. Takahashi, T; Makiguchi Y.; Hinoda Y.; Kakiuchi H.; Nakagawa N.; Imai K.; Yachi A.; (1994). J. Immunol., 153: 2102-2109.

113. Hayes, K.F.; Tondini C.; Kufe D.W.; (1992). "Clinical applications of CA 15-3 In: Serological tumor markers". S.Sell. ed. Totowa, NJ, The humana Press, pp.281-307.

114. Lamerz, R.; (1992). "CA 19-9 gastrointestinal cancer antigen In: serological cancer Markers" S.Sell. ed, Totowa, NJ, The Humana Press, pp 309-339.

115. Takasaki, H.; Uchida E.; (1987). Pancreas, 2: 398-403.

116. Furuya, N.; Kawa S.; Hasebe O.; Tokoo M.; Mukawa K.; Mukawa K.; Macjima S.; Oguchi H.; (1996). Br. J. Cancer, 73 (3): 372-376.

117. Webb, A.; Scott M. P. and Bensted J.; (1996), Eur. J. Cancer; 23A(1): 63-68.

118. Koprawski H.; Steplewski Z.; Mitchell K. and Heryn D.; (1979). Somatic Cell Cent.; 5: 957-972.

119. Magnani, J.L.; Nilsson B.; Brockhaus M.; Zopf D.; Steplewsk L.; koprowski H.; Ginsburg V.; (1982). J. Biol. Chem; 257: 14365-14369.

120. Del-Villano, B.C.; Brennan S.; Brock P.; Bucher C.; Liv V.; McClure M.; Rake B.; Space S.; Westrick B.; Schoemarker H.; Zurawski V.R.; (1983). Clin. Chem., 29 (3): 549-552.

121. Ritts, R.I. ; Del-Villano B.G.; GoV L.W.; (1984). Int.J. Cancer,33:339-345.

122. Beretta E. ; malesci A. ; Zerbi A.; (1987). Cancer, 60: 2428-2431.

123. Glenn, J.;Steinberg W.M.; Kurtzman S.H.; (1988). J. Clin. Oncol., 6: 462- 468.

124. Taniguchi, T. ; Kitamura M. ; lwasaki Y. ; Yamamoto Y. ; Igar: A. ; Toi M.; (1997). Br.J. Cancer, 75 (5): 673-677.

125. Mcknight, A.; Mannell A.; Shperling I.; (1989). Br.J. Cancer, 60: 249-251.

126. Maeta, M.; Yoshioka H.; Shimizu T.; Murakami A.; Hamazoe R.; koga S.; (1990). Oncology, 47(3): 229-233.

127. Gupta, M.K.; Arciaga R. ; Bocci L.; (1985). Cancer, 56: 277-283.

128.   Putzki, H.; Ledwoch J.; Student A.; (1988). J. Surg. Oncol., 37: 133-135.

129.   Ohuchi, N.; Takahashi K.; Matoba N.; (1989). Jpn. J. Clin. Oncol., 19: 242-248.

130.   Thomas, W.M.; Robertson J. F.R.; Price M.R.; (1991). Br. J. Cancer., 63: 975-976.

131.   Iemura, k..; Moriya Y.; (1993). Eur. J. Surg. Oncol., 19: 439-422.

132.   Kouri, M.; Pyrohonen S.; Kuusela P.; (1992). J. Surg. Oncol., 49: 78-85.

133.   Burioka, N.; Suyama S.; Tatsukawa T.; Hori S.; Kometani Y.; Kawasaki Y.; Nakada N.; Sasaki T.; (1997). Yonago. Acta. Medica., 40: 147-151.

134.   Steinberg, W.; (1990). Am J. Gastroenterol., 85: 350-355.

135.   Sherif, M.S.; A.Razek A.A.H.; (1994). The New Egyp. J. Med., 10(4): 1821-1825.

136.   Yasasever, V.; Dincer M.; Camlica H.; Karaloglu D.; Dalay N; (1997). Clin. Boichem., 30 (1): 53-56.

137.   Wojacki, J.; Bokiniec A.D.; (1995). Libri. Oncol., 24: 147-152.

138.   Van-Dalen, A.; (1999). Tumour Biol., 20 (3): 117-129.

139.   Schuurman, J.J.; Bong S.B.; Einarsson Ri; (1996). Anti Cancer Res., 16: 2169-2172.

140.   Locker, G.J.; Mader R.M.; Braun J.; Sieder A.E.; Marosi C.; Rainer H.; Jakesz R.; steger G. G.; (1995). Oncology.,l 52: 140-144.

141.   CA 15-3 as a Marker for Breast Cancer" http://www.asco org/prof./pp/html/m-Tumor 10.htm.

142.   Hayes, D.F.; Zurawski V.; kufe D.W.; (1986). J. Clin.Oncol.,4: 1542-1550.

143.   Devitu, T.V.; Helllmen S.; Rosenberg A.S.; (1996). "Important advances in oncology", Philadelphia, Lippincotl-Raven.

144.   Colomer, R.; Ruibal A.; Geuolia J.; (1989). Cancer, 64: 1674-1681.

145.   Pal, S.; Sanyal V.; Chattopadhyay V.; (1995). Int. J. Cancer, 60: 759-765.

146.   Kaplan, l.; and Pesce A.; (1989). "Clinical Chemistry", 2nd ed.; C.V.Mosby; p255.

147.   Lawry, O.H.;Rosebrough N.J.; Farr A.L.; Randell R.J.; (1951). F. Biol. Chem., 193: 265-275.

148.   Janson, J.C.; Ryden L.; (1998). "Protein purification", 2nd ed, New York, A John Wiley & Sons, Inc., Chapter 1 & 14.

149.   Al –Khayat, T.H.; (1991). "Molecular characterization of prolactin receptors in human prostate" Ph.D. Thesis supervised by Al-Mudhaffar S.A., College of Science, and Baghdad University.

150.   Scopes, R.K.; (1982). "Protein purification principles and practice", New York, Springer Verlag, pp 197, 162.

151.   Geraghty, J. G.; Coveney E.C.; Sherry B., O' Higgins N.J.; Duffy M.J.; (1992). Cancer, 70: 2831-2838

152.   Colomer, R.; Ruibal A.; Genoola J.; Salvador L.; (1989). Cancer; 64: 1674-1681.

153.   Hayes, D.F.; Zurawski V.R.; Kufe D.W.; (1986). J. Clin. Oncol., 4: 1542-1550.

154.   Nekulova, M,; Simickova M.; Pecen L.; Eben K.; Vermousek I.; Stratil P.; Cernoch M.; Lang B.; (1994). Neoplasma, 41: 113-118.

155.   Vizcarra, E. ; Lluch A. ; Cibrian R. ; Jarque F. ; Alberola V. ; Belloch V.; (1996). Breast Cancer Res. Treat., 37: 209-216.

156.   Duffy, M.J.; Sherry, F.; (1988). Ann. Clin. Biochem.; 25(Suppl.): 53s-4s.

157.   Duffy, M.J.; (1999). Ann. Clin. Biochem., 36: 579-586.

158.   Coveney, E.; Geraghty J.G.; Sherry F.; McDermott E.W.; O'Higgins NJ; Duffy M.J.; (1995). Int. J. Biol. Markers, 10: 35-41.

159.   Robertson, J.F.R.; Pearson D.; Price M.R.; Selby C.; Badley R.A.; Pearson J.; (1990). Eur. J. Cancer, 26: 1127-1132.

160.   Bon, G.S.; von Mensdorff. Povilly S.; kenemans P.; van kamp G.J.;Verstraeten R.A.; Hilgers J.; (1997). Clin. Chem., 43:585-593.

161.   Hayes, D.F.; Zurawski V.R.; kufe D.; (1986). J. Clin. Oncol., 4: 1542-1550.

162.   Ichihara, S.; Aoyamatt H.; (1994). Cancer, 73(8): 2181-2185.

163.   Pons-Anicet, D.M.F.; Krebs B.P.; Mira R.; (1987). Br. J. Cancer, 55:567-570.

164.   Crippa, F.; Bombardieri E. ; Seregni E.; (1992). J. Nucl. Biol. Med., 36:52-55.

165. Bryant, N.J.; (1986). "Laboratory immunology and serology", 2nd ed., Philadelphia, W.B.Saunders company, Chapter 5, pp 49-52.

166. Roitt, I.; Brostoff J.; Male D.; (1998). "Immunology". 5th ed, london, Mosby philadelphia st. Louis.

167. Dad liker, W.B.; and Satussure V.A.; (1970). Immunochemistry; 7: 799.

168. Steiner, A.L; Kipnis D.M.; Utiger R.; (1969). Proc. Nat. Acad. Sci. USA., 64: 367.

169. Devlin, T.M.; (1986). "Text book of biochemistry with clinical correlation", 2nd ed. John Wiley and Sons, Inc, New York, pp125, 66.

170. Scheraga, H.A.; (1961). "Protein structure", New York: Academic Press pp 365, 571.

171. Melander, W.; Horvath C.; (1977). Arch..Biochem.Biophys.,183:200-215.

172. William, E.P.; (1998). "Fundemental immunology", 4th ed. Philadelphia, Lippicott. Raven, chapter 4, pp 75-110.

173. Mellor, Maley; (1947). Nature, 159: 370.

174. Williams, R.J.P; (1959). "The Enzymes", 2nd ed., New York, Academic Press, vol I, pp391.

175. Gendler, S.J.; Spicer A.P.; (1995). Ann. Rev. Physiol., 57: 607-634

176. Webb, A.; Scott-Mackie P.; Cunningham D.; Norman A.; Andreyev J.; O'Brien M.; Bensted J.; (1996). Eur .J. Cancer, 32 A (1): 63-68.

177. Gion, M.; Mione R.; Leon A.E.; Kittadi R.; (1999). Clin. Chem., 45 (5): 630-637.

178. Stacker, S.A.; Tjandna J.J.; Xing P.X.; Walker I.D.; Thompson C.H.; Mckenzie I.F.C.; (1989). B. J. Cancer., 59: 544-553.

179. Hilkens, J.; Kroezen V.; Bonfrer J.M.G.; Brunning P.F.; Hilgers J.; Eajkeren van M.; (1985). Protides of biological Fluids; 2: 651-653.

180. Abe, M.; Dufe D.; (1987), J. Immunology, 139: 257.

181. Bonfrer, J.M.; (1995). Ned. Tijdschr. Klin. Chem., 20: 301-304.

182. Brostoff, J.; and Male D.; (1994). "Clinical immunology, an Illustrated outline", Philadelphia. Mosby, Section8, p112.

183. Shiu,R.P.C.; Friesen H.G.; (1974). J. Biol. Chem.; 249:7902.

184. Gallagher, T.S.; Voss. J r; (1969). Immuno. Chemistry, 6:573.

185.   Al-Atrakchi S.A.M.; (2002). "Protein engineering of carcinoembryonic antigen and their receptors located in malignant mammary tissues". Ph. D. Thesis, Supervised by Al-Mudhaffar S.A., College of Science, Baghdad University.

186.   Rosier, J.S.; Gokulrangan G.; Girault H.; Svojanovsky S.; Wilson G.S.; (2000). Langmuir, 16: 8489-8494.

187.   Seely, D.H.; Wang W.Y.; Salhanick H.A.; (1980). Boichem. Boiphy. Acta., 632: 535.

188.   Al- Mudhaffar, S.A.; (2000). Iraqi. J. Chem.; 26J1): 186-194.

189.   Al-Mudaffar, S.A.; (2000). Iraqi. J. Chem.; 26 (4): 892-905.

190.   Scatchard G.; (1949). Ann. N.Y. Acad. Sci, 51:660.

191.   Chamberlain J.; Jargarinece N.; Ofner P.; (1966). Boichem. J., 99:10.

192.   Adams A.; Karrott D.; (1985). Boichem. Biophy. Acta., 632:535.

193.   Weiland G.A.; Molinoff P.B.; (1981). Life Science, 29:313.

194.   Segel I.H.; (1979). "Biochemical calculation" 3rd ed., John willey & Sons, Inc. pp311.

195.   Williams, C.A.; Chase M.W.; (1971). "Methods in immunology and immuno chemistry". 5th ed.. New York: Academic Press, Vol. III, chapter 13.

196.   Nemeth, G.; Scheraga H.A.; (1962). J. Phys. Chem., 66: 1773.

197.   Waelbroeck, M.; Van-Obberghen E.; De-Meytes P.; (1979). J. Biol. chem., 254: 7736.

198.   Haro, L.S. ; Talamantes F. J.; (1985). Mol. Cell. Endocrinol, 43: 199.

199.   Blumenthal, D.K.; Stull J.T.; (1982). Biochemistry, 21:2386.

200.   Laport, D.C; Wierman E.M.; Storm D.I.; Biochemisrtry; 19:3814.

201.   Laskowski, M.; Leach S. ∂. ; Scheraga H.A.; (1960). J. Am. Chem. Soc., 5:71.

202.   Leach, S.J.; Scheraga H.A.; (1960). J. Boil. chem., 235: 2827-2829.

203.   Saif-Allah, P.H.; (2000). "Biochemical studies on prolactin and some tumor makers in breast tumors" Ph.D. thesis supervised by Al-Mudhaffar, S.A., College of Science, Baghdad University.

204.   Kiernan, J.A.; (1999). "Histological & histochemical methods theory & practice" 3rd ed., Reed Educational and Professional Publishing Ltd, Chapter 19, pp 391-398.

205.   Johustone, A.; Thorpe R.; (1996). "Immuno-Chemistry in practice", 3rd ed., Blackwell Science Ltd, pp292-311, 1-4.

206.   Williams, C.A.; Chanse M.W.; (1968). "Methods in immunology and immunochemistry", New York, Acadimic Press, Vol II, Chapter 10, pp163-174.

207.   Mathews, Ch.K.; Holde K.E.; (1990). "Biochemistry" California: The Benjamin/Cummings Publishing Company.

208.   Freifrlder, D.; (1982). "Physical biochemistry, application to biochemistry molecular biology", 2nd ed., San Francisco: W.H. Freeman & Company. Chapter 14, pp 494-591.

209.   Leach, S. J.; (1969). "Physical principles and techniques of protein chemistry", New York, Acadimic Press, Part A, Chapter 3, pp102-170.

210.   Axelsen, N.H.; (1983). "Hand book of immunoprecipitiation in gel thechniques", 3rd ed. London, W.A.Banjamin, Inc.

211.   Yang, J.T. ; Foster J.F; (1954). J. Am Chem Soc.; 76:1588.

212.   Tanforel, C.; Buzzell J.G.; Rands D.G.; (1955). J Am Soc; 77: 6421.

213.   Leach, S. J.; (1969). "Physical principles and techniques of protein chemistry", Part A. 5th ed. London, Academic Press; Chapter 3, p: 102.

214.   San, Y.; Bovey D.A; (1960). J. Am. Chem. Soc., 235: 2818.

215.   Brealy, G.J.; Kaska M.; (1950). J. Am. Chem. Soc., 77: 4462.

216.   Silvestien, R.M.; Bassler G.C.; Marril T.C.; (1981). "Spectrophotometric dentification of organic compounds", New York, John Wiley and Sons., p181.

217.   Herskowits, T.T.; Laskowski M.Jr.; (1962). J. Biol. Chem., 2481-2492.

218.   Donavan, J. W.; (1965). Boichemistry, 4:823.

219.   Scherage, H.A.; (1961). "Protein structure" New York, Academic Press, pp: 175-287.

220.   Koprowski, H.; herlyn M.; Steplewski Z.; Sears H.F.; (1981). Science,253.

221.   Takasaki, H. ; Uchida E. ; Temero M.A; (1988). Cancer Res., 48: 1435-1438.

222.   Aydiner, A.; Topuz E.; Disci R.; Yosasever V.; Dincer M.; Dincol K.; Bilge A.; (1994). Acta Oncologica, 33(2): 181-186.

223.   Barbara, A.W.; Gerald k.; (1996). Newsletter, 4 (9): 1-7.

224.   Pasquali, C.; (1994). I. J. Pancreat, 15: 171-177.

225.   Szymedera, J.J; (1986). Tumour Boil., 7: 333-342.

226.   Coreale, M.; Arnberg H.; Blockx P.; Bombardieri E.; Castelli M.; Encabo G.; Gion M.; Klapdor R.; Martin M.; Nilsson s.; (1994). Int. J. Biol Markers; 9(4): 231-238.

227.   Kim, S.M.; Kim S.H.; Choi S.Y.; Kim Y.C.; (1992). J. Korean Med. Sci., 7(4): 297-303.

228.   Reid, M.E; Lomas-Francis C.; (1997). "The Blood group antigen facts book", New York, Academic Press, pp 1-6.

229.   Shimono, R.; Mori M.; Akazawa k.; (1994). Am .J. Castroenterol., 89: 101-105.

230.   Strom, B.L.; Maislin G. and West S.L.; (1990). Int. J. Cancer; 8: 8-13.

231.   Gion, M.; Ruggeri G.; Mione R.; (1993). Int .J. Biol. Markers, 8:8-13.

232.   Filellax, Molina R. ;Pique J.M.; (1994). Tumor Biol, 15; 1-6.

233.   Encabo, G.; Ruibal A.; (1986). Bull Cancer (Paris); 73:256-259.

234.   Kovacs, I.; Toth P.; Arkosy P.; Hamori J.; Sapy P.; (1997). Acta. Chir. Hyng., 36(1-4): 172-173.

235.   Harada, H. ; Tsukada Y. ; Karasawa Y.; (1994). Clin. Chim. Acta., 228(2): 101-112.

236.   Zinser, J.W.; (1997). Rev. Gastroenterol. Mex., 62(3): 145-148.

237.   Cwiertka, K.; Dapustova M.; machacek J.; Kohoutek M.; Minarik J.; (1998). Tumor Markers. Abstracts, 2(1); 010. quoted from internet.

238.   Changeux, J.P.; (1966). Mol. Pharmacol.; 2: 369.

239.   Roitt, I.M.; (1984). "Esential immunology", 5th ed., Oxford, Blackwell Scientific Publications. Chapter 1, p 4.

240.   Haro, L.S.; Talaments F.G.; (1985). Molec. and Cellular Endoc.,43:199.

241.   Daxembichler, G.; Grill H. J.; Wiesinger H.; Wittliff J.L.; (1997). "In: Multiple molecular forms of steroid hormone receptors", Agarwal M.L., editor. Elsevier, North-Holland Biomedical Press, p163.

242.   Weiss, R.B.; (1989). Oncology, 3: 135-148.

243.   Hvidt, A.; Nielsen S.O.; (1966). Advan. Protein Chem., 21:287.

244.   Sjiu, R.P.C; Friesen H.G.; (1971). J.Biol. Chem., 294: 7902.

245.   Melander, W.; hovarth C.; (1977). Arch. Biochem. Biophys., 183:200.

Part B

Carbohydrate antigen (CA-125) in Ovarian Tumors

Prof. Dr. Sami A.AL-Mudhaffar
Dr. Majid Karbon

Contents

CHAPTER THREE	
Chromatography Purification of CA125 by Gel Filtration and Binding Characterization to its Specific Antibody.	264

CHPTER FIVE
Spectroscopic Studies   305
on Isolated (125I-anti CA125 antibody/CA125) Complex

Chapter One
Introduction
&
Literature Survey

Summary

Immunoradiomatric assay technique was used to measure the level of serum tumor markers CA125 and CEA in 30 healthy women, 24 patients with benign ovarian tumors and 34 patients with malignant ovarian tumors. Upon comparison of the results, the CA125 level was found above normal (35u.ml-1) in 80% of patients with ovarian cancer, while CEA level was elevated in 44% of patients with ovarian cancer (more than 3.0 u.ml-1). Among the pre-menopausal women, the values of CA125 and CEA in sera of patients with malignant ovarian tumors were found to be significantly higher (P<0.05) than their corresponding values in sera of healthy and that in patients with benign tumors. The mean value of CA125 tumor marker in relation to menopausal status of ovarian cancer women, was found to be significantly higher (P<0.05) in post-menopausal patients, than that in pre-menopausal patients, while there were no differences found in the CEA value between the two statuses.

Modified immunoradiometric assay (IRMA) was used to characterize the binding of 125I-antiCA125 antibody to CA125 in the supernatant fraction of ovarian tumor homogenates. Different factors affecting this binding were extensively studied such as pH, time, temperature,   concentration of salts, concentration of antibodies and concentration of antigens

CA125 of homogenate obtained from post-menopausal patients with malignant ovarian tumor was partially purified by gel filtration technique. Two forms of CA125 were found (BI and BII) with molecular weights 670 and 100 kDa respectively. The binding characteristics of the partial purified CA125 with 125I-antiCA125 antibody were investigated.

Kinetic parameters of the binding of 125I-antiCA125 antibody with CA125 of homogenate obtained from pre-menopausal patients with benign and malignant tumors, post-menopausal patients with malignant tumors, and partially purified CA125, at different temperatures were determined. The results indicated that the binding reaction was time and temperature dependent process and it follows second order rate law in all studied groups.

The thermodynamics of the binding of 125I-antiCA125 antibody with CA125 of homogenate obtained from pre-menopausal patients with benign and malignant tumors, post-menopausal patients with malignant tumors, and the partially purified CA125, at different temperatures were determined. All studied groups showed exothermic and spontaneous reactions and the participation of enthalpy was low. Thermodynamic parameters of transition state (ΔH^*, ΔG^*, ΔS^*) and activation energy (Ea) were also determined.

Spectroscopic studies, in the U.V region, were carried out on the complex (125I-antiCA125 antibody/CA125) formed of the partially purified CA125, from post-menopausal patients with malignant ovarian tumors, to its specific antibody. Different factors affecting the absorption band such as pH, polarity and denaturation agents were extensively studied. The heat stability and spectrophotometric pH titration of the complex were also included in this work.

1.1 Historical background of tumor marker

Bence jones protein which is exhibits unusual solubility in water was the first tumor marker identified in 1848, it appears in large amounts in the urine of patients with multiple myeloma. More than 100 years after its discovery the Bence-Jones protein was identified as a monoclonal light chain of immunoglobulin (1).

Between 1928-1963, many substances including (hormones, enzymes, isoenzymes and proteins) were discovered and used as tumor markers useful in the diagnosis of individual tumors, but the general application of tumor marker for monitoring cancer in patients did not start until the discovery of α-fetoprotein (AFP)(2) in 1963 and carcinoembryonic antigen (CEA) in 1965(3). The production of such markers during fetal development as well as in tumors, led to the term oncodevelopmental markers.

Monoclonal antibodies were developed in 1975(4). to detect oncofetal antigens and antigens derived from tumor cell lines such as CA125, CA 15-3, and CA 19-9.

More recent advances in molecular techniques with the use of molecular probes and monoclonal antibodies to detect chromosome or protein alteration, including the study of oncogenes, suppressor genes, and genes involved in DNA repair, have led to the rapid understanding and use of tumor markers at molecular level (5). Unlike earlier tumor markers, these new markers can be linked to specific biological processes related to the regulation of cell growth and tumor development including malignant transformation, proliferation, apoptotic cell death and metastasis.

1.2 Definition of tumor marker

A tumor marker is a substance that is present in or produced by tumor itself, or produced by the host in response to a tumor (6) that can be used to differentiate a tumor from normal tissue or to determine the presence of a tumor based on its measurement in the blood or secretions. Such a substance can be found in cells, tissue, or body fluids (7). It can be measured qualitatively or quantitatively by chemical, immunological, or molecular biological methods to identify the presence of a cancer (8).

Morphologically, cancer tissue has been recognized by pathologists as resembling fetal tissue more closely than normal adult differentiated tissue. Tumors are graded according to their degree of differentiation: as being well differentiated, poorly differentiated, or anaplastic (without form). Few markers are specific for single individual tumor (tumor-specific markers); most are found with different tumors of the same tissue type (tumor-associated markers). They are present in higher quantities in cancer tissue or in blood of cancer patients than in benign tumors or in the blood of normal subjects.

Tumor markers have been categorized as enzymes, isoenzymes, hormones, and oncofetal antigens, carbohydrate epitopes recognized by monoclonal antibodies, receptors, oncogene product and genetic changes. There are only a handful of well-established tumor markers that are being used by physicians. Many other potential markers are still being under research. Now there are many studies that are trying to find new genes involved in signaling molecules or proteins that "tell" cells to proliferate, invade or metastasize (9).

1.3 Classification of Tumor Markers

Tumor markers may be classified into chemical and genetic tumor Markers. (10)

1.3.1 Chemical tumor markers

Table (1-1) Summarizes the classification of chemical tumor markers according to biochemical characteristics, and their associated malignancy.

Table (1-1) Chemical tumor markers (11)

Marker type	Associated malignancy	Example
Enzymes	Liver	Alcohol dehydrogenase
	Bone, Liver, Leukemia, Sarcoma	Alkaline phosphatase
	Ovarian, lung, trophoplastic, gastrointestinal, seminoma, hodgkin's	Alkaline phosphatase placental
	Pancreas, Various	Amylase
	Colon, Breast	Aryl Sulfatase B
	Colon, Bladder, Gastrointestinal, Various	Galactosyl Transferase
	Lung, (small-cell) neuroblastoma, Carcinoid, melanoma, pancreatic	Neuron-Specific enolase

	Prostate, Various (large bowel, lung, ovarian)	Prostate-specific antigen (PSA) Ribonuclease
	Colorectal, Breast, etc.	Telomerase
	Colon, Breast, Lung	Sialyl Transferenase
Hormone	Gushing,s syndrome, Lung (small cell)	ACTH
Hormone	Lung (small cell) adrenal Cortex, deudonal	Antidiuretic hormone
Hormone	Medullary thyroid	Calcitonin
Hormone	Pituitary adenoma, Renal, Lung, Embryonal, choriocarinoma, Testicular (nonseminomatous)	hCG
Hormone	Torophoblastic, Gonads, Lungs, Breast	Human placental lactogen
Hormone	Liver, Renal, Breast, Lung, Various	Parathyroid hormone
Hormone	Pituitary adenoma, renal, lung, breast.	prolactin
Oncofetal Antigen	Hepato cellular, germ line (non seminoma)	□-feto protein
Oncofetal Antigen	Colon	β- oncofetal antigen
Oncofetal Antigen	Liver	Carcino fetal ferritin
Oncofetal Antigen	Colorectal, Gastrointestinal, Pancreatic, Lung, Breast	CEA
Oncofetal Antigen	pancreatic	Pancreatic oncofetal
Oncofetal Antigen	Cervical, Lung, Skin, Head& neck (Squamous)	Squamous cell antigen
Oncofetal Antigen	Colon,Gastrointestinal, Bladder	Tennesse antigen
Mucin	Ovarian, endometrial, Lung	CA125
Mucin	Breast, ovarian	CA15-3
Mucin	Breast	CA27-29
Mucin	Breast, ovarian	MCA
Mucin	Pancreatic, Ovarian, Gastrointestinal, Lung	Du-PAN-2
protein	Multiple Myeloma, β-Cell lymphpoma chronic	β- 2 microglobulin

		Insulinoma	C-peptide
		Liver, Lung, Leukemia	Ferritin
		multiple myeloma, Lymphomas	Immunoglobulin
		Pancreatic, Stomach	Pancreas associated antigen
		Trophoplastic, Germ cell	Pregnancy specific protein
		Hepatocellular	Prothrombin precursor
		Ovarian	Tumor associated trypsin inhibitor
Blood Group Related antigen		Pancreatic, Hepatic, Gastrointestinal,	CA19-9
		Pancreatic, Gastrointestinal, Ovarian	CA19-5
		Colon, Pancreatic Gastrointestinal,	CA50
		Ovarian, Breast, Colon ,Gastrointestinal,	CA72,4,CA242
Others		Breast	Estrogcn&progesterone receptors
		Brain, Various	polyamine
		Bone Metastasis (Breast), (multiple myeloma)	Hydroxy proline
		Neuroblastoma, pheochromocytoma	Catecholamine metabolites
		Gastroitestinal, Lung, Rhenmatoid	Lipid-associated sialic acid

1.3.2 Genetic tumor markers

A simple definition of cancer is "a relatively autonomous growth of tissue". Understanding the cause of autonomous growth would clearly facilitate the search for care. Advance in molecular genetics have provided a better understanding of the genesis of human cancer. The proliferation of normal cell is thought to be regulated by growth – promoting oncogenes and counterbalanced by growth – constraining tumor suppressor genes. The development of cancer appears to involve the activation or altered expression of oncogenes, and the loss or inactivation of tumor suppressor genes.(11)

Oncogenes (cell activation genes) are derived from proto- oncogenes (normal celluler genes) which may be activated by dominant mutations. The type of mutation might be point mutation, insertion, deletion, translocation, or inversion. Most oncogenes are associated with haematological malignancies such as leukemia and to lesser extent, solid tumors. (12)

Suppressor genes (genes involved in the recognition and repair of damaged DNA) have mostly been isolated from solid tumors. p53 tumor suppressor gene is the most frequently mutated gene in human cancer, indicating its important role in the conservation of normal cell cycle progression (13). One of p53'S essential roles is to arrest the cells in G1 after genotoxic damage, to allow DNA repair prior to DNA replication and cell division. In response to massive DNA damage, p53 triggers the apoptotic cell death pathway (14). The loss of function of this gene may result in the inability of DNA repair process and may lead to the development of tumorgensis (15).

The exciting promise of using the detection of oncogenes and suppressor genes, for diagnosis, determining the prognosis, and predicting the response to the chemotherapy remains to be realized. Oncogens detection remains an experimental approach to human cancer.

1.4 Ideal Tumor Marker

An ideal tumor marker should be specific for a given type of cancer and sensitive enough to detect small tumors for early diagnosis or during screening, provide an estimation of tumor burden, and serve for monitoring effects of therapy and detecting recurrence of tumors (7). It can be measured qualitatively or quantatively by chemical, immunological, or molecular biological methods to identify the presence of a cancer (8).

1.5 Clinical Applications of Tumor Markers

Clinical applications of tumor markers depend on specificity and sensitivity. Specificity refers to the detection of specific tumors by specific markers. Sensitivity, in this instance, has to do with detecting all patients with the specific tumor.

The potential uses of tumor markers are (16):

- Screening in general population.
- Differential diagnosis of symptomatic patients.
- Clinical staging of cancer
- Estimating tumor volume.
- Prognostic indicator for disease progression
- Evaluating success of treatment.
- Detecting response to therapy
- Radioimmunolocalization of tumor marker.
- Determining direction for immunotherapy.

In general tumor markers may be used for diagnosis, prognosis, and monitoring effect of therapy, as well as a target for tumor localization and therapy. Monitoring treatment with tumor markers is an accepted application and generally indicates successful treatment; such monitoring is seen after both invasive and noninvasive treatment.

The use of tumor markers for screening the presence of cancer in asymptomatic individuals in a general population has been limited because most tumor markers are present in normal, benign and cancer tissues and are not specific enough to be used for screening cancer (17). However if the incidence of cancer is high among certain population, screening is feasible (18). Potential uses of some tumor markers are summarized in table (1-2).

Table (1-2) Clinical Uses of some tumor markers (19)

Tumor marker	Biochemical properties	Molecular weight	Primary clinical applications
Alpha–fetoprotein (AFP)	Glycoprotein, 4% carbohydrate; considerable homology with albumin	~70kDa	Diagnosis and monitoring of primary hepatocellular carcinoma and germ cell tumors. Prognosis of germ cell tumors.
Cancer antigen 125 (CA125)	Mucin identified by monoclonal antibodies	~ 200kDa	Monitoring ovarian carcinoma. Prognosis after chemotherapy
Cancer antigen 15-3 (CA15.3)	Mucin identified by monoclonal antibodies	>250 kDa	Monitoring breast cancer

Cancer antigen 72.4 (CA 72.4)	Glycoprotein identified by monoclonal antibodies	~48 kDa	Monitoring gastric carcinoma
Cancer antigen 19-9 (CA19-9)	Glycolipid carring the Lewis a blood group determinate	~1,000 kDa	Monitoring pancreatic carcinoma
Carcinoembri - yonic antigen (CEA)	Family of glycoproteins, 45%-60% carbohydrate	~180 kDa	Monitoring gastrointestinal and other Adenocarcinomas
Estrogen receptor	Nuclear transcription	65 kDa	Predicting response to endocrine therapy in breast cancer
Human chorionic gonadotrophin (hCG)	Glycoprotein hormone consisting of tow non- covalently bound subunits (α and β)	~36 kDa	Diagnosis and monitoring non-seminomatous germ cell tumors, Prognosis of germ cell tumors.
Placental alkaline phosphatase (PLAP)	Heat – stable isoenzyme of alkaline phosphatase	~86 kDa	Monitoring of germ cell tumors (seminomas)
Progesterone receptor	Nuclear transcription factor	A from : 94 kDa B from :120 kDa	Predicting response to endocrine therapy in breast cancer.
Prostate specific antigen (PSA)	Glycoprotein serine protease	~ 36 kDa	Diagnosis, screening and Monitoring prostatic carcinoma
Tissue polypeptide antigen (TPA)	Fragments of cytokeratin 8,18 and 19	~22 kDa	Monitoring bladder and lung carcinoma
Tissue polypeptide specific antigen (TPS)	Fragments of cytokeratin 18	~22 kDa	Monitoring metastatic breast carcinoma

1.6 Tumors of Ovary

Classification

The pathological conditions of the ovary may be classified as (20, 21):

1.6.1 Non-neoplastic Functional Cysts

Follicular cyst

Corpus luteum cyst.

Theca lutein and granulose lutein cysts.

Polycystic ovarian disease.

Endometriomatous cysts.

1.6.2 Ovarian Neoplasm's.

The classification of ovarian neoplasm's given in table (1-3), is a simplified version of world health organization (WHO) histological classification, which separates ovarian neoplasm's according to the most probable tissue of origin. (22)

Table (1-3) Derivation of various ovarian neoplasms' and some data on their frequency and age distribution (22)

Origin	Surface Epithelial cells (surface Epithelial – stromal cell tumor)	Germ cell	sex cord - stroma	Metastasis to ovaries
overall frequency	65-70%	15-20%	5-10%	5%
Proportion of malignant ovarian tumors	90%	3-5%	2-3%	5%
Age group affected	20 + years	0-25 + years	All ages	Variable
Types	- Serous tumor - Mucinous tumor	- Teratoma - Dysgerminoma	- Fibroma - Granulos -theca cell	

	- Endometrioid Tumor - Clear cell Tumor - Transitional cell Tumor - Undifferentiated carcinoma	- Endodermal sinus tumor - Chorio carcinoma	tumor - Sertoli – leydig cell tumor	

1.7 Epithelial Ovarian Tumors

The most common group of ovarian neoplasm originates from the coelomic mesothelium that covers the ovary, which after neoplastic transformation seems to retain the capacity to recapitulate the epithelial components of the mullerian ducts. According to the (WHO) classification of ovarian tumors, surface epithelial-stromal tumors can be divided into serous tumors, mucinous tumors, endometrioid tumors, clear cell tumors, transitional tumors and undifferentiated carcinoma (23, 24,25) table (1-3).

Serous tumor is the most frequent of the ovarian tumors and the most common epithelial ovarian carcinoma, accounting for 40-50% of all such tumors. (26)

According to histopathological classification of ovarian tumors, serous tumors can be classified into. (27)

Benign

- Cystadenoma and papillary cystadenoma.

- Surface papilloma

- Adenfibroma and cyst adenofibroma .

Borderline malignancy (of low malignant potential)

- Cystic tumors and papillary cystic tumor.

- Surface papillary tumor.

- Adenofibroma and cystadenofibroma.

Malignant.

- Adenocarcinoma, papillary adenocarcinoma.

- Cystadenocarcinoma.

- Surface papillary adenocarcinoma.

- Adenocarcinofibroma & cystadenocarcinofibroma.

Evidence is lacking about whether ovarian carcinoma may go through a borderline phase during its development and whether borderline tumors always shift into invasive ovarian carcinoma (28-29).

In the overall spectrum of serous tumors, about 60% are benign, 15% of low malignant potential, and 25% malignant (22). Benign serous cystadenomas occur slightly more often than benign mucinous tumors, but in their malignant form serous cyst adenocarcinomas are three to four times more common than mucinous cystadenocarcinomas. Serous and mucinous borderline tumors are seen but other types of epithelial tumors of borderline malignancy, such as the variant of Brenner and endometrioid tumors are rare (30).

1.7.1 Incidence

Ovarian cancer is the leading cause of death from gynecological malignancies (31) worldwide, the highest incidence of disease is found in America and northern Europe, the lowest incidence is found in Asia and Latin Amarica(32). In United States approximately 23000 cases occur annually leading to 13900 death each year (33), rate among blacks are lower than among whites, but rates for women of Chinese and Japanese are higher than rates in their countries of origin (32). In Iraq, ovarian cancer forms 38% of all gynecological malignancies, it was the seventh most common cancer among females with an incidence of 0.8 per 100,000 woman (34). It is the most common cancer to occur at an advanced stage (35).

1.7.2 Etiology and Risk Factors of ovarian cancer

Although the exact etiology of ovarian cancer is unknown, there are many risk factors which have been associated with the developing of ovarian cancer, such as Genetic, environmental, hormonal, and nutritional.

1.7.2.1 Genetic factors

The strongest known risk factor for ovarian cancer is family history which is present in about 10-15 % of women who develop the disease (36). Family history in one relative increased the lifetime probability of ovarian cancer in a 35- years old women from 1.5 to 5%; the probability increased to 7% if she had two relatives with the disease.

The rare familial ovarian cancer syndromes are accounting for less than 1% of ovarian cancer cases. The most common hereditary syndrome is the breast-ovarian cancer syndrome. Most of these families have germ- line mutation in one of the breast cancer susceptibility genes, BRCA-1 (37) or BRCA-2. (38)

1.7.2.2 Increasing Ages

The incidence of ovarian cancer increases with age, the highest proportion of cases is diagnosed in women 50 to 59 of age. In women 50 to 75 years of age, the annual incidence is 50 per 100,000 (adjust for prior oophorectomy), approximately twice the rate in young women (39, 40), while benign tumors occur mostly in young women between the ages of 20-40 years old. (22)

1.7.2.3 Reproductive factors

Several potentially modifiable reproductive factors appear to reduce the risk of ovarian cancer

- Pregnancy reduces the odds of ovarian cancer by 25 to 50 percent (41,42) the decrease in risk is associated with an increasing number of pregnancies.

- Use of the oral contraceptive pill is associated with a 35 % reduction in the risk of ovarian cancer, increasing the duration of use is associated with decreasing risk, (41,42) ten years of use by women with a positive family history can reduce their risk to a level below that for women with no family history who never used oral contraceptives. (43)

- Breast feeding is associated with a more modest effect on risk, reducing the odds of ovarian cancer by 20 % (41,42).

Certain gynecological surgical procedures are also associated with a lower likelihood of ovarian cancer. The risk of ovarian cancer is reduced by about 15% after tubal ligation or hysterectomy with ovarian preservation (41,42).The protective mechanism of these procedures may relate to impairment of ovarian function, causing an ovulation, or protection from exposure to exogenous carcinogens that enter the peritoneal cavity through the vagina. Talcum powder may be one of the carcinogen materials, studies have shown that woman who use talcum powder as part of their perineal hygiene are at increased risk. (43) Talc is found in soap powders, and deodorants, and is used in packing of condoms and (30, 44, 45) contraceptive diaphragms, talc might then migrate through vagina to reach the ovaries.

Infertility may increase the risk of ovarian cancer (46, 47). An increased risk of ovarian cancer has also been reported with infertility treatment, particularly prolonged use of clomiphene citrate. (48)

1.7.3 Staging

Staging of ovarian cancer is based on the finding at the time of surgery and pathological review. Because of the clinically occult spread, surgery is mandatory. The clinical staging of cancer is intended to provide means by which information related to the progress of the disease, the methods and success of treatment modalities is obtained.

Ovarian malignancies are staged according to the international federation of gynecology and obstetrics (FIGO), basing on the finding of surgical exploration(49)   see table (1-4).

Table (1-4) Staging of ovarian cancer according to FIGO. (49)

Stage I
In stage I, cancer is found in one or both of the ovaries. Stage I is divided into

Stage I

In stage I, cancer is found in one or both of the ovaries. Stage I is divided into

→ Stage IA: Cancer is found in a single ovary.

→ Stage IB: Cancer is found in both ovaries

→ Stage IC: cancer is found in one or both ovaries and one of the following is true:

• Cancer is found on the outside surface of one or both ovaries.

• The tumor has ruptured the ovary wall.

• Cancer cells are found in fluid from the peritoneal cavity (the body cavity that contains most of the organs in the abdomen). The fluid may already be in the peritoneal cavity or it may be added by the doctor to wash the peritoneum (tissue lining the peritoneal cavity).

Stage II

In stage II, cancer is found in one or both ovaries and has spread into other areas of pelvis. Stage II is divided into

→ Stage IIA: Cancer has spread to the uterus and / or the fallopian tubes.

→ Stage IIB: Cancer has spread to other tissue within the pelvis.

→ Stage IIC: cancer has spread to the uterus and/or fallopian tubes and /or other tissue within pelvis and one of the following is true:

• Cancer is found on the outside surface of one or both ovaries.

• The tumor has ruptured the ovary wall.

• Cancer cells are found in fluid from the peritoneal cavity.

Stage III

In stage III, cancer is found in one or both ovaries and has spread to other parts of the abdomen. Cancer has spread to the surface of the liver. Stage III is divided into:

→ Stage IIIA: The tumor is found only in the pelvis, but cancer cells have spread to the surface of the peritoneum.

→ Stage IIIB: Cancer has spread to the peritoneum but is not larger than 2 centimeters (less than 1 inch) in diameter.

↪ Stage IIIC: Cancer has spread to the peritoneum and is larger than 2 centimeters in diameter and/or has spread to lymph nodes in the abdomen.

STAGE IV

In stage IV, cancer is found in one or both ovaries and has metastasized (spread) beyond the abdomen to other parts of the body .Cancer is found in the tissues of the liver.

1.7.4 Diagnosis

Ovarian tumors are occasionally detected on pelvis examination, although early stage tumors are rarely found due to deep anatomic location of the ovary. Thus tumors detected by pelvic examination are usually at an advanced stage and associated with poor prognosis (50), more than 56-70% of the patients are diagnosed as having stage III or IV disease. (51)

Tests that examine the ovaries, pelvic area, blood, and ovarian tissue are used to help diagnose ovarian cancer.

These include the following. (49)

↪ Pelvic exam: A procedure to check the uterus, Vagina, ovaries, fallopian tubes, bladder, and rectum to find any abnormality in their shape or size.

↪ Ultrasound test: Transvaginal sonography (TVS) is capable of detecting more than 95% of stage I ovarian cancers, it also detects large numbers of patients with benign disease who subsequently undergo surgery to rule out malignancy, the predictive value was only 1.5%. (52)

↪ CA125 Test: A blood test used to measure the level of CA125 (53), a substance sometimes found in an increased amount in the blood, other body fluids or tissues.

→ Computerized axial tomography (CAT scan): A series of detailed pictures of areas inside the body, taken from different angles. This method fails to differentiate benign disease from stage I disease. (54, 55)

→ Intravenous pyelogram: A series of x-ray of the kidneys, Ureters, and bladder to help determine if cancer has spread outside the ovaries.

→ Biopsy: Removal of tissue for examination under microscope.

1.7.5 Treatment

There are treatments for all patients with ovarian epithelial cancer. Some treatment are standard, and some are being tested in clinical trials. A treatment clinical trial is a research study meant to help improve current treatments or (49) obtain information on new treatments for patients with cancer.

1.7.5.1 Standard treatment: three kinds of standard treatment are used, these include the following:

→ Surgery

Most patients have surgery to remove as much of the tumor as possible. Different types of surgery may include

• Hysterectomy (removal of the ovaries, fallopian tubes, and uterus).

• Unilateral Salpingo-oophorectomy (removal of one ovary and one fallopian tube).

• Bilatera salpingo-oophorectomy (removal of both ovaries and both fallopian tubes).

• Omentectomy (partial removal of the lining of the abdominal cavity).

• Lymph node biopsy (removal of the lymphnodes for examination under a microscope to check for cancer cells).

→ Radiation therapy

Radiation therapy is the use of x- ray or other types of radiation to kill cancer cells and shrink tumors. Radiation therapy may use external or internal radiation.(49)

➜   Chemotherapy

Chemotherapy is the use of drugs to kill cancer cells. Chemotherapy may be taken orally or injected into a vein or muscle. Another way to give chemotherapy is intraperitoneal chemotherapy. With this method, most of the drug remains in the abdomen; this technique is effective in advanced disease with minimal residual disease. (44)

➜   Biological therapy

➜   High-dose chemotherapy with bone marrow transplantation.

Biological therapy is the treatment to stimulate the ability of the immune system to fight cancer. Substances made by the body or made in laboratory are used to boost, direct, restore the body's natural defense against disease.

Biological therapy is sometimes called biological response modifier (BRM) therapy or immunotherapy. (49)

Within the last few years, different immunotherapeutic strategies based on immunization with tumor specific antibody constructs or immunogenic peptides have been developed (56, 57). Alternative concepts include the application of genetically modified tumor cells for the expressions of cytokines or consitimulatory molecules as well as dentritic cells for the effective presentation of immunogenic peptides in the extent of MHC and the activation of cellular immune responses, (57) in this context, ovarian cancer cells express a mutated form of the P53 (58, 59, 60) and/or BRCA1 (61, 62) (Tumor suppressor gene).

Ovarian tumors also over express the CA125 (63) and DF3/MUCI (64) carcinoma-associated antigens. In addition, these tumors over express the HER2/neu (c-erbB2) (65, 66) thus certain targets for immunotherapy of cancer are already known and others although remain undefined presumably exist.

Stage I: Treatment of stage I may include hysterectomy, unilateral or bilateral salping-oophoretomy and omentectomy. It also may include radiation therapy, chemotherapy and clinical trail conservative unilateral salpingo oophorectomy is adequate. It appears that ovarian preservation and women's fertility is safe and reasonable in women of reproductive age.(44, 67)

Stage II: treatment of stage II may include surgery to remove the tumor (hysterectomy, bilateral salpingo-oophorectomy, and omentectomy). Combination with chemotherapy or radiation therapy gives approximately 85-90% five years survival. (44, 68)

Stage III: treatment of stage III may include surgery to remove the tumor (hysterectomy, bilateral salping - oophorectomy, and omentectomy) followed by chemotherapy or chemotherapy followed by second look surgery.

Stage IV: Treatment of stage IV ovarian epithelial cancer is combination chemotherapy with or without surgery to reduce the size of the tumor. Extensive surgery is often insufficient to eliminate the intra-abdominal tumor and response to chemotherapy is only partial in many of these patients(44).

1.8 Ovarian Tumor Markers

Ninety percent of ovarian malignancies are epithelial. (25, 69) There are quantitative and qualitative changes in numerous circulating substances which have been associated with epithelial ovarian cancer. These may reflect an alteration in ovarian function, surface molecular structure or general responses to malignancy.

Expression of specific antigens associated with epithelial ovarian cancer is useful for establishing a diagnosis, classification and providing prognostic information. Monitoring the appropriate antigen titers is very useful in the identification of occult metastasis, monitoring of therapeutic response and detection of asymptomatic recurrence at an early stage. (70, 71, 72)

The antigens defined on ovarian tumors are regarded as tumor-associated rather than tumor-specific (73). Several tumor markers have been investigated for one or more clinical use in ovarian cancer as shown in table (1-5).

Table (1-5): Tumor markers that have been investigated in ovarian cancer (10).

Marker type		Example
Hormones		Progesterone (74), Estrogene , urinary gonodotrophin fragment.
Enzymes		Placental alkaline phosphatase(75,76) creatine kinase, amylase glactosyl transferase, ribonuclease
Oncofetal antigens		Tissue polypeptide antigen(77) alpha-fetoprotein ,carcinoembryonic antigen(CEA) (78) .
Carbohydrate markers		A:Mucin tumor markers: CA125, CA15-3 B. blood group antigens related cancer marker. CA72-4 (79) .
Genetic markers	Oncogene products	C- erb B-2 amplification HER-2/neu (80)
	Tumor suppressor genes	BRCA1(37) ,BRCA2 (38)

There are several tumor markers that correlate with the incidence of ovarian cancer, but the most important markers are:

1.8.1 CEA

Carcinoembryonic antigen (CEA), one of the onco-fetal proteins, is a cell surface glycoprotein, with a high molecular mass of 150-300 kDa. It is normally expressed in the early embryonic development and tends to disappear with the onset of differentiation of fetal tissue into adult ones. CEA has been studied extensively in ovarian cancer and has been reported to be elevated in 30-65% of epithelial tumors, mainly in patients with advanced stage disease. This antigen has been shown not to correlate well with status of disease. (81)

1.8.2 CA 19.9

CA19.9 is a carbohydrate antigen that is measured by a monoclonal antibody and can be found elevated in only 17-25% of patients with epithelial malignancies (82,83).

1.8.3 CA 15-3

CA15-3 is a mucin-like membrane glycoprotein recognized by a pair of monoclonal antibodies: the murine antibody DF-3 and 115D8 (64). Distinct epitopes of this high molecular weight antigen (300-400kDa) (84) is the carbohydrate side chain which accounts for about 50% of its structure (85).

CA15.3 is found in adenocarcinoma of breast, lungs, ovaries and pancreas(86, 87). Its level is elevated in 64% of ovarian cancer, it is most useful tumor marker for breast cancer (88).

1.8.4 IL.6 and IL.10

The interleukins, IL-6 and IL-10, have been shown to be present in very high levels in the ascites and serum of women with advanced stage epithelial cancers (89, 90). IL-6 correlates well with the stage and status of disease, but is elevated in only about 66% of patients, and its complementarily with CA125 is only modest.

1.8.5 M-CSF

Macrophage colony stimulating factor (M-CSF) has been found to be measurable in the serum of 68% of patients with clinically detectable disease(91,92).

Interestingly, some complementarities with CA125 has been documented. Patients with clinically evident tumor and a negative CA125 (< 35 u.ml-1), 56% had an elevated M-CSF serum level (92).

1.8.6 LSA

Lipid-associated sialic acid (LSA) can be measured in the sera of about 60% of patients with ovarian cancer, mostly those with advanced stage disease. A combination of LSA and CA125 improve sensitivity for detection of advanced disease but does not improve specificity (82).

1.8.7 OVXI

OVXI antigen is a high molecular weight mucin. The antigenic determinate of OVXI antigen was raised by immunization of mice with human ovarian cancer cell line. OVXI antigen is elevated in 67%of patients with clinically evident ovarian cancer who are CA125 negative. The OVXI is elevated however, in only 45%of patients with ovarian cancer. In patients with residual disease at second-look surgery and a negative CA125, 27% had an elevated OVXI level in the serum.(93)

1.8.8 NB 70 K

NB70K antigen appears to be present in most major types of epithelial ovarian cancer, with an apparent molecular weight of 70 kDa (94). Among sera samples from ovarian cancer patients ,elevated NB70K levels were found in 87% of samples that contained elevated CA125 levels. No quantitative correlation was found, however, between levels of NB70K and CA125.(94,95)

1.8.9 TAG 72

Tumors associated glycoprotein (TAG-72) level is elevated in 50% of ovarian carcinoma cases and only in 4% of benign disease cases with the highest level of expression in mucinous cystadenocarcinoma and its measurement may be useful as a confirmatory tumor marker for the presence of ovarian cancer in those patients with elevated CA125 serum levels. Combined TAG-72 and CA-125 test increase the sensitivity for the detection of primary ovarian cancer to 73% with no significant change in specificity (96).

1.9 Cancer Antigen 125(CA125)

1.9.1 Biochemistry

Cancer antigen 125(CA125) was first defined by monoclonal antibody (OC125) more than 20 years ago (53). It was associated with a family of high molecular weight glycoproteins, that differed from classical mucins by means of carbohydrate conversion(less than 50%) and presence of both N and O linked carbohydrate residues (97,98). Size exclusion chromatography of native CA125 antigen material from body fluids results in at least two broad peaks of antigen reactivity with approximate relative molecular mass of 200 and >1000 kDa,(99) but lower molecular weight species have also been reported .

Chemical study has revealed sensitivity of CA125 to proteases; low pH, high temperature, and high ionic strength, properties consisted of conformational peptide determinant. However, CA125 activity can also be destroyed with relatively high concentration of periodate and blocked with different lectins, suggesting a close association with carbohydrate. (97)

1.9.2 Structure

Although CA125 biochemical nature has long been elusive, its primary structure was established four years ago, indicating that it is trans-membrane protein with a short intracellular and a giant extracellular domain, the latter is with 22,097 amino acid residues. The extracellular part is composed of an amino-terminal part spanning 12,070 residues (100), followed by more than 60 tandem repeats of 156 amino acid motif and 229-residues linker to trans-membrane domain (101). Both the amino terminal part and the repeat domains are rich in serine and thereonine residues and are highly glycosylated. The carbohydrate content was estimated to be 24-28%, with O-linked and N-linked glycans (102). Because highly O-glycosylated repeats are the landmark of the mucin family of glycoproteins, CA125 was also named MUC 16 to reflect the nature of CA125 as a new member of protein family of mucins (103). The mucin-like repeats contain a domain that was reported to be susceptible to proteolytic cleavage (104). An additional potential proteolytic cleavage site in CA125 was reported to be located immediately membrane-proximal (101). Figure (1-1) represents a proposed structure of CA125 antigen.

1.9.3 FUNCTION OF CA125

Although primary structure of CA125 has been elucidated, a functional role for this molecule in physiological context or in cancer remains unknown.

However, a number of publications have pointed out several properties of CA125 that may be of relevance for its biological function.

First, because of its expression in embryonic membranes and adult derivatives of the fetal periderm, CA125 has been suggested to play a role as a lubricant, preventing adhesion of membranes (105). Anti adhesive properties have also been assigned to other mucins (106).

Second, close analysis of glycans present on CA125 protein revealed the presence of several glycan structures that have been implicated in immune suppression (102) raising the possibility that CA125 might help protect the embryo from maternal immune rejection and play an immunovasive role in ovarian cancer. Furthermore mucin can bind to various sugar-binding molecules, such as galectins (107). CA125 was found to be a novel counter receptor for galectin-1(108). The known cellular responses to the cell-surface recruitment of galectin-1 include a change in proliferation activity, regulation of cell survival and regulation of cell adhesion. Depending both on the cellular context and its local concentration, galectin-1 exerts both inhibitory and stimulatory effects on these processes (109).

Third Gaetje et al. found that CA125 from human peritoneal fluid was shown to enhance the invasiveness of a benign endometriolic cell line EEC145, but it did not affect the invasiveness of a variety of non-endometrioid cell lines, raising the possibility that CA125 plays a role in endometriosis (110).

Recently, Rump et al. in 2004 (111) have demonstrated that mesothelin (a glycoprotein which is present in peritoneal fluid of ovarian cancer patients) (112) is a novel CA125-binding protein and they (CA125 and mesothelin) are co-expressed in advanced grade ovarian adenocarcinoma, which indicates that CA125 might contribute to the metastasis of ovarian cancer to the peritoneum by initiating cell attachment to the mesothelial epithelium via binding to mesothelin.(111)

1.9.4 Expression

CA125 is derived from celomic epithelium (pleura, peritoneum and pericardium), amnion and Mullerian duct during embryonic development. Trace amounts of CA125 are found in adult tissues derived from the epithelial lining of the pleura, peritoneum, pericardium, fallopian tube, endometrium and endocervix (98, 113).

Relative to the expression levels of CA125 found in normal tissues, CA125 is often overexpressed from epithelial ovarian cancer tissue and other tumors of non-gynecological malignances.(53, 114)

Although CA125 is expressed both by normal and tumor cells, cell surface expression and release of soluble proteolytic fragments of CA125 into the extracellular space (115) appear to be associated with the conversion from benign to cancer cells (116).

1.9.5 Developing The CA 125 Assay

The development of an assay for the CA125 tumor marker grows out of attempts of Bast et al (117) which aimed to obtain monoclonal antibodies for serotherapy of patients in ovarian cancer. In this attempt, mice were repeatedly injected with a human ovarian cancer cell line and hybridomas were prepared from immune spleen cells and the P3NS-1 plasmacytoma. From these hybridomas, clones were isolated based on the production of antibodies that bound to the ovarian cancer cell line used for immunization, but not to a B lymphocyte cell line developed for the tumor cell donor. The one hundred twenty-fifth promising clone produced an IgG1 antibody of the desired specificity and was designated as OC (ovarian cancer). (117)

Using immunohistochemical analysis, the OC 125 antibody was found to bind to antigen expressed by approximately 80% of epithelial ovarian cancer as well as by other gynecologic, breast, lung, and colon carcinomas: this antigen was designated as CA (cancer antigen) 125.(117)

The first monoclonal antibody radioimmunoassay for monitoring epithelial ovarian cancer, using OC125 antibody, was reported in 1983 by Bast et al. (53). After that several different formats for the assay have been developed using radiolabeled or enzyme-labeled OC 125 as a probe. Over the last decade, a number of monoclonal antibodies have been developed that react with one or two distinct epitopes on molecules expressing CA125. One of these antibodies, M11, has permitted the development of a second generation assay, CA125II, in which M11 is used to trap antigen, followed by OC125 to detect antigen that has been captured on a solid phase (118).

1.9.6 Clinical Applications of CA125

The best available marker for epithelial ovarian cancer is CA125. The normal range most frequently quoted for CA125 is 0-35 u.ml-1, although 99% of apparently healthy post-menopausal women have levels below 20 u.ml-1. In apparently healthy pre-menopausal women, levels of 100u/ml or higher can occur during menses.(75) Elevation was also observed with the first trimester of normal pregnancy.(119) Although elevated CA125 levels are found in approximately 80% of all patients with epithelial ovarian cancer, high levels are found in only about 50% of stage I disease. (120)

This lack of sensitivity for early disease, and the fact that CA125 can be elevated in multiple benign disease such as endometriosis (121,75) , limits the use of CA125 for the diagnosis of early epithelial ovarian cancer. Further limitation is that CA125 can be elevated in adenocarcinomas other than ovarian cancer. Although CA125 can also be elevated in germ cell tumors of ovary (120), the markers of choice for this type of ovarian cancer are $\alpha\beta$-fetoprotein (AFP) and human chorionic gonadotrophin (hCG) and its β-subunite (β-hCG).

1.9.6.1 Screening

The lack of early symptoms means that approximately 70% of the patients with ovarian cancer present with advanced disease. While the overall five-year relative survival rate is of the order of 30%, the survival rate for stage III and IV disease combined is only 10% (122). In contrast, a five year survival of 90% may be achieved for patients with early stage disease confined to the ovary (123).

As a screening test, the main problems with CA125 are lack of sensitivity for early stage disease (only about 50% of patients with stage I have elevated levels) and lake of specificity. Thus, a single measurement of CA125 is not an adequate screening tool for ovarian cancer (124). The rate of change in CA125 levels over time appears to be more specific screening method. In one study, the specificity reached 99.9% after redefining a positive test as CA125 concentration greater than 35 u.ml-1 was doubles within six months.(124)

CA125, however, in combination with transvaginal ultrasound may have the role in the early detection of ovarian cancer. This screening strategy achieved a specificity of 100%, and an apparent sensitivity of 81.7% (125). Other reports have found that the use of tumor markers complementary to CA125 (eg. OVX1) is useful to achieve a specificity of 99.9% and an apparent sensitivity of 80%. Measurement of complementary serum markers can be used as primary screening technique followed by transvaginal ultrasongraphy. This could provide cost-effective means of early detection and could significantly decrease the probability of surgical intervention for false-positive test results.(126)

1.9.6.2 Diagnosis

The diagnosis of ovarian cancer is usually carried out by surgery followed by histopathology. However, pre-operative serum levels of CA125 especially in post-menopausal women, may be useful in the differential diagnosis of benign and malignant pelvic masses. Among post menopausal patients with a pelvic mass, a CA125 level   greater than 65 u.ml-1 has distinguished malignant disease with greater than 90% accuracy. The accuracy of CA125 (cut-off concentration 35 u.ml-1) in differentiating between benign and malignant masses was 77%, which was almost identical to accuracy achieved with pelvic examination and Ultrasound (76% and 74% respectively) (127). The combination of Ultrasound, CA125 and pelvic examination, however, improved the accuracy. Significantly, no cancer was found in any subject in which all three tests were negative. (127)

1.9.6.3 Prognosis (chance of recovery)

The traditional prognostic factors for ovarian cancer include tumor stage, grade, histological type and size of residual tumor after primary debulking (cytoreductive surgery). However multiple studies have shown that CA125 levels after either 1,2 or 3 courses of chemotherapy is one of the strongest available indicators of disease outcome (128).

A prolonged half life for CA125, or decrease in CA125 concentration of less than 7 folds of pretreatment concentration, during the early month of treatment, has been suggested to be an indicator for a poor outcome. CA125 concentration >70 u.ml-1 before the third course of chemotherapy was the single most important factor for predicting disease progression at twelve months (128).

1.9.6.4 Monitoring

The most important application of CA125 is in the monitoring of patients with epithelial ovarian cancer. Serial CA125 levels can pre-clinically detect recurrent disease with lead times of 1-17 months (median 3-4 months)(75,120), Doubling of initially elevated CA125 levels has been associated with disease progression in more than 90% of cases (75). Furthermore, longitudinal monitoring with this marker has the potential to detect recurrent disease earlier and more cost-effectively than radiological procedures (128). While early detection of recurrent disease may lead to altered patient management, no study has yet shown that this leads to enhanced survival. The use of CA125 and other markers for monitoring, will attain greater importance, as more effective treatment becomes available for previously - treated ovarian cancer.

1.9.6.5 Treatment

Induction of specific immune responses by vaccination with murine monoclonal anti-idiotypic antibody (Anti-CA125), which imitates the tumor-associated antigen CA125, has a positive influence on the survival of patients with recurrent ovarian carcinoma. Patients subjected to this immunotherapy technique showed increased concentration of human anti mouse antibodies. Specific anti-anti-idiotypic antibodies, as a marker for induced immunity, were detected in 66% of treated patients. Survival of patients with a positive immune response was 19.9 ± 13.1 months in contrast with 5.3 ± 4.3 months in those patients without detectable Anti CA125-immunity.(129)

The explanation of this specific immuno response caused by vaccination with anti-ioditypic antibody is that the variable antigen binding regions of antibodies (Ab1) contain idiotypic determinants that are immunogenic and induce the formation of so-called anti-idiotypic antibodies (Ab2), some of these antibodies are able to functionally mimic the three dimensional structure of original antigen, thus selective immunization with Ab2 could induce specific immune reaction directed against the original antigen. (129)

Antitumor vaccines were also developed by fusions of tumor associated antigens with dendritic cells. Human ovarian carcinomas express the CA125, HER2/neu, and MUC1 Tumor associated antigens which are potential targets for the induction of active specific immunotherapy. Fusions of ovarian cancer cells to dentritic cells resulted in the formation of heterokaryons that express the CA125 antigen and dendritic cells-derived costimulatory and adhesion molecules. The fusion cells have been shown to stimulate proliferation of autologous T cell that induce cytolytic T-cell activity and lysis of autologous tumor cells. (130)

Chapter Two

Preliminary studies for the binding of 125I- antiCA125 antibody to the CA125 in Human

Sera and homogenates of benign and malignant ovarian tumors.

Abstract

Measurements of the two biochemical tumor markers CA125 and CEA were carried out in serum samples obtained from 30 healthy donors, 34 ovarian cancer patients (20 post-menopausal patients with malignant ovarian tumors (OI)and 14 pre-menopausal patients with ovarian tumors (OII) and 24 ovarian benign patients (OIII) using Immunoradiometric assay (IRMA) technique.

Mean values of CA125 in pre-menopausal patients with benign and malignant ovarian tumors and CEA in pre-menopausal patients with ovarian cancer were found to be significantly higher (P<0.05) than their corresponding values in sera of healthy control, while insignificant differences (P>0.05) between CEA values in patients with benign tumor and healthy control were found. In comparison between post-menopausal and pre-menopausal patients with ovarian cancer tumor, values of CA125 and CEA in post-menopausal were significantly higher (P<0.05) than those found in pre-menopausal group. The tumor marker CA125 shows the best sensitivity 80% for detecting ovarian cancer patients, than CEA, which gave 44% sensitivity. Also CA125 gave the highest specificity 100% for the ability of this marker to exclude normal individuals while CEA gave a specificity of 90%. The mean value of the ratio of CA125 level to CEA level in sera of ovarian cancer patients was found to be 87 in those patients with elevated CA125 concentration.

The binding of CA125 to 125I-anti CA125 antibody in the tissue of benign and malignant ovarian tumors was preliminarily tested. The results showed that the supernatant fraction of the tissue homogenates contains higher CA125 level than the pellet fraction in all studied groups.

The effects of protein concentration, 125I-anti CA125 antibody concentration, pH of the reaction medium, time of reaction and temperature were studied for the binding of CA125 to 125I-anti CA125 antibody, in the tissue homogenates of malignant and benign ovarian tumors. The optimum conditions observed for the binding were as follows:

Optimum protein concentration in tissue homogenate was (225, 150 and 175 μ.ml-1) for (OI, OII and OIII) respectively.

125I-anti CA125 antibody optimum concentration was (450,360 and 450 μ.ml-1) for (OI, OII and OIII) respectively. Optimum pH was (7.2, 6.2 and 6.4) for (OI, OII and OIII) respectively. The optimum time and temperature was 240 minute at 4°C for all studied groups.

The use of different halides was shown to cause promotion effects on the binding of 125I-anti CA125 antibody to CA125 in groups OI, OII and OIII except I^- in group OI. The studies also show that the use of different mono and divalent cations increases the binding in all groups except NH_4^+ in group OIII.

2.1 Introduction

The role of ovarian tumor markers is to enhance the clinician's ability to provide more effective management of the disease. CA125 was found to be the best available marker for epithelial ovarian cancer. This oncofetal antigen is found in the embryonic coelom epithelium and, later, in the derived fetal tissues. CA125 is not expressed, or barely expressed, on the epithelial tissues of the ovary but is found in serous adenocarcinomas of the ovary from which it is shed and can then be assayed in the blood (131).

CA125 has limited specificity. It has been reported that CA125 is elevated in approximately 1% of healthy women (27), 6-40% of women with benign masses (e.g. , uterine fibroids, endometriosis, and pancreatic pseudocyst) (121) and 29% of women with non-gynecologic cancers (e.g., pancreas, lung, stomach, colon and breast) (53,108), while generally reported specificity in screening studies should be about 99% (132). It has been reported that it may be possible to improve the specificity of CA125 measurement by either selective screening of post – menopausal women (124), modifying the assay technique, measuring other tumor markers beside CA125 (126), persistent elevation of CA125 level over time, or combining CA125 measurement with ultrasound. (125)

Serum CA125 concentration was determined by several methods including Immunoradiometric assay (IRMA) (53), Enzymeimmunoassay (EIA), Immunoflorometric assay (IFMA) (133) and enzyme-linked immunosorbent assay (ELISA) (134). Today in commercially available CA125 assays, two monoclonal antibodies directed against different protein determinants in the CA125 protein core are used. Such antibodies seem to be less influenced by differences in glycosylation between different individuals and conditions (118).

CA125 has been used in the management of patients with ovarian cancer. It has been evaluated for its ability to determine diagnosis, prognosis, monitor therapy, predict recurrence of disease following curative surgery and treatment of ovarian cancer using immunotherapeutic strategies (135).

The objective of the present study was to evaluate the clinical application of biochemical tumor markers CA125 and CEA in the diagnosis of ovarian cancer. Also, this study was carried out in order to develop an immunoradiometric assay technique to determine optimum condition of

125I-antiCA125 antibody binding with CA125 in ovarian tumor tissue homogenates.

Materials and Methods

2.2 Materials

2.2.1 Chemicals

All chemicals in this study were of analar grade, the specification of these chemicals are tabulated in table (2.1)

Table 2-1: Specification of the Used Chemicals

No.	Chemical	Company
1.	Immunoradiometric kit for CA125 antigen level. Immunoradiometric kit for CEA antigen level.	Immunotech (France)
2.	Tris buffer, Bovine serum albumin, ZnCl2, CaCl2, MgCl2, EDTA, NH4CL, urea and NaN3	Fluka (Switzerland)
3.	CuSO4.5H2O, Na, K –Tartarate, NaOH, HCl, Na2CO3, NaF, NaCl, NaBr, NaI, MnCl2 , polyethylene glycol 6000 (PEG 6000) and Folin Ciocalteaue reagent	BDH (U.K)
4.	Blue dextran, Sepharose CL-6B	Pharmacia Fine Chemicals (Sweden)

2.2.2 Instruments

Table (2-2) Instruments Used and Companies

Instruments	Company
Gamma counter type 1270 rack Gamma II	LKB
Double Beam spectrophotometer	Shimadzu
pH meter	Pyeunicam
Sartorius analytical balance	Germany
Cooling centrifuge with maximum speed 5000 rpm	Hettich
SM shaker	England
Memmert water bath, Memmert incubator	Germany

2.2.3 Patients

This is a prospective study from November 2002 to September 2004 for 58 women admitted for surgical management of ovarian masses in different gynecological centers in Baghdad and southern Iraq matched with 30 healthy individuals.

Several points were taken into consideration, related to individual used throughout this study which includes the following:

(1)   No evidence of liver disease.

(2)   Not pregnant.

(3)   Un smokers.

(4)   Not taken any type of treatment.

(5)   No oral contraceptive pill used.

(6)   The time of taking the samples out of ministration period.

Patients included in this study were divided into three groups:

Group 1 consisted of 20 post – menopausal patients with ovarian cancer, group 2 consisted of 14 pre menopausal patients with ovarian cancer and group 3 consisted of 24 patients with Benign ovarian tumor. In addition to group 4 consisted of 30 healthy individuals.

The host information of all patients and normal healthy subjects is summarized in table (2-3).

Table (2-3): The host information of ovarian tumors patient and healthy subjects Studied.

Group	Patients	No.	Age	Type of tumor
OI	Post-menopausal malignant ovarian tumor	20	55-72	Serous cystadenocarcinoma
OII	Pre-menopausal malignant ovarian tumor	14	19-45	Serous cystadenocarcinoma
OIII	Benign ovarian tumor	24	22-46	Benign epithelial cyst (serous cystadenoma)
Control	healthy individuals	30	20-50	control

All patients were admitted for the treatment to (Medical City, Baghdad Teaching Hospital), AL- Habbibia General Hospital, Ibn Ghaswan Hospital (Basrah) and AL-Saadun private hospital (Basrah).

All surgical operations of tumor were carried out under the supervision of surgeons Dr. Fouad Al Dahhan, Dr. Luay Edward Kury and Dr. Amal Fatoohi.

2.2.4 Preparation of Blood Samples

Five milliliters of blood sample were obtained from patients by vein puncture just before surgery. Blood samples were left for 20 min at room temperature after coagulation; sera were separated by centrifugation at 1500 g for 10 min. Serum specimens were then frozen at -20°C until time of analysis.

2.2.5 Specimens Collection

The tumor tissues were surgically removed from ovarian tumor patient by either unilateral salpingo oophorectomy or total abdominal hysterectomy with bilateral salpingo oophorectomy. The specimens were cut off and immediately rinsed with ice-cold isotonic saline solution. They were collected individually in plastic receptacles and stored at -20°C until homogenization.

2.2.6 Preparation of phosphate Buffered Saline

Phosphate buffered saline (PBS) 0.1 M, pH 7.2 was prepared as the following:

A: Disodium basic phosphate (0.1 M); 1.419 g Na_2HPO_4 and 0.9 g of NaCl were dissolved in a final volume 100 ml deionized distilled water.

B: Monobasic sodium phosphate (0.1M); 1.1998 g of NaH_2PO_4 and 0.9 g of NaCl were dissolved in a final volume 100 ml deionized distilled water.

Phosphate buffer saline pH 7.2 was prepared by mixing a volume of solution A with appropriate amounts of solution B to obtain the required pH.

2.2.7 Preparation of Ovarian Tumors Tissues Homogenates

The frozen tissue was weighed, sliced finely and scalped in Petri dish standing on ice bath, and then homogenized with three fold volumes of PBS buffer pH 7.2, using manual homogenizer . The homogenate was filtered through four layers of nylon gauze in order to eliminate fibers connective tissues, and then centrifuged at 1500 g for 30 min at 4°C in order to precipitate the remaining intact cells and the intact nucleus. The supernatant fraction at this speed was separated and divided in a liquots and freezed at -20°C until use

2.3 Methods

2.3.1 Determination of protein concentration

Solutions
1. Standard bovine serum albumin (BSA), (0.2 mg/ml) as stock solution.
2. Reagent A: Alkaline carbonate solution (2% Na_2CO_3 in 0.1 N NaOH).
3. Reagent B: copper sulphate- sodium potassium tartarate solution (0.5% $CuSO_4. 5H_2O$ in 1% Na, K tartarate)
4. Reagent C: Alkaline copper solution, Mixing (50ml of reagent A with 1 ml of reagent B), discard after one day
5. Reagent D: Folin Ciocaltean reagent (1N) was prepared by the dilution of the commercial reagent (2N) with an equal volume of distilled water on the day of use.

Total homogenate protein's content was determined by the method of Lowry (136), using bovine serum albumin (BSA) as the standard solution. The details of the method are according to the following steps:

1. A volume of 1 ml of each of standard BSA (zero, 20,40, 60, 80,100, 120, 140, 160, 180, and 200) µg/ml was pipetted in a set of test tubes the experiment was carried out in duplicate.

2. A volume of 100 µl of ovarian tumors homogenate was also pipetted in test tubes and the volumes were made up to 1 ml with distilled water.

3. A volume of 5 ml of reagent C was added to all assay tubes. Then the contents were mixed by vortexing and allowed to stand for 10 min at room temperature.

4. A volume of 0.5 ml of reagent D was added drop by drop with mixing to all assay tubes the mixture was left to stand for 30 min at room temperature.

5. The absorbance of the developing color was read at 600 nm against the appropriate blank.

6. The standard curve was obtained by plotting the absorbance against the corresponding concentrations of standard protein and used to determine the unknown protein concentration of the sample (ovarian tumors homogenate) Fig (2-1)

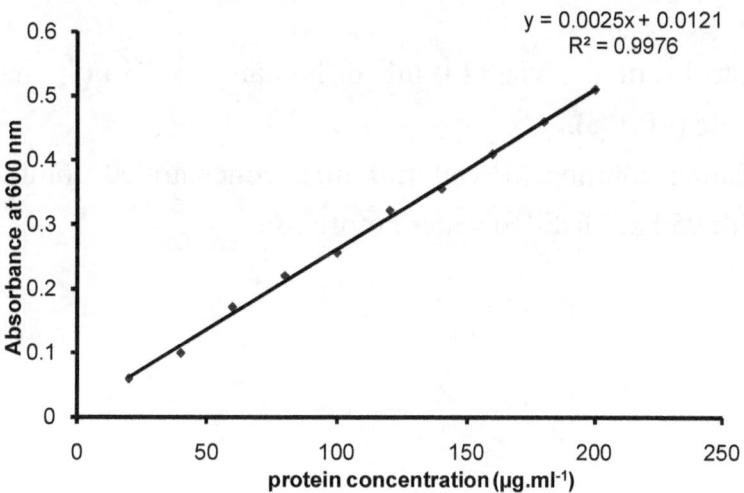

Figure (2-1) standard curve of protein determination
(All other details are explained in the text)

2.3.2 Determination of Cancer Antigen CA125 level in Sera of Patient with Benign and Malignant Ovarian Tumors

Serum CA125 levels were measured by immunoradiometric assay kit (IRMA) supplied by Immunotech (France).

IRMA – CA125 is a solid phase two-site "sandwich assay", utilizes to mouse monoclonal antibodies (OC125 and M11)directed against to different epitopes on the CA125 molecule. The M11 antibody is couted on polystyren tube (solid phase) while OC125 antibody is used as tracer after being radiolabelled with iodine 125. The CA125 antigen molecule present in the two antibodies.

Following the formation of the coated antibody/antigen/iodinated antibody sandwich, the unbound tracer is easily remove by a washing step. The radioactivity bound to the solid phase is proportional to the concentration of CA125 present in the sample.

Reagents

The following reagents were equipped with the kit:

1. Tracer: One vial (33 ml) contains less than 480 kBq of 125I- labeled anti-CA125 in liquid form with buffer, BSA, NaN3 (<0.1%).

2. Coated Tubes: Anti CA125 monoclonal antibody-coated tubes (100 plastic tubes).

3. Standard: 5 vials contain (0, 15, 50, 200 and 500 u.ml-1 of human CA125 antigen).

4. Control serum: 1 vial (1.0 ml) of human CA125 in human serum with sodium azide (<0.1%).

5. Washing solution: 1 vial (50 ml): concentrated solution should be diluted with 950 ml distilled water before use.

Procedure

The assay protocol is described in table (2-4).

Table (2-4) IRMA assay protocol of CA125 u.ml-1

	0	15	50	200	500	control	unknown 1	2 etc.
coated tubes no.	1,2	3,4	5,6	7,8	9,10	11,12	13,14	15 etc.
standard (µl)	100	100	100	100	100			
Control or sample (µl)						100	100	100
125I-anti-CA125 antibody* (µl)	300	300	300	300	300	300	300	300
	All tubes were incubated for 4 hrs at 25°C in horizontal shaker.							
	The contents of each tube were aspirated, and tubes were washed twice with 2 ml diluted washing solution except total count tubes.							
	The radioactivity bound in each tube were measured in gamma counter for 1 min.							

* 300 µl of tracer were added to 2 additional tubes to obtain total c.p.m

Note: Samples having concentrations greater than the highest standard were diluted with zero standard before assay.

Calculations

The specific binding of each concentration was measured by dividing the counts of each concentration on the total counts

$$(B/T \%) = \frac{\text{standard or sample mean count}}{\text{total activity mean count}} \times 100$$

The standard curve was generating by plotting the B/T% on vertical axis and the CA125 concentration of the standards on the horizontal axis (u.ml-1)

2.3.3 Determination of Cancer Antigen CEA level in Sera of Patient With Benign and Malignant Ovarian Tumors

Serum CEA levels were measured by immunoradiometric assay kit (IRMA) supplied by Immunotech .

Principles of the assay

IRMA – CEA is a solid phase two-site "sandwich assay ", utilizes to mouse monoclonal antibodies directed against to different epitopes on the CEA molecule. The samples or calibrators are incubated in tubes with the first monoclonal antibody in the presence of the second monoclonal antibody labeled with iodine 125.

After incubation, the content of tubes was aspirated and the tubes were rinsed so as to remove 125I- antiCA125 antibody. The bound radioactivity was then determined in gamma counter. The CEA concentration in the samples was obtained by interpolation from the standard curve and was directly proportional to the radioactivity measured.

Reagents

The following reagents were equipped with the kit:

1. Tracer: one vial (22 ml) contains less than 640 kBq of 125I- labeled anti-CEA in liquid form with buffer, BSA, NaN3 (<0.1%).

2. Coated Tubes: Anti CEA monoclonal antibody-coated tubes (100 plastic tubes).

3. Standard: 5 vials contain (0, 1, 5, 20, 100 and 400) ng.ml-1 of human CEA antigen.

4. Control serum: 2 vials contain CEA lyophilized in human serum.

5. Washing solution: 1 vial contains (50 ml): concentrated solution should be diluted with 950 ml distilled water before use.

Procedure

The assay protocol is described in table (2-5).

Table (2-5) IRMA assay protocol of CEA ng.ml-1

	CEA standard in ng.ml-1						Control		Unknown samples	
	0	1	5	20	100	400	Level 1	Level 2	1	2 etc.
coated tubes no.	1, 2	3, 4	5, 6	7, 8	9, 10	11, 12	13, 14	15, 16	17, 18	19, etc.
standard (µl)	50	50	50	50	50	50				
Control or sample (µl)							50	50	50	50
125I-anti-CA125 antibody* (µl)	200	200	200	200	200	200	200	200	200	200
	All tubes were incubated for 2 hrs. at 25°C in horizontal shaker.									
	The contents of each tube were aspirated and tubes were washed twice with 2 ml of diluted washing solution except total counts tubes.									
	The radioactivity bound in each tube were measured in gamma counter for 1 min.									

* 200 µl of 125I-antiCEA antibody were added to 2 additional tubes to obtain total count c.p.m

Calculations

The specific binding of each concentration was measured by dividing the counts of each concentration on the total counts

$$(B/T \%) = \frac{\text{standard or sample mean count}}{\text{total activity mean count}} \times 100$$

The standard curve was generating by plotting the B/T% on vertical axis and the CEA concentration of the standards on the horizontal axis (ng.ml-1)

Figure (2-3): Standard curve of CEA determination in human sera by IRMA method (All details are explained in the text).

2.3.4 Preliminary Test of CA125 Binding to 125I-anti CA125 antibody in Ovarian Tumor Homogenate

Reagents

Tris buffer of 0.05 M, pH 7.4 for binding experiments was prepared according to the following:

Tris (hydroxyl methyl amino methan) 0.6075g, 0.1816g of EDTA, 1g Bovine serum albumin (BSA) and 0.02g sodium azide (NaN3) , were dissolved in 80 ml deionized distilled water and the pH was adjusted with HCl (1M) at pH 7.4 then the solution was completed to 100 ml with deionized distilled water.

Polyethylenglycol (PEG 6000) was prepared by dissolving 2 g in 10ml of Tris buffer (pH = 7.4, 0.05 M).

Procedure

1-   Five clean and dry tubes were counted for their background using Gamma counter.

2-   Twenty five microliter (450 µg.ml-1) of 125I-anti CA125 antibody (tracer) was added to each of five tubes denoted as

→   First tube   : Non specific binding without precipitating agent.

→   Second tube: Non specific binding with precipitating agent.

→   Third tube : Binding without precipitating agent

→   Fourth tube : Binding with precipitating agent

→   Fifth tube   : Total c.p.m (T)

3-   Filtrate of homogenate, 50 µl (337 µg)   was added to third and fourth tubes.

4-   The volume of all tubes was completed to 400 µl using Tris-buffer pH 7.4, 0.05 M except the T tube.

5-   The tubes were incubated at 25°C for 4 hrs.

6-   After incubation 400 µl of 20% polyethyleneglycol 6000 (PEG 6000) was added to the second and fourth tubes and the incubation was continued for further 30 min.

7-   After incubation all tubes were centrifuged at 1500 g for 30 min. at 4°C except (T) tube.

8-   The supernatant was aspirated, except (T) tube

9-   The radioactivity in each tube was counted using gamma counter for 1 min.

10-   The pellet of the homogenate was suspended in 1:3 Tris-buffer pH 7.4, 0.05 M, and the same steps mentioned above were repeated for the suspended pellet to determine the radioactivity of the complex.

236

Calculations

1. The counts radioactivity in tubes number 2, 1 (expressed in c.p.m.) represents the non specific binding (NSB) with and without using precipitating agent respectively.

2. The counts radioactivity in tubes number 4, 3 (expressed in c.p.m.) represents the sample count with and without using precipitating agent respectively.

3. (Sample counts-non specific binding counts) represents bound fraction (B).

4. The counts radioactivity in the tubes containing 125I-anti CA125 antibody only represents the total counts (T). The (B/T) ratio counted as follows:

$$\frac{B}{T}\% = \frac{\text{Sample counts} - \text{non specific binding counts (NSB)}}{\text{Total counts (T)}} \times 100$$

2.3.5 Factors Affecting the Binding CA125 to 125I-anti CA125 antibody in ovarian tumor Homogenate.

2.3.5.1 Effect of Different Amount of protein concentration of the tumor Homogenate on the Binding of CA125 with 125I-anti CA125 antibody.

Reagents:

All reagents were prepared as described previously in section (2.3.4).

Procedure

1. Twenty five microliters (450 µg.ml-1) of 125I-anti CA125 antibody were read for their radioactivity and added to an increasing amounts of protein (37.5, 75, 150, 175, 225 and 300 µg.ml-1) of the supernatant of (post-menopausal malignant ovarian tumors "OI", pre-menopausal malignant ovarian tumors "OII", and benign ovarian tumors "OIII").

Then all volums were completed to 400 µl with Tris buffer (0.05M, pH 7.4).

2. The assay tubes were then incubated for 4 hrs at 25°C.

3. At the end of the incubation 400 µl of 20% polyethyleneglycol 6000 (PEG 6000) was added and the incubation was continued for further 0.5hr.

4. At the end of incubation, the assay tubes were centrifuged at 1500 g for 30 min at 4°C.

5. Supernatant was aspirated carefully.

6. The radioactivity of the complex was counted using gamma counter.

Calculations

1. The B/T % was calculated as described in section (2.3.4).

2. The B/T% was plotted against the increasing amount of protein of ovarian tumor homogenate

2.3.5.2 Effect of 125I-anti CA125 antibody concentration on its binding to CA125

Reagents

All reagents were prepared as described previously in section (2.3.4).

Procedure

1. Increasing concentrations of 125 I-anti CA125 antibody (90, 180, 270, 360, 450, and 900 µg.ml-1) were read for their radioactivity and then added to homogenate (OI, OII, OIII) containing (225, 150, 175 µg.ml-1) respectively. Then all tubes were completed to 400 µl with Tris-buffer (0.05M, pH 7.4).

2. Steps 2, 3, 4, 5 and 6 mentioned in the experiment (2.3.5.1) were repeated.

Calculations

1. The B/T% was determined using the same mathematical equation mentioned in section (2.3.4).

2. The percent of binding was plotted against 125I-anti CA125 antibody concentrations.

2.3.5.3 The Effect of pH on Binding of CA125 to 125I- anti CA125 antibody

Reagents

All reagents were prepared as mentioned in section (2.3.4), except PEG 6000. PEG 6000 which was prepared in a set of different pHs (6.0-8.0) by dissolving 2 g of PEG 6000 in 10 ml of Tris-buffer of different pHs (6.0-8.0).

Procedure

1. Tracer (450, 360, 450 µg.ml-1) were added to (225, 150, 175 µg.ml-1) of OI, OII and OIII homogenate respectively.

2. Each reaction mixture was completed to 400 µl with Tris-buffer at different pH (6.0-8.0).

3. Steps 2, 3, 4, 5 and 6 of the experiment 2.3.5.1 were repeated.

Calculations

1. Values of B/T % were calculated as described in section (2.3.4)

2. B/T % was plotted against their pH values.

2.3.5.4 Time course of the binding of CA125 with 125I-antiCA125 antibody in

ovarian tumor homogenate

Reagent

All reagents were prepared according to the experiment in section (2.3.4) except 20% PEG 6000 solution which was prepared according to the optimum pH of each group (i.e. OI, OII and OIII).

Procedure

1. Tracer (450, 360, 450 µg.ml-1) were added to (225, 150, 175 µg.ml-1) of OI, OII and OIII homogenate respectively.

2. Each mixture was completed to 400 µl with Tris -buffer at the optimum pH of each group

3. All tubes were incubated at 25°C at different time intervals (0.5, 1, 1.5, 2, 2.5, 3, 3.5, 4, 4.5, and 5) hrs.

4. Steps 3, 4, 5 and 6 in the experiments (2.3.5.1) were repeated.

5. To determine the time course of CA125 binding to 125I-anti CA125 antibody at different temperatures.

Steps 1, 2, 3, 4 and 5 in this experiment were repeated at different temperature (5, 37 and 45) °C.

Calculations

1. The same mathematical equation mentioned in section (2.3.4) was used to calculate (B/T) % at each time and temperature.

2. The (B/T) % values were plotted against the time of incubation at different temperatures.

2.3.5.5 Effect of Different Halides on the Binding of CA125 to 125I-anti CA125
        antibody.

Reagents

1. Tris buffer, that was prepared as described in section (2.3.4), was adjusted to corresponding pH for each group of tissue homogenate.

2. Halides solution was prepared in concentration of (0.01M) in Tris buffer at pH (7.2, 6.2 and 6.4) individually, by dissolving each of 0.021 gm of NaF, 0.0292 gm of NaCl , 0.0515 gm of NaBr, and 0.075 gm of NaI in final volume of 50 ml of Tris buffer and the pH was adjusted.

3. The ovarian tumor homogenates were prepared as described in section (2.2.7), except phosphate buffer was used instead of phosphate buffer saline at the same pH and concentration was used as homogenizer buffer.

Procedure

1. Tracer (450, 360, 450 µg.ml-1) were added to (225, 150, 175 µg.ml-1) of protein of (OI, OII and OIII) homogenate respectively.

2. Fifty micro liters of the following halides (0.01 M) (NaI, NaBr, NaCl and NaF) were added in each assay tube. (A sample without the addition of any salt was used as a control).

3. The volume of the mixture was completed to 400 µl with Tris-buffer at the optimum pH of each group.

4. The assay tubes were then incubated for 240 minute at 5°C for all studied groups.

5. Steps 3, 4, 5 and 6 mentioned in section (2.3.5.1) were repeated.

Calculations

1. The values of (B/T) % were calculated as described in section (2.3.4).

2. (B/T) % was plotted against the halide type.

2.3.5.6   Effect of Monovalent and Divalent Cation on the binding

Reagents

1. Tris buffer was prepared as described in section (2.3.4) was adjusted to corresponding pH for each group of tissue homogenate.

2. Monovalent and divalent cations salts were prepared in concentration of (0.025M) in Tris buffer at pH (7.2, 6.2 and 6.4) individually, by dissolving each of 0.0931 gm of KCl, 0.0668 gm of NH4Cl, 0.2541 gm of MgCl2.6H2O, 0.1388 gm of CaCl2.2H2O, 0.2474 gm of MnCl2 4H2O, 0.315 gm of CuSO4. 5H2O and 0.1703 gm of ZnCl2) in a final volume 50 ml of Tris and the pH was adjusted.

Procedure

1. Step (1) of effect of halide experiment was repeated.

2. Fifty micro liters of (0.25 M) of the following monovalent and divalent cations (KCl, NH4Cl, MgCl2 6H2O, CaCl2.2H2O, MnCl2.4H2O, CuSO4.5 H2O and ZnCl2) were added to each group of tissue homogenate.

3. Steps 3, 4, 5, and 6 in effect of halide experiment were repeated.

Calculations

1. The values of (B/T) % were calculated as described in section (2.3.4).

2. B/T % was plotted against each monovalent and divalent cations.

2.4. Result and Discussion

Three groups of ovarian tumors were included in this study. These groups were classified according to the type of ovarian tumors (benign and malignant) and the malignant ovarian tumors were again classified into sub groups (pre-menopausal and post-menopausal). Each type was examined histologically according to WHO classification system.

Homogenization of tissue samples was carried out in cold medium (40C) to avoid protein denaturation and to decrease the proteolytic enzymes activity. The filtration of the tissue homogenate through several layers of nylon gauze was used to remove any suspended piece of unhomogenized fragments and blood vessels, while the centrifugation of homogenate at 1500 g removed the unruptured cells and intact nuclei of ruptured cells .

2.4.1 Determination of Cancer Antigen CA125 level in Sera of Patient with Benign and Malignant Ovarian Tumors

CA125 levels in sera were measured with an Immunoradiometeric assay (IRMA) in three groups of ovarian tumors matched with one group of control subjects. Group I consisted of twenty post-menopausal patients with malignant ovarian tumors, group II consisted of fourteen pre-menopausal patients with malignant ovarian tumors and group III consisted of twenty four pre-menopausal patients with benign ovarian tumors.

The data of CA125 measurements in normal healthy individuals, benign ovarian tumors and malignant ovarian tumors will be presented separately.

Normal controls

Low levels of CA125 were observed in the sera of 30 apparently healthy women used as a control (Table 2-4) . The mean CA125 levels (±SD) in this group was (11.9 ± 6.6 u.ml-1) with an upper normal value of   35 u.ml-1 .

Table (2-6): Sera CA125 levels (u.ml-1) in patients with benign and malignant ovarian tumors compared to the control group

Group	Patients	No.	Age range	CA125 assay u.ml-1			P values
				Range	Median	mean ± SD	
OI	Post-menopausal malignant ovarian tumor	20	55-72	12-2300	288	512± 621	P<0.05
OII	Pre-menopausal malignant ovarian tumor	14	19-45	10-610	161	212± 200	P<0.05
OIII	Benign ovarian tumor	24	22-46	5-50	13	19.7± 13.93	P<0.05
Control	Healthy individuals	30	20-50	3-28	11	12.9± 6.6	

P – value ≤ 0.05 is consider significant.

A positive scoring or an abnormal level was indicated by those values of CA125 which exceeded the 35u.ml-1 limited (53). All normal controls had CA125 concentration lower than 35u.ml-1 suggesting a test specificity of 100% for the ability of this marker to exclude normal individuals.

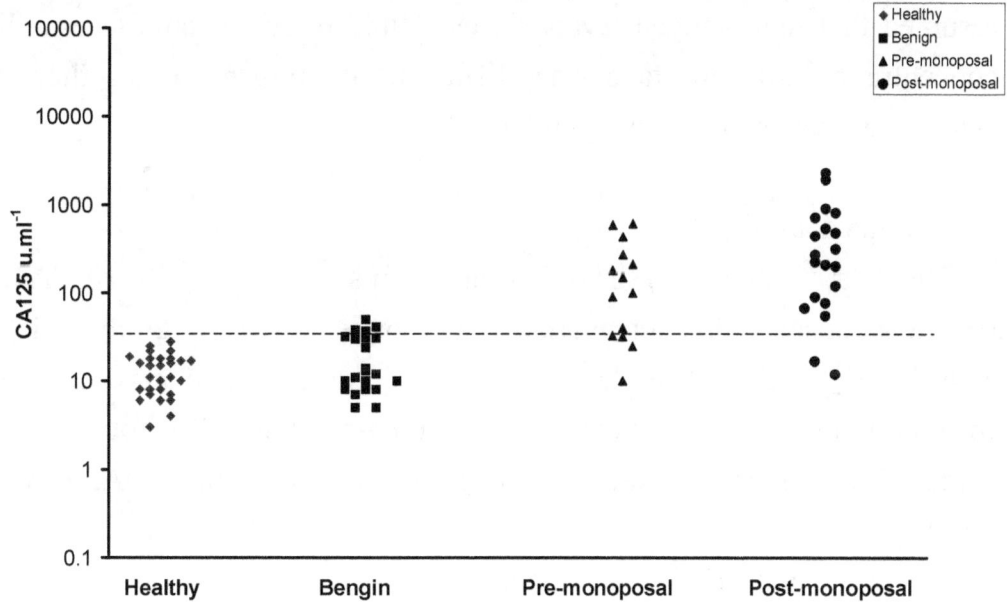

Figure (2-4): Distribution of CA125 value over different groups of patients and healthy individuals.

(All other details are explained in the text).

Benign ovarian tumor

Figure (2.4) shows that of 24 samples of patients with histological confirmed benign ovarian cases, four had level of CA125 above the cutoff value >35u.ml-1 (about 16%). The mean level of CA125 antigen (19.7±13.93) observed in these patients (Table 2-6) was significantly different from normal controls (P<0.05). Fleurn et al (137) explained why most benign cases have CA125 level below 35u.ml-1 as that in benign ovarian tumor there might be an effective barrier between the antigen-producing neoplastic cells and the serum. Such barriers may play a role in the distribution of tumor antigens over various body compartments whereas in malignant tumors infiltrative growth   lead to the release of antigen into the circulation (137).

Another explanation suggests that peritoneum serves as a barrier for high molecular weight tumor antigens, and lag in the transfer of CA125 from Cyst fluid through the cyst wall might be increased by the high molecular weight of this glycoprotein which has been estimated to exceed 200 kDa (137).

Slight elevation of CA125 serum levels in   few patients with benign ovarian tumors may be explained by the observations of Bast et al which assumed that high antigen levels in cyst fluid might be able to establish a concentration gradient favouring diffusion of antigen into the lymph vessels and veins of the ovary(117).

Ovarian Cancer

The data in table (2-6) show that the mean serum value ±SD of CA125 in pre-menopausal malignant ovarian tumor patients (212 ± 200u.ml-1), was significantly higher than that in healthy control or patients with benign ovarian tumor. These results are in agreement with that found by AL-Barazanji (138) who obtained the same results using Mini VIDAS CA125 II kit.

Result in table (2-6) also indicates that there is significant difference between mean serum value ±SD of CA125 in post- menopausal ovarian cancer patients (512 ± 621 u.ml-1) and that found in pre- menopausal ovarian cancer patients (P<0.05) that is the same finding of Malkasione et al study (139).

Data in table (2-6) indicate that determination of CA125 serum levels may be useful as a prognostic factor in the differentiation between malignant and benign ovarian cancer especially in postmenopausal patients. These results were in agreement with the observations reported by other investigators which suggested that among postmenopausal patients with pelvic mass, CA125 level greater than 65u.ml-1 indicated the presence of malignant disease with greater than 90% accuracy (134).

In table (2-7) the percentage of positive scoring of CA125 is presented in relation to menopausal status of ovarian cancer women. The post menopausal patients gave the highest percentage 90% of CA125 positive scoring, in comparison to the pre- menopausal patients with 71% sensitivity.

Table (2-7): positively of CA125 in relation to menopausal status

Menopausal state	No. of patients	No. of elevated CA125 level	% Patients with elevated CA125
Pre-menopausal	14	10	71
Post-menopausal	20	18	90

2.4.2 Determination of CEA level in sera of ovarian tumor patients

Tumor markers complementary to CA125 were mentioned as a useful method to improve the specificity of CA125 assay. A specificity of 99.6% and sensitivity of 80% were reported to be achieved using OVXI antigen as a complementary tumor marker to CA125 in the diagnosis of ovarian cancer. (126) CEA levels have been reported to be elevated in a high percentage of ovarian cancer cases (30-65%).(53) High ratio of CA125 to CEA in serum was suggested to be a useful method to differentiate ovarian from non-ovarian malignant diseases when both sera contain increased CA125 concentrations. (140)

Normal Controls

Low levels of serum CEA were observed in normal women (n=30) who had a mean value (±SD) 1.2±0.82 ng.ml-1 with the cut off value of 3.0 ng.ml-1 (Table 2-8), and a percentage specificity of 90%. These values are close to those obtained by other investigators. (141, 142)

Ta ble (2-8): Sera CEA Levels (ng.ml-1) in Patients with Benign and Malignant Ovarian Tumors Compared to the Control Group.

Gro up	Patients	No.	Age range	CEA assay ng.ml-1			P values
				Range	Median	mean ± SD	
OI	Post-menopausal malignant ovarian tumor	20	55 -72	0.9-15	2.8	4.1± 3.66	P<0.05
OII	Pre-menopausal malignant ovarian tumor	14	19 -45	0.8-10	2.85	3.39± 2.35	P<0.05
OIII	Benign ovarian tumor	24	22 -46	0.5-5.5	1.45	1.6 ± 1.37	P>0.05
Control	Healthy individuals	30	20 -50	0.3-3.6	0.9	1.2± 0.82	

P – value ≤ 0.05 is consider significant.

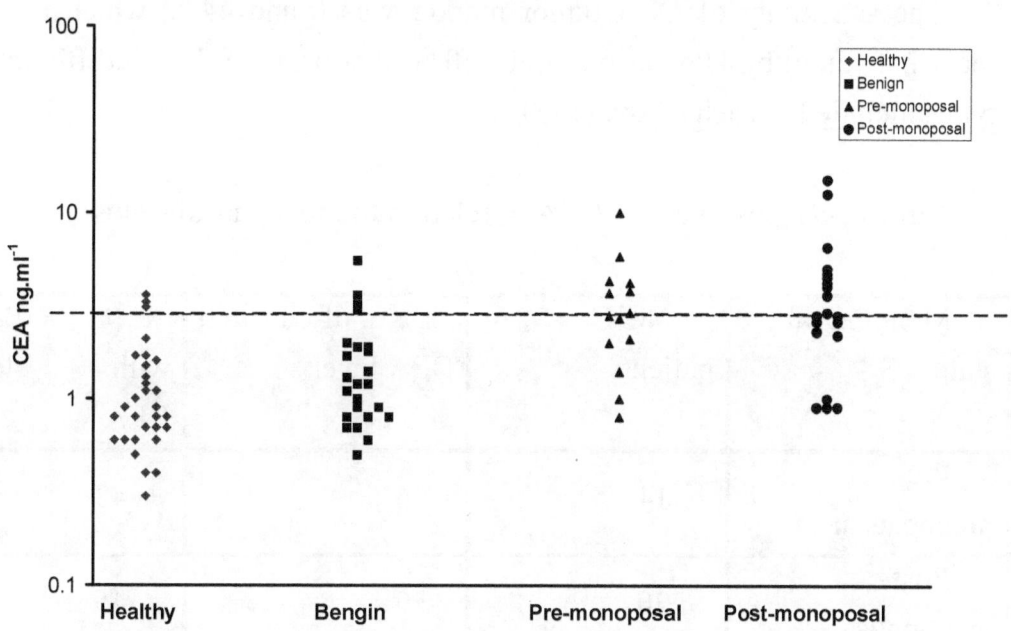

Figure (2-5): Distribution of CEA value over different groups of patients and healthy individuals.

(All other details are explained in the text).

Benign Ovarian Tumor

Of 24 samples from patients with histologically confirmed benign ovarian cases(Fig 2-5), four of them had CEA >3.0 ng.ml-1. The other 20 patients gave CEA value <3.0 ng.ml-1, which is not significantly different from normal controls (P>0.05).

Ovarian Cancer

The data in table (2-8) show that the mean serum value (±SD) of CEA in pre-menopausal patients with ovarian cancer is (3.39±2.35 ng.ml-1) which is significantly higher (P<0.05) than their correspondent values in sera of healthy and that in patient with benign tumors, while there were insignificant differences (P>0.05) between CEA values in patients with benign tumor in comparison to their values in healthy control.

Table (2.9) shows that the rate of positive scoring was found not remarkably affected by menopausal states. It was 45% in post-menopausal states in comparison to 43% in pre-menopausal states.

The sensitivity of CEA tumor marker was found 44%, which is lower than that found by Donaldson et al. (60%) that may be due to different cell types included in each study. (143)

Table (2-9): positively of CEA in relation to menopausal status

Menopausal state	No. of patients	No. of elevated CEA level	% Patients with elevated CEA
Pre-menopausal	14	6	43
Post-menopausal	20	9	45

2.4.3 Determination of the ratio of CA125 level to CEA level in Sera of ovarian cancer patients

Of 34 samples from patients with histologically confirmed malignant ovarian cases, 29 samples contain increased CA125 concentration (85%). High ratio of CA125 level to CEA level in sera of patients with increased CA125 concentration were found 87, in comparison to 0.94 for non-ovarian malignances (colorectal, breast, lung, and pancreatic carcinomas), reported by James et al. (140)

This observation confirms the results found by James et al. which suggest that high ratio could be used to differentiate ovarian from non ovarian malignant diseases when both sera contain increased CA125 concentration, and that will really improve the specificity of the CA125 test for ovarian cancer.

2.4.4 Preliminary test of the binding of CA125 to 125I-anti CA125 antibody in Ovarian tumor homogenate.

This part of the work was carried out to check the assay method in order to be able to find out the optimum conditions for CA125 binding to its specific antibody in our studied women. Supernatant and pellet formed at speed 1500 g in the three groups of human ovarian tumor homogenate (benign ovarian tumor, pre and post-menopausal malignant ovarian tumors) were used in this experiment. Table (2-10) shows the results of the preliminary test for the binding.

Ta   Table (2-10):   Incidence of CA125 in Supernatant and Pellet fractions in the three fferent Ovarian homogenate

Group	B/T %							
	supernatant				Pellet			
	N	(NS B⁻)	B⁻	B	N	(NS B⁻)	B⁻	B
Post-menopausal (OI)	1.2	1.21	2.1	12.2	1.25	1.19	1.9	4
Pre-menopausal (OII)	1.07	1.1	1.1	5.3	1.1	1.1	1.13	1.6
Benign(OIII)	1.17	1.2	1.7	3	1.7	1.18	1.15	1.1

NSB⁻   : nonspecific binding in absence of precipitating agent.

(NSB) + : non specific binding in presence of precipitating agent.

B⁻   : binding in absence of precipitating agent.

B+   : binding in presence of precipitating agent.

The results reveal that the supernatant fraction contains higher CA125 content than the pellet fraction according to the (B/T%) values, therefore the pellet fraction was discarded. Complex (125I-antiCA125 antibody/CA125) formed did not precipitate in the absence of the precipitating agent . So it is necessary to use (20% PEG 6000) in the reaction mixture to precipitate this complex .

2.4.5 Factors Affect of 125I-anti CA125 antibody binding to CA125
      in ovarian tumor homogenates

2.4.5.1 The Effect of different amounts of protein concentration of the tumor homogenate on the binding with 125I- anti CA125 antibody.

To obtain the optimum concentration of homogenates for the binding of CA125 with 125I-anti CA125 antibody, the supernatant of the homogenate containing increasing amounts of CA125 were incubated with a fixed amount of 125I-anti CA125 antibody, according to the details in section (2.3.5.1).

Figure (2-6) represents the quantities precipitation curve in which the amount of (125I-antiCA125 antibody/CA125) complex in three groups (benign ovarian tumors, pre-and post-menopausal ovarian tumors) was plotted as a function of CA125 concentration.

The results revealed that the binding of CA125 to 125I-antiCA125 antibody increases with increasing CA125 homogenate until a point of maximum binding was reached, thus the increase in protein concentration which would increase the number of binding sites until the saturation state. After this point as the amount of CA125 increased the amount of complex formed diminished that means the reaction behaves according to Hook effect which has ascending and descending phases at low and high antigen concentration (144). The decrease in binding after reaching the maximum binding may be due to the conformational changes in CA125 and 125I-antiCA125 antibody (145).

According to the results obtained in this experiment the amount of (225, 150, 175 µg.ml-1) of tissue homogenate in groups OI, OII and OIII respectively were used in all subsequent experiments.

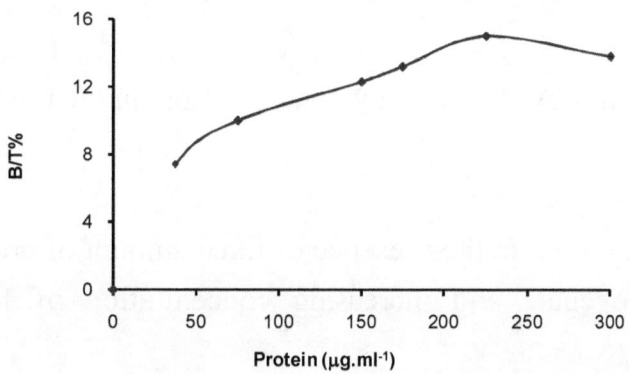

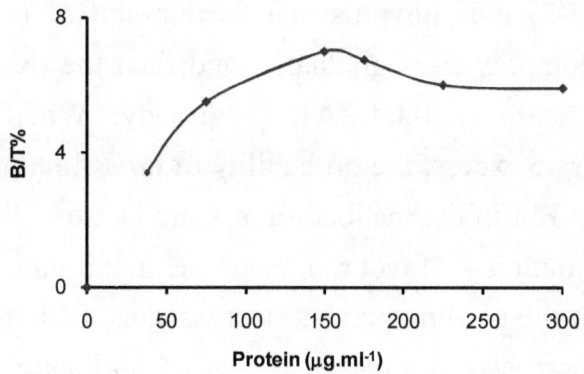

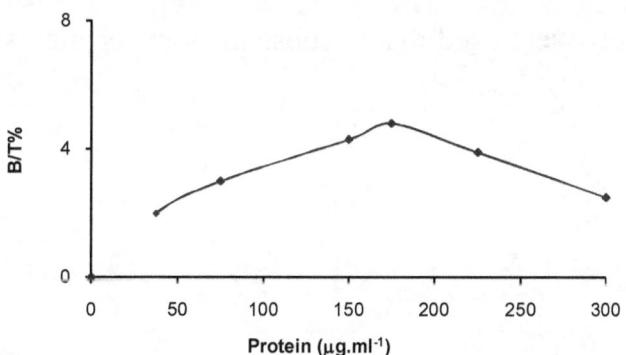

Figure (2-6): The effect of protein concentration on the binding of CA125 to its 125I-antiCA125 antibody in ovarian tumors homogenates OI, OII and OIII (All other details are explained in the text).

251

2.4.5.2 Effect 0f 125I-antiCA125 antibody concentration on the binding to CA125.

The experiment was carried out in the presence of fixed amount of protein concentration of the homogenate and increasing concentration of 125I-antiCA125 antibody.

The results are illustrated in figure (2-7) which represents 125I-antiCA125 antibody binding with supernatant fraction of the three studied groups. As shown in figure (2-7) it is obvious that the amount of (125I-antiCA125 antibody/CA125) complex rises gradually, and then the ovarian tumor protein was saturated with 125I-antiCA125 antibody. When the amount of antibody is in moderate excess, the probability of cross-linking of 125I-antiCA125 antibody to CA125 in the incubation mixture is more likely, and hence large complex formation is favoured then the maximum B/T percent was detected. After that the binding percent decreased as the amount of 125I-antiCA125 antibody increased, the reason is that all antigenic sites covered with antibody and complex formation is inhibited (146).

According to the results obtained in this experiment the amount of (450, 360, 450, µg.ml-1) of 125I-antiCA125 antibody in the three studied groups (OI, OII and OIII) respectively were used in all   subsequent experiments.

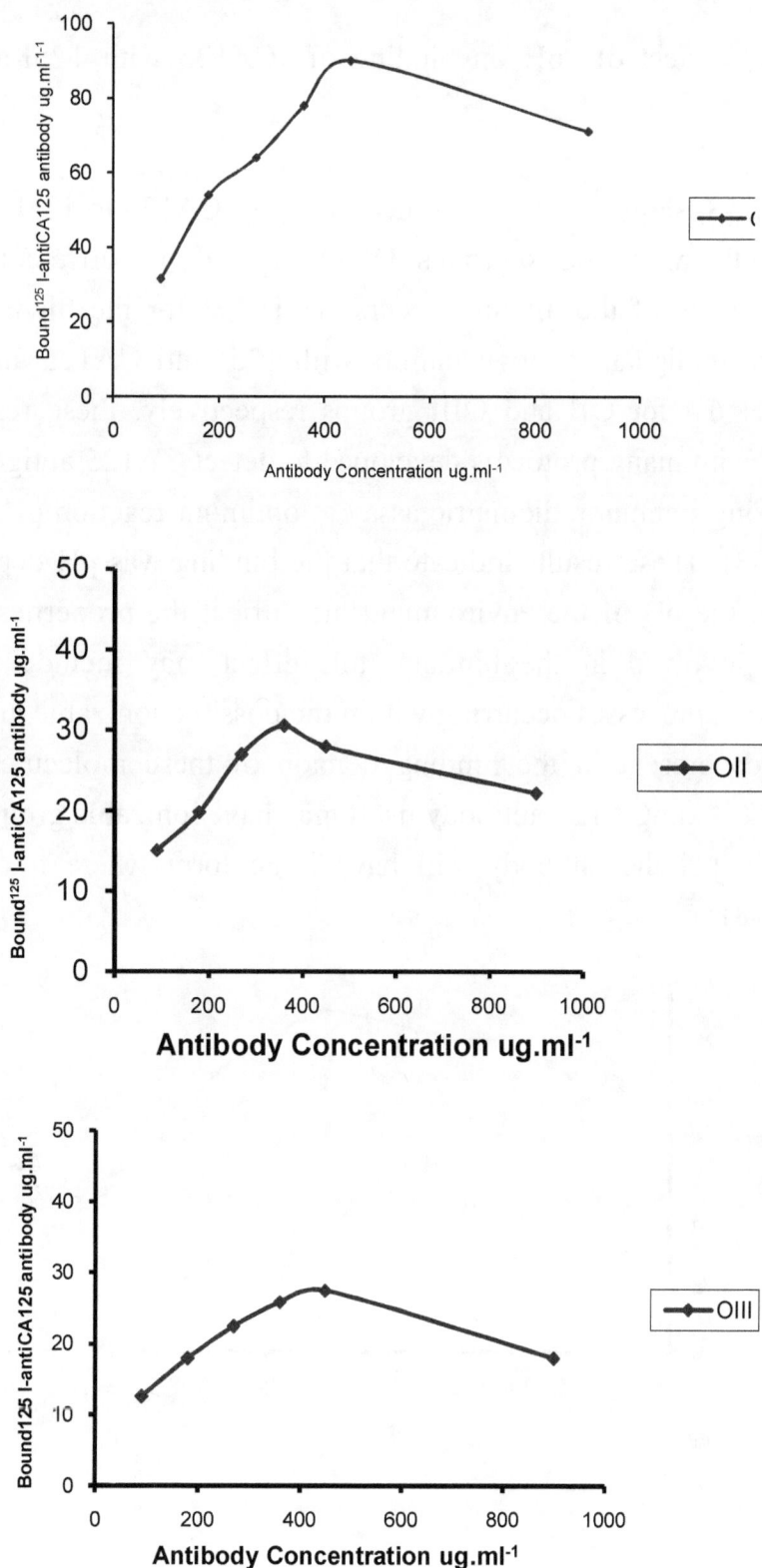

Figure (2-7): The effect of 125I-antiCA125 antibody concentration on the binding with CA125 Antigen in ovarian tumors homogenates OI, OII and OIII (All other details are explained in the text).

2.4.5.3   Effect of pH on binding of CA125 with 125I-anti CA125 antibody

Figure (2-8) shows the value of the binding of CA125 to 125I-anti CA125 antibody in the three studied groups (OI, OII and OIII) at different pH values. Maximum value of the binding occurs at pH 7.2 for the binding of post-menopausal malignant ovarian tumors with 125I-anti CA125 antibody and pH 6.2, pH 6.4 for OII and OIII groups respectively, these results are in agreement with many protocols developed to detect CA125 antigen in serum samples using immunoradiometric assay at optimum reaction pH around 6.0 (53, 97, 133). These results indicate that the binding was pH dependent and the shift in the pH of the environment may affect the properties of CA125 molecules involved in the binding, this effect may include protonation deprotonation processes occurring within the possible ionizable groups of the amino acids present in the binding domain of these molecules (147). In addition, 125I-antiCA125 antibody itself may have ionizable groups and only at a certain pH the antibody will have ionic form where it can bind to CA125.(148)

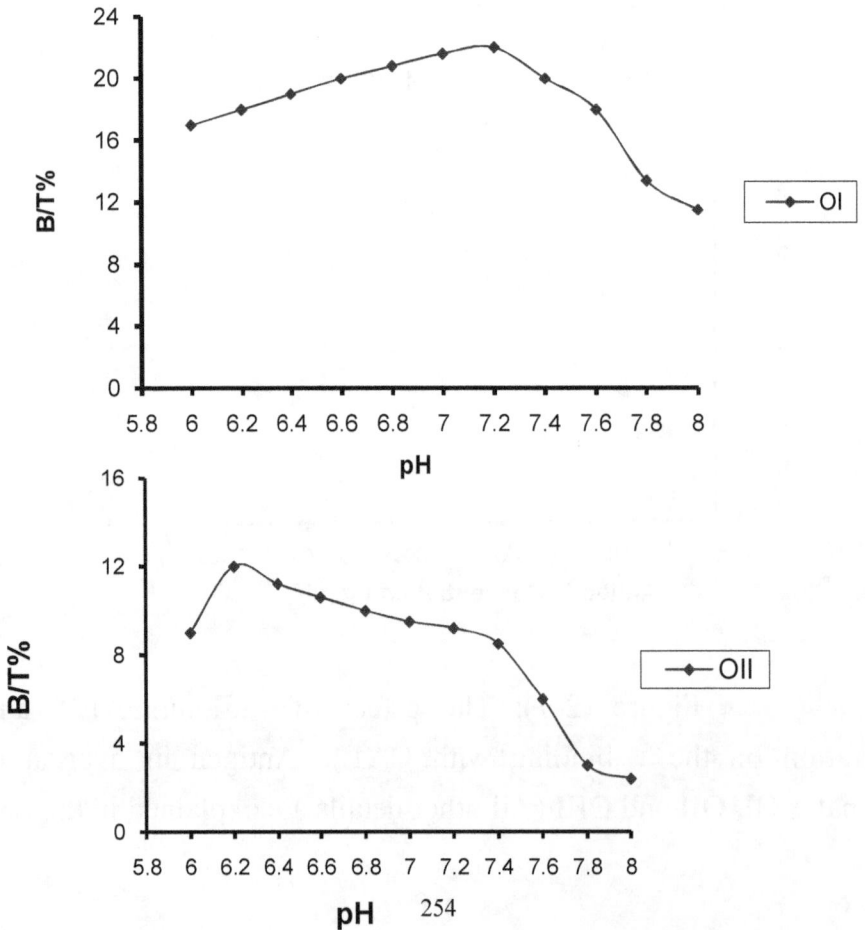

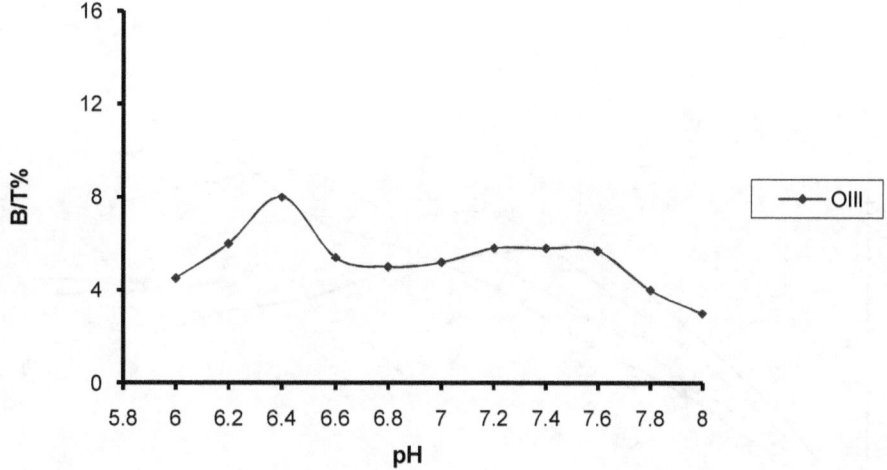

Figure (2-8): The effect of pH on the binding with CA125 to its 125I-anti CA125 antibody in ovarian tumors homogenates OI, OII and OIII (All other details are explained in the text).

2.4.5.4 Time course of the binding of CA125 to 125I-antiCA125 antibody in

ovarian tumor homogenate

Figure (2-9) shows the time course of binding of CA125 to 125I-antiCA125 antibody at different temperatures (5, 20, 37 and 45°C). The maximum binding occurred at 5°C after incubation for 4 hrs in crude fractions of post and pre menopausal malignant ovarian tumor and at 5°C after incubation for 4.5 hrs for benign ovarian tumor homogenate, in these states it seems that the energy is enough to overcome the energy barrier and give maximum binding(149).

The results indicate that 125I-antiCA125 antibody binding to crude fraction of CA125 is temperature and time dependent process.

The decrease in the binding as temperature increase may be due to either degradation of CA125 or irreversible dissociation of the (125I-antiCA125 antibody/CA125) complex at higher temperature, denaturation and destruction tertiary structure may occur leading to conformational changes and loss of activity.

255

The results obtained in these experiments were used in all subsequent experiments.

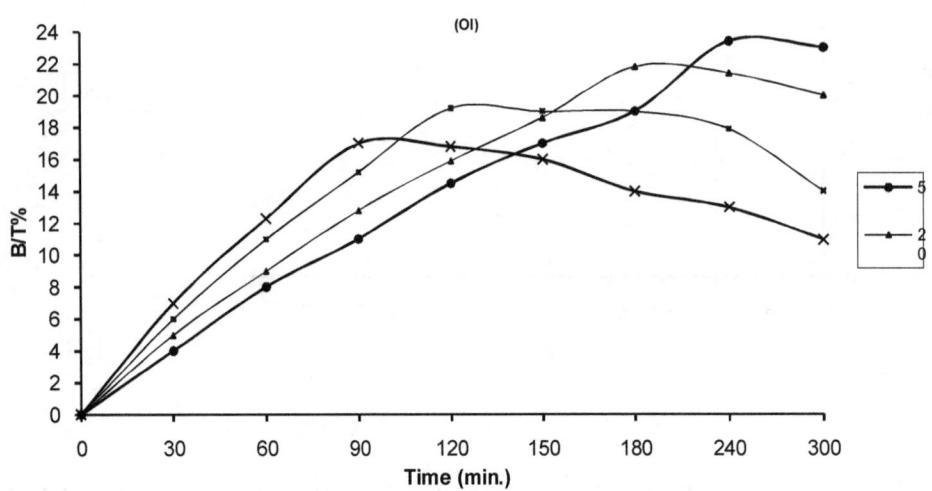

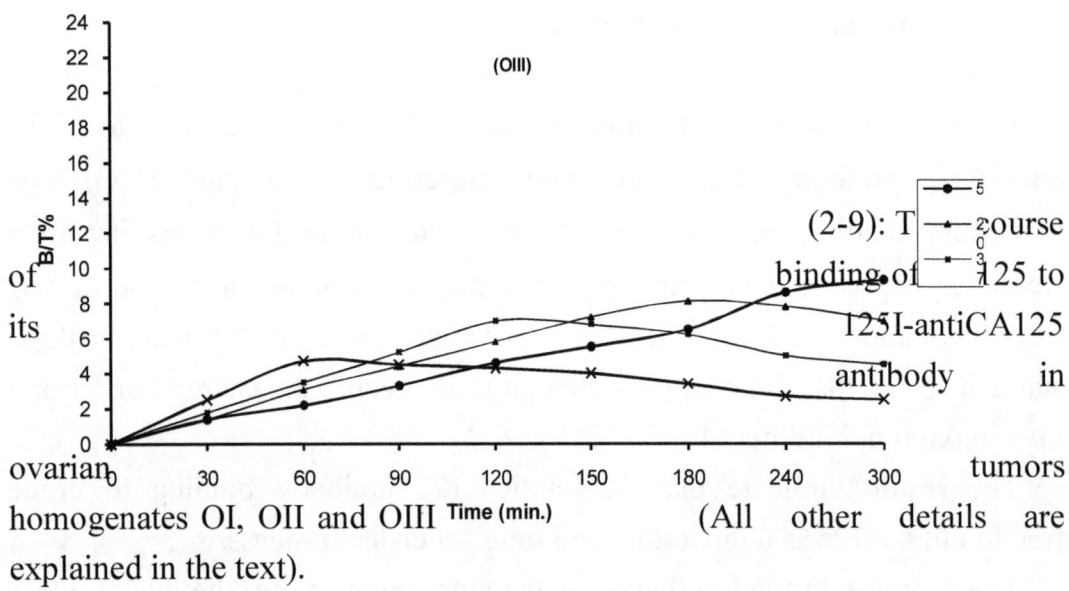

Figure (2-9): The time course of binding of I125 to its 125I-antiCA125 antibody in ovarian tumors homogenates OI, OII and OIII (All other details are explained in the text).

2.4.5.5 The Effect of Different Halides on the Binding

Figure (2-10) shows the effect of different sodium halides (i.e NaF, NaCl, NaBr, and NaI) at 0.01 M concentration on the binding of 125I-antiCA125 antibody with CA125 in benign ovarian tumors and pre and post-menopausal malignant ovarian tumors.

It seemed that the sodium halides promoted the binding according to the following order:

NaI < NaBr < NaCl < NaF

The order corresponds to the decreasing ionic radius and increasing radius of hydration presumably, the lesser degree of hydration permits greater interaction of the salt with an ionic group located in the antigen or antibody. (11)

Melander and Horvath (150) reported that the capacity of the halides salt was due to the influence of hydrophobic interaction and dependence on the molal surface tension increment (MSTI), the halides with higher MSTI strengthens the hydrophobic interaction, while halide with lower MTSI values reverses this effect.

The magnitude of surface-tension increment depends on the interaction of salt ions with the surrounding water. High – lytropic series salts (kosmotropes) interact with water strongly; water molecules surrounding the salt ions are more structured relative to bulk water. Low-lyotropic series salts (chaotropes) break the structure of the surrounding water molecules (relative to the bulk water) as a result of the large size of the ion and its weak interaction with water. (151)

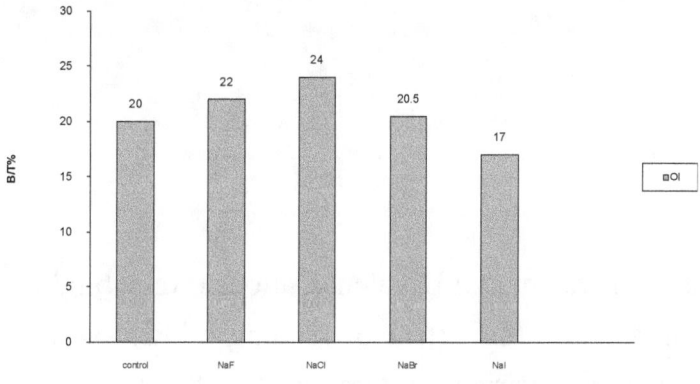

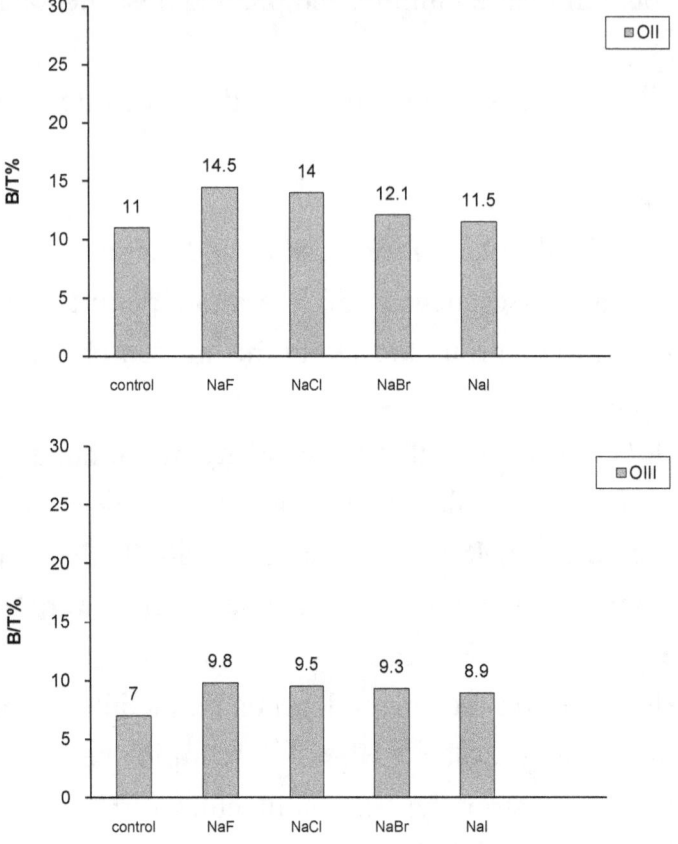

(2-1   0): The effect of different halides on the binding of CA125 to its 125I-antiCA125 antibody in ovarian tumors homogenates OI, OII and OIII (All other details are explained in the text).

2.4.5.6 The Effect of Monovalent and Divalent Cations on the binding.

The effect of different salts on the extent of binding of 125I-antiCA125 antibody to CA125 in benign ovarian tumors, post and pre-menopausal malignant ovarian tumors are shown in figures (2-11) and (2-12).

The result indicates that the presence of divalent cations (i.e. MgCl2.6H2O, CaCl2, MnCl2.4H2O, CuSO4.5H2O and ZnCl2) at 25mM concentration increases the binding in different ratios in comparison to the control as shown in figure (2-11). Cu(II) increases the binding more than other divalent cations for the three tissues homogenates the reason may be due to electrostatic interactions.

In general, the mechanism by which these salts effect protein-protein interactions is not completely clear, one hypothesis assumes that salt may alter the nature of the hydrophobic forces controlling the stabilization of protein-protein complex formed and these vary depending on the nature of the interacting groups (152). Results illustrated in figure (2-11) suggested that these salts may provide some conformational changes in the CA125 and charge groups of the binding domain of the antibody and antigen molecules.(153)

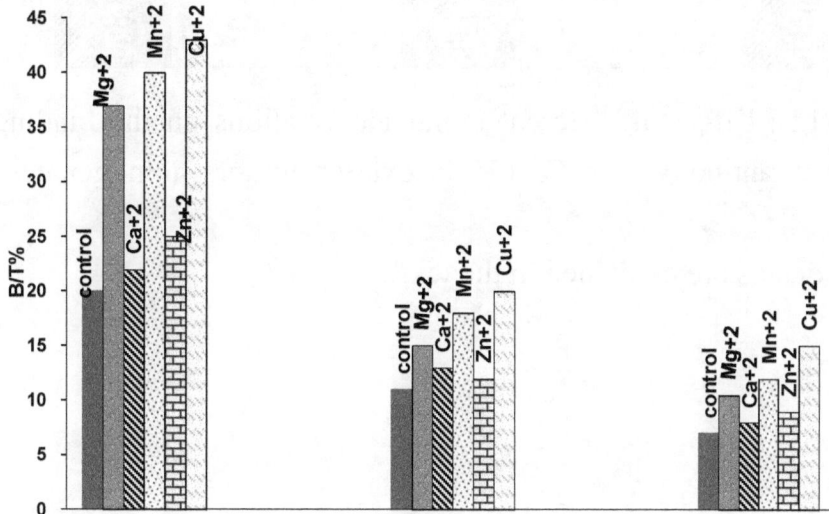

Figure (2-11): Effect of different divalent cations on the binding of 125I-anti CA125 antibody with CA125 in ovarian tumors homogenates OI.OII and OIII (All other details are explained in the text).

Figure (2-12) illustrated the effect of monovalent cations (KCl and NH4Cl) on the binding of 125I-antiCA125 antibody to its antigen. KCl at 25 mM concentration was shown to increase the binding of the three tissues homogenates. While NH4Cl at the same concentration seemed to increase the binding of post and pre-menopausal malignant ovarian tumor homogenates and slightly inhibited the binding 0f benign ovarian tumor which may be due to the presupposition that the lesser degree of hydration permits greater interaction of the salt with an ionic group located in the antibody combining site and then inhibits the complex formation. (11)

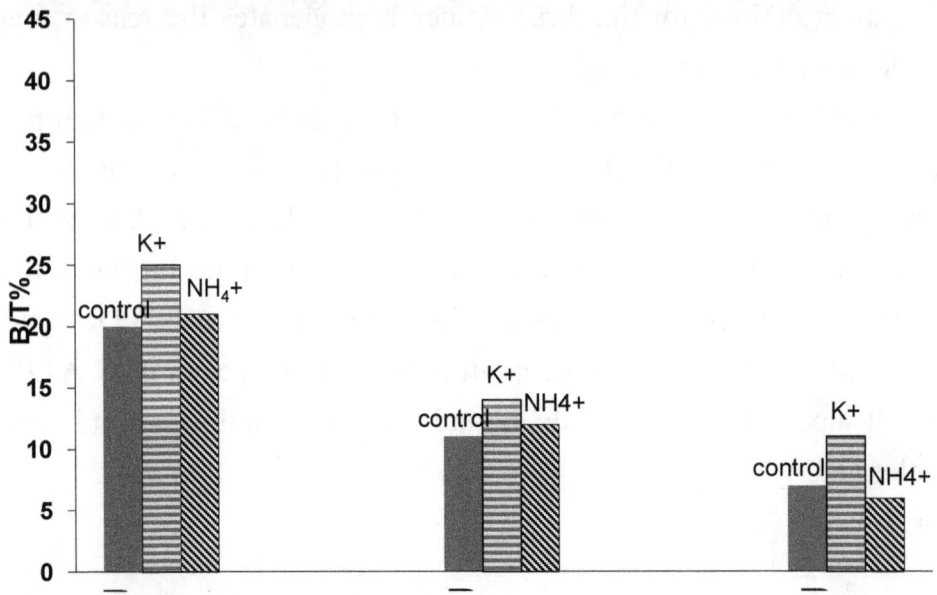

Figure (2-12): Effect of different monovalent cations on the binding of 125I-antiCA125 antibody with CA125 in ovarian tumors homogenates OI, OII and OIII.

(All other details are explained in the text).

Chapter Three

Chromatographic purification of CA125 by Gel Filtration and Binding Characterization to Its Specific Antibody.

Abstract

Cancer antigen CA125 was partially purified from homogenate of malignant ovarian tumor by Gel filtration chromatography technique.

The results revealed   presence of two forms of CA125 antigen (BI) and (BII) with molecular weight 670 and 100 KD respectively. (BI)   form possesses a high affinity for the binding to its antibody 125I-antiCA125 in comparison to (BII) form.

The elution volume (Ve) and the Kav values for elution of CA125 from Sepharose CL-6B column were calculated. The experiments of optimum conditions of binding between the two forms of CA125 antigen and 125I-anti CA125 antibody were determined.

3.1 Introduction

CA125 antigen has been characterized as a high molecular weight glycoprotein aggregate with notable size heterogeneity ranged from 200 - 1000 kDa.

Many authors tried to isolate and purify CA125 from different sources like sera of ovarian carcinoma patients (94), ovarian cancer cell line (OVCA433) (97) and human milk, using size exclusion chromatography, affinity chromatography, gel electrophoresis and buoyant density ultracentrifugation techniques (97). Another study found that CA125 antigen isolated from amoniotic fluid using gel filtration and anion exchange chromatography was composed of two subunits of approximately 240 and 180 kDa as detected by iodine 125-lablled OC125 monoclonal antibody. (154)

In this present study, post-menopausal malignant ovarian tumor tissue was used as a source for partial purification of CA125. The factors affecting the binding of partial purified CA125 to 125I-antiCA125 antibody was also studied.

Materials and methods

3.2 Materials

3.2.1 Chemicals

All chemicals and reagents mentioned in section (2.2.1) were used in the experiments of this chapter.

3.2.2 Instruments

All instruments mentioned in section (2.2.2) were also used in the experiments of this chapter.

3.2.3 Patients

The tissues homogenates of post-menopausal patients with ovarian cancer (OI) were used in the following experiments.

3.3 Methods

3.3.1 Partial Purification of CA125 by Sepharose CL-6B Column.

3.3.1.1 Preparation of the Column

The dimensions of the column were chosen according to the following equation. (155)

$$\text{Diameter} = 3\sqrt{\frac{m}{10}}$$

Where m = amount of protein in mg.

L = 30 x diameter

L = length of the column.

3.3.1.2 Preparation of the Buffer

Tris-HCl buffer of 0.05M, pH=7.2 containing 0.02% Sodium azide was prepared as mentioned previously in section (2.3.4).

3.3.1.3 Preparation of the Gel

Sepharose CL-6B gel was prepared by allowing the pre-swollen gel to swell again in Tris-buffer (0.05M pH 7.2) then left to settle and the excess of buffer was decanted. The step was repeated several times. The gel was degassed using evacuation pump and slurry was left for 24 hrs to equilibrate with buffer.(97)

The swollen gel was suspended and carefully poured into a vertical glass column (1.0x27cm) down the wall using a glass rod. After the gel has settled, the column was equilibrated with Tris-buffer for 24 hrs.

3.3.1.4 Void Volume Determination

The void volume of the column was determined by using blue dextran 2000 at a concentration of 2mg.ml-1 dissolved in Tris-buffer pH 7.2, and then the elution was carried out with the same buffer at a flow rate of 12 ml /1 hr at 10°C.

Fractions of 1 ml were collected and their absorbance was measured at 600 nm. Figure (3.1) shows the elution profile of blue dextran 2000. The volume of the buffer required to elute the blue dextran, which represents the void volume, was (10ml).

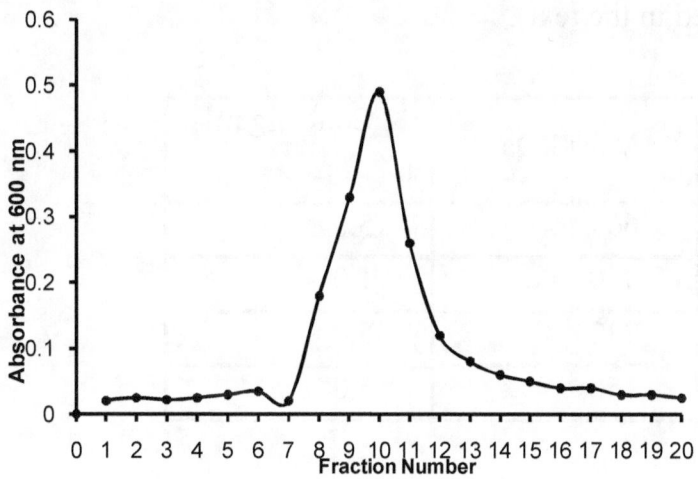

Figure (3-1): The elution profile of blue dextran 2000 using sepharose CL-6B gel, 12 ml/hr flow rate, Tris-buffer pH 7.2 and 10°C. (All other details are explained in the text).

3.3.1.5 Determination of the Molecular Weight by Gel Filtration Chromatography:

Pharmacia calibration kit for determination of M.wt by gel filtration was used. The kit comprises highly purified proteins individually packed. Each protein was reconstituted in 1.0 ml. Tris buffer pH 7.2. The standard proteins and their M.wt are detailed in table (3.1).

Table (3-1): Standard proteins and their molecular weights (All other details are explained in the text).

Protein	M.wt kDa	Conc.mg.ml-1
Thyroglobulin	669	5.0
Ferritin	440	1.0
Catalase	232	5.0
Aldolase	158	5.0

Procedure

The same sepharose CL-6B column used in this section (3.3.1) was calibrated for molecular weight determination. Standard protein solutions were prepared according to the manufacturer instruction, then applied through two portions (0.5ml/portion), thyroglobulin and catalase in the first, Ferritin and Aldolase in the second. Elution was carried out with Tris buffer pH 7.2 at a flow rate 12 ml/hr at 10°C. The absorbencies of the fractions collected were measured at 280 nm to evaluate the elution volume (Ve) of the standard proteins.

Calculations

The Kav of the proteins eluted were determined using the following equation (156)

$$Kav = \frac{Ve - V_O}{Vt - V_O}$$

Where:

V0 = void volume

Ve = Elution volume

Vt = Total gel bed volume, which was calculated according o the following:

$$Vt = \left(\frac{d}{2}\right)^2 \times 3.14 \times h \qquad (d=1.0 \text{ cm}, h= 27 \text{ cm})$$

The calibration curve of Kav against log M.wt of the proteins was plotted.

3.3.1.6 Separation of CA125 from Malignant postmenopausal Ovarian Tumor

Homogenate

Tris-buffer (0.05M, pH7.2) containing 0.02% Sodium azide was prepared as described previously in section (2.3.4.).

Procedure

The sample of tissue homogenate (500µl) containing approximately 7.8mg protein was applied to the surface of the gel, equilibrated with Tris-buffer 0.05M, pH 7.2 the sample was eluted using the same buffer with flow rate of 12ml/hr and fractions volume of 1ml each were collected. Gel filtration was carried out at 10°C and the absorbance of each fraction was measured at 280 nm.

The fractions that contained CA125 antigen was identified by the assay method as follows:

1-   Twenty five micro liters (450 µg.ml-1) of 125I-antiCA125 antibody was added to 100µl of each fraction number of post-menopausal malignant ovarian tumor homogenate. Then all tubes were completed to 400µl with Tris-buffer (0.05M, pH 7.2).

2-   Steps 2, 3, 4, 5, and 6 mentioned in experiment (2.3.5.1) were repeated.

Calculations

1- The absorbance of each fraction was determined at 280 nm.

2- The value of B/T ratio for the eluted fractions was calculated as mentioned in section 2.3.4.

3- The values of B/T ratio and the absorbencies at 280nm were plotted against the fraction number.

3.3.1.7 Dialysis for Concentration

After preparing dialysis tube, the fractions that contained high level of the binding activity were pooled and concentrated by dialyzing against sucrose at 4°C for 3hrs to get the required concentration to be used in the next experiments.

3.4 Determination of the optimum Reaction Conditions for the Binding of the partially purified CA125 antigen to 125I-antiCA125 antibody.

The optimum reaction conditions for the binding of partially purified CA125 to its 125I-antiCA125 antibody were studied using the same experiments mentioned for the factors affecting the binding in chapter 2.

3.5 Results and Discussion

3.5.1. Partial Purification of CA125

Partial purification of CA125 was performed by gel exclusion chromatography technique. Post-menopausal malignant ovarian tumor homogenate (OI) was applied to sepharose CL-6B (1.0x27cm) column. The void volume (Vo) of this column was (10ml) as predicted from the elution profile of the blue dextran figure (3-1).

Figure (3-2) shows the elution profile for (OI) homogenate after measuring the absorbance of collected fractions at 280 nm. It gave three main peaks separated according to their molecular weight, their fractions number were 10, 19 and 28.

The binding reaction that was carried out for the collected fractions gave two peaks (BI&BII) at fraction number 11 and the fraction number 21 for BI & BII respectively, as shown in figure (3-2). The resultant fractions containing the binding activity of CA125 were collected, pooled and concentrated then subjected to protein determination as described in section (2.3.1).

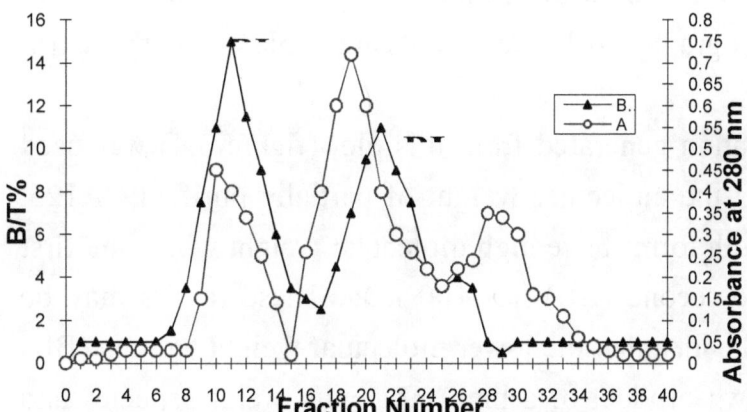

Figure (3-2): The elution profile of human CA125 from post-menopausal malignant ovarian tumor using sepharose CL-6B gel, 12ml/hr flow rate, Tris-buffer pH 7.2, at 10°C.(All other details are explained in the text).

Different standard proteins of known molecular weights were used to determine the molecular weight of the isolated antigens. The elution volumes (Ve) of standard proteins are shown in figure (3-3). The Kav values for these standard proteins were calculated by using the formula represented in section (3.3.1.4) and the calibration curve was plotted between Kav values of the standard proteins versus their logarithmic molecular weight as shown in figure (3-4).

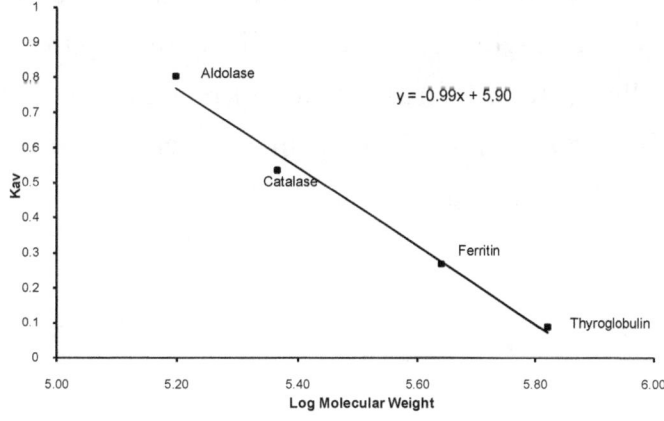

Figure (3-4) Calibration curve for determination of M.wt by gel filtration chromatography (All other details are explained in the text).

The straight line equation generated from this plot (figure 3.4) was used for the determination of the molecular weight of partially purified CA125. The results shows that both forms have high molecular weight where the first BI has 670 kDa and the second (BII) has 100 kDa. These results may be explained according to the idea that the lower molecular weight antigen (BII) is considered a breakdown product of a high molecular weight species and therefore contains the same antigenic determinants (154,157). On the other hand high molecular antigen (BI) may be explained according to that CA125 has high molecular mass aggregate. The size exclusion of native CA125 from body fluids gave at least two broad peaks reactivity of 200 and > 1000kDa molecular weight. (99)

3.5.2 Determination of the Optimum Reaction Conditions for the Binding of Partially Purified CA125 to125I- antiCA125 antibody

3.5.2.1. Optimum protein concentration

Figure (3-5) shows the effect of increasing amount of partially purified CA125 (BI & BII) to fixed amount of 125I-anti CA125-antibody to produce (125I-antiCA125 antibody/ CA125) complex. The shape of the curve is similar to that obtained for the crude CA125, the figure shows that the amount of partially purified CA125 needed to reach maximum binding with 125I-antiCA125-antibody as 90, 110 µg.ml-1 which is less than the amount needed for crude extract (225 µg.ml-1).

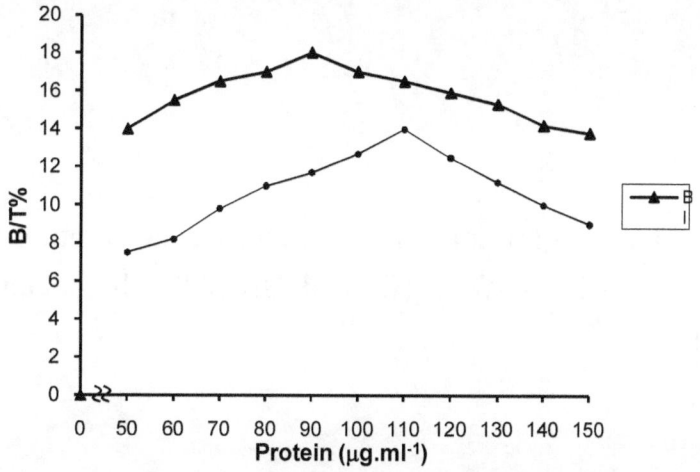

Figure (3-5): The effect of protein concentration on the binding of 125I-anti CA125 antibody with partially purified CA125 (BI and BII) (All other details are explained in the text).

3.5.2.2. Optimum 125I- anti CA125-antibody Concentration.

Figure (3-6) illustrates the effect of increasing 125I-antiCA125 antibody concentration on the binding with partially purified forms of CA125 (BI & BII). The maximum binding obtained when 360 µg.ml-1 for (BI) and 450 µg.ml-1 for (BII) were used. From these result it was found that partially purified CA125 (BI) form was saturated with small concentration of 125I-antiCA125 antibody than those required for BII. Thus it was concluded that BI has higher affinities at low concentrations toward 125I-antiCA125 antibody than BII.

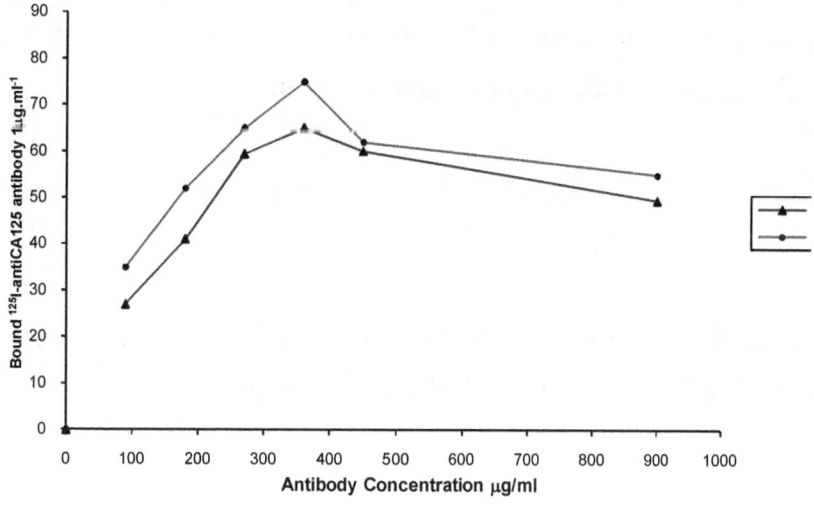

Figure (3-6): The effect of 125I-antiCA125 antibody concentration on the binding with partially purified CA125 (BI and BII)(All other details are explained in the text).

3.5.2.3. Optimum pH

Figure (3-7) shows the effect of pH on binding of 125I-antiCA125 antibody to partially purified CA125 (BI&BII) of post-menopausal malignant ovarian tumor homogenate. The results revealed that the optimum pH for (BI) and (BII) was 6.8 and 7.2 respectively. These results indicate that the binding was pH dependent and the differences in the optimum pHs may suggest the differences in the binding sites of these partially purified antigens (158).

Figure (3-7): The effect of pH on the binding of 125I-antiCA125 antibody with partially purified CA125 (BI and BII)

(All other details are explained in the text).

3.5.2.4 The time course of the binding of partially purified CA125 (BI &BII)

to 125I- antiCA125 antibody.

The optimum time and temperature for partially purified CA125 (BI and BII) was studied. Figures (3-8) and (3-9) show that the (BI) form antigen binds to its specific antibody in highest state after 180 min at 5°C, while BII form reach the maximum binding after 210 min at 5°C .

Figure (3-8): Time course of binding of 125I-antiCA125 antibody with partially purified CA125 (BI) (All details are explained in the text).

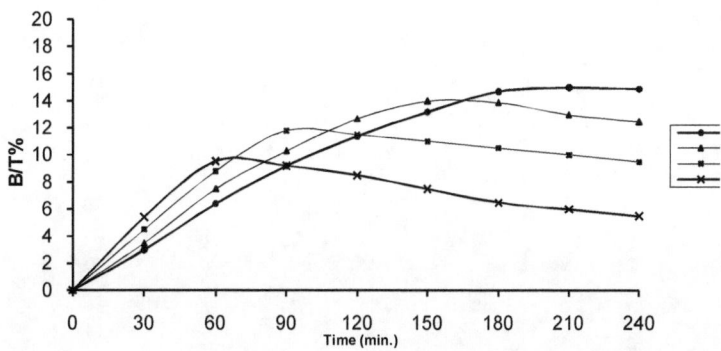

Figure(3-9): Time course of binding of 125I-antiCA125 antibody with partially purified CA125 (BII)(All details are explained in the text).

In comparison with crude homogenate, the time was shortened for both BI & BII from 240 minutes for the crude homogenate to 180 and 210 minutes for BI & BII respectively. A possible explanation for the fast kinetics of complex formation with partial purified antigen may be due to losing of inhibitory factors, by exclusive gel filtration process. This in turn affects the rate of complex formation between CA125 and its specific antibody

Chapter Four
Kinetic & Thermodynamic Studies of the Binding of CA125 with   125I-antiCA125 antibody in Ovarian Tumor Homogenates

Abstract

Kinetic and thermodynamic parameters associated with the binding of 125I-anti125 antibody to crude CA125 of benign, post and pre-menopausal malignant ovarian tumors and with partially purified CA125 (BI) and (BII) forms of post-menopausal malignant ovarian tumor were carried out using different rate equations. Then the order of the reactions were tested. It was showed that the reaction in all groups follow second rate law. In addition, the kinetic parameters K_a, K_d, $k+1$, $k-1$, $t\frac{1}{2}$ of association and dissociation were determined at 5, 20, 37 and 45°C. In all studied groups the affinity constant (K_a) and maximum binding capacity (B_{max}) decrease and their rate constant ($k+1$) values increase with increasing temperature. Scatchared plots of all groups showed no curvature in the plotted lines, where the data obeyed the straight line equation suggested that the CA125 has a single binding site or more than one site with identical affinities. The thermodynamics of the binding of 125I-antiCA125 antibody with CA125 for all groups were studied using Van't Hoff and Arrhenius equations, the thermodynamic parameters of standard state ($\Delta H°$, $\Delta G°$ and $\Delta S°$) were determined. The data showed that the binding reactions were exothermic ($\Delta H° < 0$) and spontaneous ($\Delta G° < 0$) and the binding reactions were entropically and enthalpically driven ($\Delta S° > 0$ and $\Delta H° < 0$). Arrhenius plot indicated that there was a linear- relationship between log $k+1$ and $1/T$. The transition state thermodynamic parameters (E_a, ΔH^*, ΔG^* and ΔS^*) for the formation of (125I-anti CA125 antibody/CA125) were determined.

4.1 Introduction

Molecular interactions involve cooperative, independent and contiguous binding regions. Molecular interaction generates dynamic structural changes, which increase the complexity of these interactions. The rate of the reaction and equilibrium conditions is the algebraic sum of the energies involved in reversible macromolecular interactions (160). The specific reaction between antibody and antigen, as a type of these interactions, is usually driven by electrostatic forces between oppositely charged amino acids, hydrogen bonding, and hydrophobic interactions. The equilibrium reaction termed "biospecific interaction" is characterized by the affinity of the reaction to form Antibody- Antigen complex. (161)

The analysis of temperature dependence of kinetic and equilibrium constants allows determination of the energetic of binding. The changes in Gibes free energy, enthalpy and entropy that are associated with the binding of antibody to its antigen can be calculated mathematically using such constant (162).

In other words, thermodynamic measurements of reactions interactions under equilibrium conditions provide information about differences between the initial and final states of each reactant, while kinetics studies supplement the information on the differences between these states and an intermediate activated complex state, (i.e. the pathway taken by the reactants to reach the final product).(163,164)

The elucidation of biomolecular interactions is of steadily increasing importance. Exact knowledge of the principles governing the strengths and formation of molecular interaction is of highest importance for a huge number of applications in widely different areas, such as : The design of new drugs, the understanding of cross-reactions of antibodies used in medical diagnosis or medical treatment, the improvement of our understanding in diseases, the understanding and regulation of biocatalytic activity, the understanding cell-cell communication and cell differentiation, ...etc.

In this chapter, the basic mathematical analysis was described and used to explain the mechanism, through kinetics and thermodynamic, of binding of CA125 antibody to its CA125 antigen in benign, post-and pre-menopausal malignant ovarian tumor homogenates and to its partially purified forms (BI) and (BII) to form (125I-antiCA125 antibody/CA125) complex.

Materials and Methods

4.2 Materials

4.2.1 Chemicals

All chemicals and reagents mentioned in section (2.2.1) were used in the experiments of this chapter.

4.2.2 Instruments

All instruments mentioned in section (2.2.2) were also used in the experiments of this chapter.

4.3 Methods

4.3.1. Kinetic Studies

4.3.1.1 Time course of Binding

A. The time course of the binding of 125I-antiCA125 antibody with CA125 in ovarian tumor homogenate

Reagents

All reagents were prepared according to section (2.3.4) except 20% PEG6000 which was prepared according to the optimum pH of each group.

Procedure

1. Tracer (450, 360and 450) µg.ml-1 were added to (225,150 and 175 µg.ml-1 protein) of OI, OII and OIII respectively.

2. Each mixture was completed to 400µl with Tris-buffer at the optimum pH of each group.

3. All tubes were incubated at 5°C at different time intervals (30, 60, 90, 120, 150, 210, 240, 270 and 300) minutes.

4. Steps 3, 4, 5, and 6 in the section (2.3.5.1.) were repeated.

5. To determine the time course of CA125 binding to 125I-antiCA125 antibody at different temperatures. Steps 1, 2, 3 and, 4 in this experiment were repeated at (20, 37 and 45°C).

Calculations

The B/T% values were calculated as described in section (2.3.4.) and plotted against incubation time at different temperatures.

B. The time course of binding of 125I-antiCA125 antibody with partially purified forms (BI) and BII of malignant ovarian tumor.

Reagent

All reagents were prepared according to the section (2.3.3.) except for 20% PEG 6000 which was prepared according to optimum pH of each group.

Procedure

1. Tracer (360 and 450) µg.ml-1 were added to 90 and 110 µg.ml-1 protein) of BI and BII respectively.

2. Each mixture was completed to 400µl with Tris-buffer at optimum pH of each group.

3. The (125I-antiCA125 antibody/CA125) complex for each group were estimated by following steps 3 and 4 in section 4.3.1.1.A

4. The experiment was repeated at different temperatures (20, 37 and 45°C).

Calculations

The B/T% values were calculated as described in section (2.3.4) and plotted against incubation time at different temperatures.

4.3.1.2. Determination of Kinetic parameters

A. Determination of the affinity constant (Ka) and maximal binding capacity (Bmax) of 125I-antiCA125 antibody associated with CA125 in ovarian tumor homogenates.

1. Increasing volumes (4, 8, 12, 16 and 20 µl) of 125I-antiCA125 antibody containing (72, 144, 216, 288, and 360 µg.ml-1 protein) respectively was added to each (150 µg.ml-1) of pre-menopausal malignant ovarian tumor homogenate. Then the final reaction volume was completed to 400µl with the same buffer.

2. All tubes were incubated at 5°C for 240 minutes.

3. The (125I-antiCA125 antibody/CA125) complex was estimated by following the steps 3, 4, 5, and 6 in the section (2.3.5.1.)

4. The previous steps were performed at different temperature (20, 37 and 45°C).

5. The experiment was repeated using increasing volumes (5, 10, 15, 20 and 25µl) of 125I-antiCA125 antibody containing (90, 180, 270, 360 and 450) µg.ml-1 protein respectively, were added to (225 and 175) µg.ml-1 of each of the post-menopausal malignant ovarian tumor homogenate and

benign ovarian tumor homogenate respectively, instead of pre-menopausal ovarian tumor homogenate (in step 1 above). Tris-buffer at optimum pH of each group was used to complete the volume of the reaction and to prepare 20% PEG 6000.

6. The times of incubation needed to get the equilibrium state for all cases are reported in table (4-1) .

Ta   Table (4-1):   The time of incubation for Benign and malignant post and pre-menopausal ovarian tumor homogenates at different temperature.

Temp. oC	Time		
	Post. Menopausal malignant ovarian tumor homogenate	Pre-menopausal malignant ovarian tumor homogenate	Benign ovarian tumor homogenate
5	240	240	270
20	180	150	180
37	120	90	120
45	90	60	60

Calculations

1. The B/F ratio was computed for each tube, where:

B: is the bound radioactivity (mean counts in c.p.m.) which represent the formation of (125I-antiCA125 antibody/CA125) complex.

F: is the free radioactivity (mean counts in c.p.m.), which represents the (unbound or unreacted), 125I-antiCA125 antibody.

T : is the total activity (mean counts in c.p.m.)

F : T (total counts)-B (bound radioactivity)

2. The concentration of (125I-antiCA125 antibody/CA125) complex in mg.ml-1 which found after time (t) was calculated from the following equation:

$$B \ (\text{mg.ml-1}) \ = \ \frac{B(c.p.m.)}{T(c.p.m.)} \text{ x concentration of }^{125}\text{I - antiCA125 antibody} \quad \text{in}$$

incubation medium in mg.ml-1

3. The affinity constant and maximal binding capacity was determined according to scatchared equation (165).

$$\frac{B}{F} = \frac{1}{K_d} \ X \ (Bmax-B)$$

$$Ka = \frac{1}{K_d}$$

Where Ka = affinity constant

Kd = dissociation constant

Bmax = maximal binding capacity

4. The plot of B/F ratio Vs. the B values in mg.ml-1 gives a linear relationship. The value of affinity constant of the binding (Ka) at each temperature can be calculated from the slope of the straight line, while the value of the total concentration of CA125 (Bmax) in ovarian tumor homogenate of each group was calculated from the intercept of the x-axis.

B. Determination of the affinity constant (Ka) and maximal binding capacity (Bmax) of 125I-antiCA125 antibody associated with partially purified CA125 (BI) and (BII) of post-menopausal ovarian tumor homogenate.

1. Increasing volume (4, 8, 12, 16 and 20 μl) of 125I-antiCA125 antibody containing (72,144,216,288 and 360) μg.ml-1 protein respectively were each added to (90 μg.ml-1) of partially purified CA125 (BI) form. Then final reaction volume was completed to 400 μl with the same buffer.

2. All tubes were incubated at 5°C for 180 minute

3. The (125I-antiCA125 antibody/CA125) complex was estimated by following the steps 3, 4, 5, and 6 in the section (2.3.5.1).

4. The previous steps were performed at different temperature (20, 37 and 45°C).

5. The experiment was repeated using increasing volumes (5, 10, 15, 20 and 25μl) of 125I-antiCA125 antibody containing (90,180,270,360 and 450μg protein) respectively were each added to (110 μg) of partially purified CA125 of post-menopausal ovarian tumor homogenate (BII) form instead of

(BI) (in step 1 above). Tris-buffer at pH = 6.8 was used to complete the volume of the reaction and to prepare 20% PEG6000.

6.   The times of incubation needed to get the equilibrium state for both cases are reported in table (4-2) .

Table (4-2): The time of incubation for partially purified CA125 of postmenopausal ovarian tumor homogenate at different temperatures.

| Temp.°C | Time   min. | |
	Partially purified CA125 (BI) form	Partially purified CA125 (BII) form
5	180	210
20	120	150
37	90	90
45	60	60

Calculations

The method outlined in experiment (4.3.1.2A) was followed exactly to out line the values of Ka and B max at each temperature.

4.3.2 The thermodynamic Studies

4.3.2.1 The thermodynamic studies of the interaction of 125I-antiCA125 antibody with CA125 in ovarian tumor homogenates.

The same steps mentioned in section (4.3.1.1. A) and (4.3.1.2. A) were performed using protein fraction of Benign, malignant post-menopausal and pre-menopausal ovarian tumor homogenates.

Calculations

1. The thermodynamic parameters of standard state were obtained from Van't Hoff plot, the values of the natural logarithm of equilibrium constant (affinity constant Ka) obtained at different temperatures were plotted against the reciprocal values of the absolute temperature in kelvin (1/T), according to the following equation:

$$\ln Ka = \frac{\Delta S^{\circ}}{R} - \frac{\Delta H^{\circ}}{RT}$$

Where:

$\Delta H° =$ The enthalpy change of the standard state.

$\Delta S° =$ The entropy change of the standard state.

R $\quad =$ The gas constant (8.314 J.K-1.mol-1)

ΔH value was obtained from the slope of the linear relationship of the plot.

The change in Gibbs free energy of the standard state ($\Delta G°$) was obtained from the following equation:

$\Delta G° = $-RT ln Ka

where Ka is the affinity constant, while the standard state entropy ($\Delta S°$) change was obtained from.

$$\Delta S° = \frac{\Delta H° - \Delta G°}{T}$$

2. The thermodynamic parameters of the transition state were obtained from Arrhenius plot of ln k+1 values against (1/T) values, that given a linear relationship according to the following equation

$$\ln k{+}1 = \ln A{-}[\frac{Ea}{RT}]$$

Where:

A: Arrhenius constant.

The value of the activation energy (Ea) of the binding reaction can be determined from the slope of the straight line.

The enthalpy of transition state ΔH^* was obtained from

$\Delta H^* = $Ea-RT

Transition state of free energy change ΔG^* is calculated from the following equation

$$\Delta G^* = \text{-RT ln k+1} + RT \ln \frac{KT}{h}$$

where K and h were boltzman and Blank's constants which are equal to (1.38 x 10-23 J.K-1), (6.62 x 10-34 J.sec-1) respectively.

The change in entropy of the transition state ΔS^* was calculated from the following equation:

$$\Delta S^* = \frac{\Delta H^* - \Delta G^*}{T}$$

4.3.2.2 The thermodynamic studies of the interaction of 125I-antiCA125 antibody with partially purified CA125 (BI) and (BII) of post-menopausal ovarian tumor homogenate.

The experiment was performed as described in section (4.3.1.1.B) and (4.3.1.2.B) using partially purified CA125 (BI) and (BII) forms of malignant post – menopausal ovarian tumor homogenate.

Calculations

The method outlined in the experiment (4.3.2.1.) was followed exactly for estimating the thermodynamic parameters of the standard and transition state.

4.4. Results and Discussion

4.4.1 Determination of kinetic parameters of CA125 Associated with 125I-antiCA125 antibody.

The time course of (125I-antiCA125 antibody/CA125) complex formation was carried out to describe the kinetic parameters of the binding. The simplest proposed model representing this interaction is:

125I-antiCA125antibody + CA125 $\underset{k_{-1}}{\overset{k_{+1}}{\rightleftharpoons}}$ [125I-antiCA125 antibody/CA125]

Where

k+1: is the association rate of 125I-antiCA125 antibody to CA125.

k-1: is the dissociation rate of 125I-antiCA125 antibody/CA125) complex formed.

At equilibrium

$$Ka = \frac{\left[^{125}I\text{-antiCA125 antibody}/CA125\right]}{\left[^{125}I\text{-antiCA125antibody}\right]\left[CA125\right]} \quad \cdots\cdots (1)$$

$$Kd = \frac{\left[^{125}I\text{-antiCA125 antibody}\right]\left[CA125\right]}{\left[^{125}I\text{-antiCA125 antibody}/CA125\right]} \quad \cdots\cdots (2)$$

Thus:

$$Ka = \frac{1}{K_d} = \frac{k_{+1}}{k_{-1}} \quad \cdots\cdots (3)$$

The value of Ka and maximal binding capacity (Bmax) were calculated from scatchared plot at four different temperatures for all studied groups [OI, OII, OIII and partially purified CA125 (BI & BII) of malignant post-menopausal ovarian tumor homogenate. The experiment was carried out at the optimum conditions that were obtained in previous experiments and was repeated at different temperatures (20, 37 and 45°C).

Scatchared plots were analyzed according to their linearity as shown in figures (4.1 A, B and C) and (4.2.A & B), all groups showed no curvature in the plotted lines where the data obeyed the straight line equation, indicating that CA125 has a single binding site or more than one site with identical affinities.

Table (4.3) shows that the affinity constant (Ka) and (Bmax) depended on the type of tumor (benign or malignant) and on the temperature. Ka decreases with the increased temperature in all studied groups. The highest value of Ka occurred in OI group at 5°C, it is about (5.432 mg.ml-1) which suggest the highest affinity for binding among the two rest groups. The increase in temperature may affect the protein conformation which leads to decrease the affinity of binding. On the other hand, determination of (Bmax) of CA125 to each type of tissue homogenate shows similar result for Ka value, it is temperature depended, Bmax decreased with increasing temperature.

The results in table (4-4) also reveal that there is a decrease in Ka and Bmax values for partially purified CA125 (BI) and (BII) forms with increasing temperature. Ka for BI and BII was (7.092 mg-1.ml and 3.333mg-1.ml at 5°C respectively, while it was 3.20 mg-1.ml and 2.080 mg.ml-1 at 45°C for the two groups respectively. In comparison of Ka and Bmax values for BI and BII, BI show higher affinity and lower binding capacity than BII.

In general, it can be concluded that partially purified CA125 (BI) form interacts with its specific antibody with higher affinity than the interaction of crude CA125 antigen.

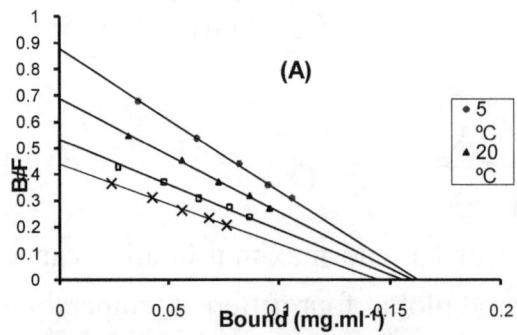

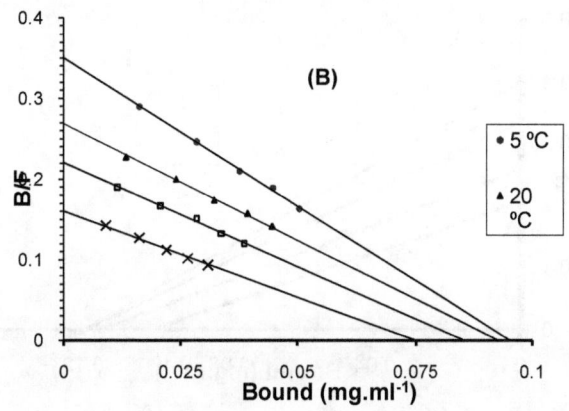

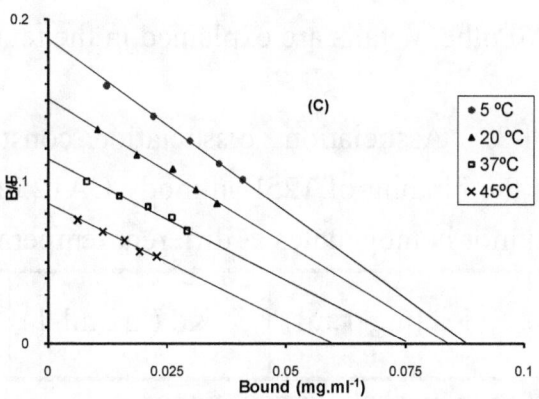

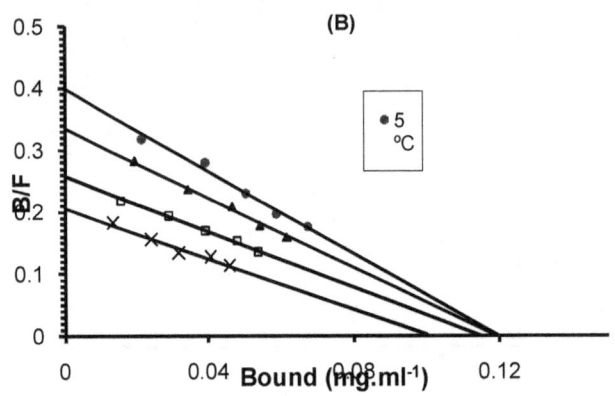

Figure (4-2): Scatchard Plot for partially purified CA 125, A) BI, B) BII, at different

temperatures. (All other details are explained in the text).

Table 4-3: Association, dissociation constants and maximal binding capacity of the binding of 125I-antibody CA125 antibody to CA125 antigen in ovarian tumor homogenates at different temperatures

Temperature °C	Ka (mg-1.ml)	Kd (mg.ml-1)	B max(mg.ml-1)
Malignant post-menopausal ovarian tumor			
5	5.432	0.184	0.162
20	4.367	0.228	0.158
37	3.419	0.292	0.155
45	3.034	0.329	0.145
Malignant pre-menopausal ovarian tumor			
2	3.684	0.271	0.095
20	3.027	0.330	0.092
37	2.588	0.386	0.085
45	2.133	0.468	0.075
Benign ovarian tumor			
5	2.148	0.465	0.087
20	1.800	0.555	0.083
37	1.554	0.643	0.074
45	1.433	0.697	0.060

Table (4-4): Association, dissociation constants and maximal binding capacity of the binding of 125I-antiCA125 antibody to partially purified CA125 BI and BII of malignant post-menopausal ovarian tumor homogenates at different temperatures.

Temperature °C	Ka mg-1.ml	Kd (mg.ml-1)	Bmax(mg.ml-1)
Partially purified (BI)			
5	7.092	0.141	0.141
20	5.000	0.200	0.140
37	3.676	0.272	0.137
45	3.2	0.312	0.125
Partially purified (BII)			
2	3.333	0.300	0.120
20	2.750	0.363	0.120
37	2.263	0.441	0.110
45	2.080	0.480	0.100

However the time course data could be used to determine the reaction order of CA125 binding to its specific antibody using the graphical method. Attempts were carried out using pseudo first order and second order graphs.

For second order graph the following equations (163) were used

$$\ln [AbAg]\ e \left[\frac{[Ab]_T - [AbAg]_t\ [AbAg]_e\ /[Ag\ ]_T}{[Ab]_T\ ([AbAg]_e - [AbAg]_t)} \right] = k+1t \left[\frac{[Ab]_T [Ag]_T - [AbAg]_e}{[AbAg]_e} \right] ...4$$

Where:

K+1: is the association rate constant.

[AbAg]e: is the concentration of (125I-antibodyCA125 antibody/CA125)complex formed at equilibrium.

[AbAg]t: is the concentration of (125I-antibodyCA125 antibody/CA125)complex after time t.

[Ab]T: is the initial antibody concentration at time 0.

[Ag]T: is the initial antigen concentration at time 0.

Or by using another second order kinetic equation from:

$$\frac{1}{[Ab]_T - [Ag]_T} .\ln \left(\frac{[Ab]_T - [AbAg]_t}{[Ag]_T - [AbAg]_t} \right) = K_{+1}t + \frac{1}{[Ab]_T - [Ag]_T} \ln \frac{[Ab]_T}{[Ag]_T} ....5$$

287

For first order graph as the percent of binding was in some cases small (166) and must be labeled antibody remains free and only small fractions binds even at equilibrium ,ie. $[Ab]T \gg [AbAg]e$

Thus

$$[Ab]T \gg \frac{[AbAg]_t [AbAg]_e}{[Ag]_T}$$

So the following equation could be used in order to fit the pseudo-first order kinetics:

$$\ln \frac{[AbAg]_e}{[AbAg]_e - [AbAg]_t} = K_{+1}.t \frac{[Ab]_T [Ag]_T}{[AbAg]_e} \quad \ldots\ldots 6$$

On the other hand figure (4-3 A, B &C) and (4-4 A&B) show the plot of

$$\frac{1}{[Ab]_T - [Ag]_T} \ln\left(\frac{[Ab]_T - [AbAg]_t}{[Ag]_T - [AbAg]_t}\right)$$

Against time give a straight line for all studies groups OI, OII, OIII and partially purified CA125 (BI and BII form).The association rate constant k+1 was determined at each temperature from the slope of the plot.

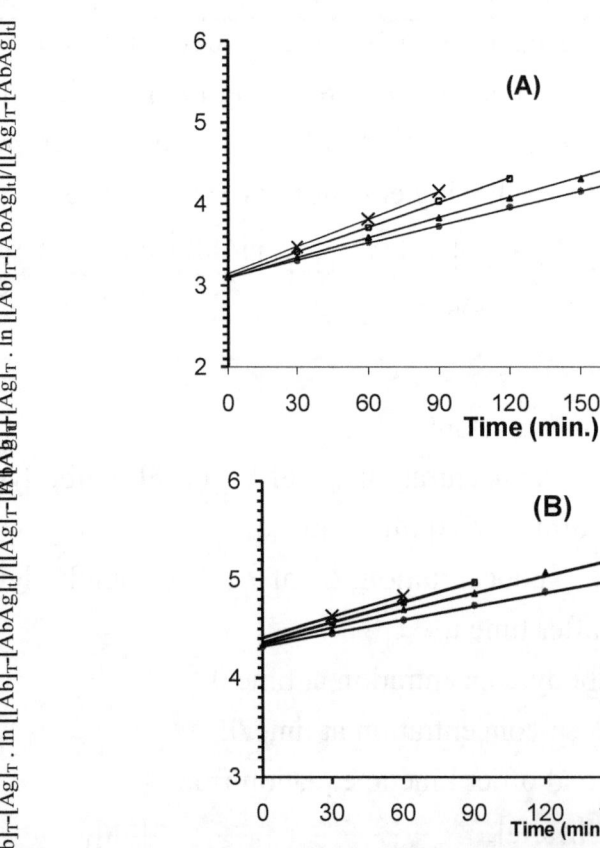

288

Figure (4-3): Kinetics of the binding of 125I-anti CA125 antibody to CA125 of

A: Malignant post-menopausal ovarian tumor homogenate.

B: Malignant pre-menopausal ovarian tumor homogenate.

C: Benign ovarian tumor homogenate. At different temperature using second order rate law (All other details are explained in the text).

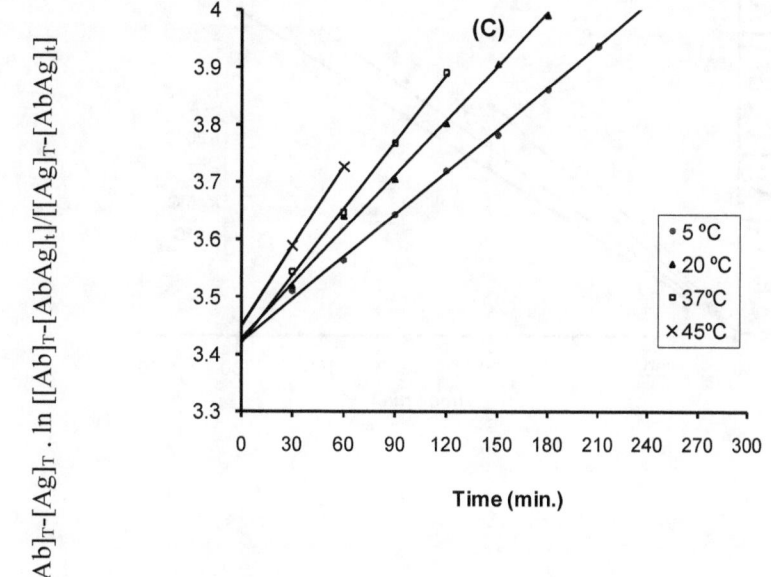

Figure (4-3) continued

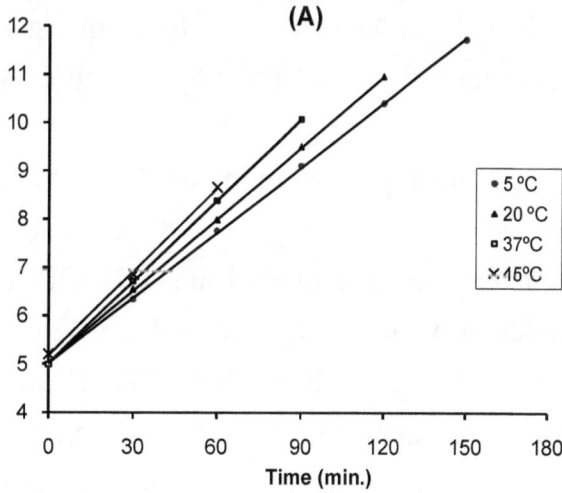

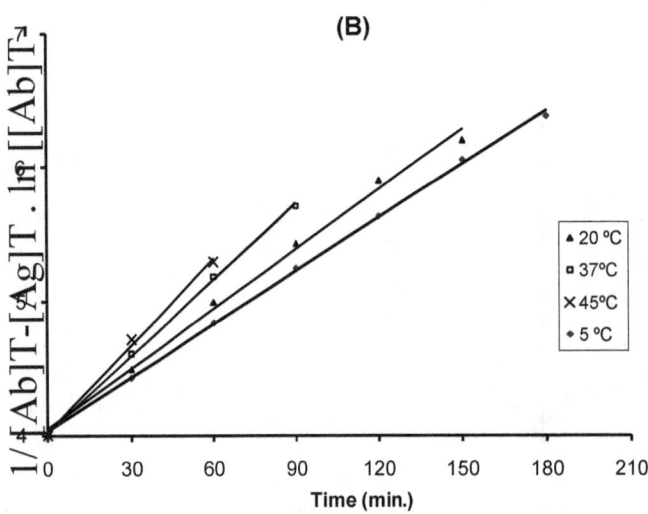

(B)

Figure (4-4): Kinetics of the binding of 125I-anti CA125 antibody with partially purified CA125 BI and BII from malignant post- menopausal ovarian tumor homogenate. At different temperature using second order rate law

(All other details are explained in the text).

Kinetic parameters for all studied groups (OI, OII, OIII, BI and BII) were illustrated in tables (4-5) and (4-6). The value of k_{+1} indicates that highest rate of association of CA125 with 125I-antiCA125 antibody occurs at 45oC, whereas the lowest rate occurs at 5°C. Thus when the reaction temperature was increased from 5 °C to 45°C, the values of the association constant increased approximately (1.6, 1.6, 1.8, 1.3 and 1.6 folds) in group OI, OI, OIII, BI and BII respectively.

According to k_{+1} values, the rate of reaction in OI is faster than in OII and OIII which may relate to the origin of CA125 tumor marker.

Table (4-6) also shows that reaction rate of the interaction of partially purified CA125 to 125I-antiCA125 antibody is faster than that in crude CA125 (OI group). The increase in reaction rate is associated with decrease in the reaction time from 240 min. for crude antigen to 180 min and 210 min for BI and BII respectively.

The value of k-1 was also determined from the values of Ka (equation 3), which has been estimated at the four temperatures investigated. The results showed that k-1 increased with elevation of temperature. The increase in k-1 value was about 2.8 folds for all studied groups when the temperature increased from 5 °C to 45 °C.

Table (4-5): Kinetic parameters for the binding of 125I-antibodyCA125 antibody with CA125 in ovarian tumor homogenates at different temperatures using second order rate law (All other details are explained in the text).

Temperature °C	k+1 (mg-1.ml.min-	k-1 x10-3 (min-1)	t1/2ass (min)	t1/2 diss
Malignant post-menopausal ovarian tumor				
5	0.0070	1.288	93	538
20	0.0083	1.900	72	364
37	0.0101	2.954	52	235
45	0.0110	3.625	36	191
Malignant pre-menopausal ovarian tumor				
5	0.004410	1.1970	81	578
20	0.005580	1.8434	51	375
37	0.006722	2.5973	27	26
45	0.007250	3.3989	18	203
Benign ovarian tumor				

5	0.002470	1.150	123	602
20	0.003172	1.7622	84	393
37	0.003925	2.5257	60	274
45	0.004510	3.1447	27	220

Table (4-6): Kinetic parameters for the binding of 125I-antibodyCA125 antibody to partially purified CA125 BI and BII form of malignant post-menopausal ovarian tumor homogenate at different temperature using second order rate law. (All other details are explained in the text).

Temperature °C	k+1 (mg-1.ml.min-1)	k-1 x10-3 (min-1)	t1/2ass (min)	t1/2 diss (min)
Partially purified (BI)				
5	0.04500	6.3450	48	109
20	0.04965	9.9300	35	74
37	0.05620	15.288	27	45
45	0.05937	18.550	24	37
Partially purified (BII)				
5	0.01356	4.0680	72	170
20	0.01583	5.7560	55	120
37	0.01860	8.2450	38	84
45	0.02266	10.894	25	63

4.4.2. The thermodynamic studies of the interaction of 125I-antiCA125 antibody with CA125.

4.4.2.1 Thermodynamic parameters of standard state

Figures (4-5 and 4-6) represents the dependence of equilibrium constant (affinity constant) for binding of 125I-antiCA125 antibody to crude CA125 of benign, pre-and post-menopausal and partially purified CA125 in ovarian tumor homogenates on the temperature (Van't Hoff plot).

Figure (4-5): Van't Hoff plot for the binding of CA125 to 125I-antiCA125 antibody in ovarian tumor homogenates at different temperature for OI, OII and OIII (All other details are explained in the text)

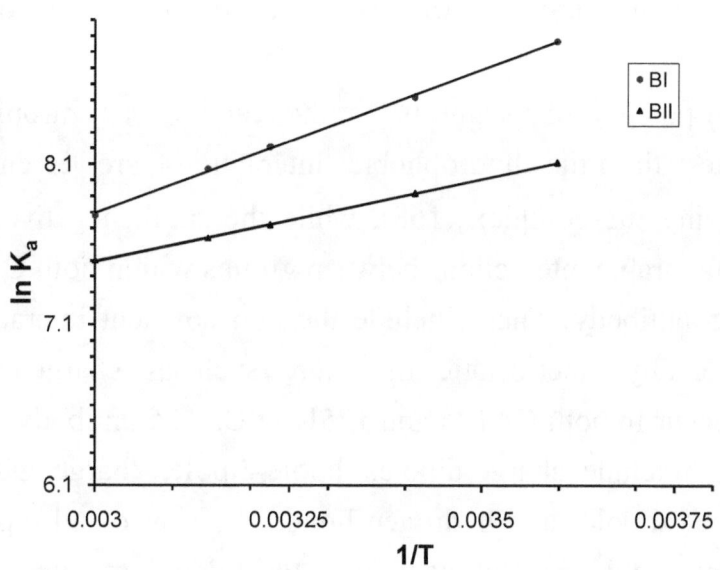

Figure (4-6): Van't Hoff plot for the binding of partially purified CA125 with 125I-antiCA125 antibody at different temperatures

(All other details are explained in the text).

Tables (4-7 and 4-8) summarize the calculated thermodynamic parameters for all studied groups (OI, OII, OII, BI and BII) respectively. The results obtained revealed that $\Delta H0$ in general has small negative value for all groups; their negative sign suggested an exothermic CA125-125I-antiCA125 antibody interaction reaction.

The other values of thermodynamic parameters of the standard state such as ΔG° and ΔS° at four temperatures, are summarized in the same tables (4-7 and 4-8).

A high value of positive ΔS° suggests that the reaction spontaneity was entropically driven.

The high negative value of ΔG° reflects the stability of complex, hence, the high affinity of the reactants. The high negative values of ΔG° for the binding reaction are controlled by high positively ΔS° and low negatively ΔH°. (167) so our CA125-125I-antiCA125 antibody interaction system is characterized by the contribution of ΔS° and ΔH° to the stability of the complex formed.

The high value of positive ΔS° suggests that the reaction was entropically driven and indicates that the hydrophobic interactions are essentially important in stabilizing the complex (168), while the small negative ΔH° value may indicate favorable interactions between groups within both CA125 and 125I-antiCA125 antibody. These include the non covalent interactions which are fundamentally electrostatic in nature such as charge-charge interactions which occur in both CA125 and 125I-antiCA125 antibody, other types of interactions include charge-dipole, dipole-dipole, charge induced dipole, dipole induced dipole and hydrogen bond. The sum of all types of these interactions can yield sum stabilization to the folded structure of the complex. So the negative value of ΔG° showed that the overall reaction was energetically favorable in the direction of complex formation.

Table (4-7): Thermodynamic parameters for standard state of the binding of 125I-antiCA125 antibody with CA125 in ovarian tumor homogenates at different temperatures.

(All other details are explained in the text).

Temperature 0C	ΔH°(KJ.mol-1)	ΔG°(KJ.mol-1)	ΔS°(J.mol-1 K-1)
Malignant post-menopausal ovarian tumor			
5	-10.808	-19.877	32.622
20	-10.808	-20.416	32.791
37	-10.808	-20.928	32.645
45	-10.808	-21.177	32.6069
Malignant pre-menopausal ovarian tumor			
5	-9.342	-18.978	34.616
20	-9.342	-19.524	34.750

37	-9.342	-20.232	35.125
45	-9.342	20.267	34.355
Benign ovarian tumor			
5	-7.407	-17.732	37.140
20	-7.407	-18.270	37.075
37	-7.407	-18.938	37.196
45	-7.407	-19.2128	37.125

Table(4-8): Thermodynamic parameters for standard state of the binding of 125I-antiCA125 antibody with partially purified CA125 at different temperatures.

(All other details are explained in the text)

Temperature 0C	ΔH^{o}(KJ.mol-1)	ΔG^{o}(KJ.mol-1)	ΔS^{o}(J.mol-1 K-1)
Partially purified BI			
5	-15.121	-20.491	19.316
20	-15.121	-20.754	19.225
37	-15.121	-21.157	19.470
45	-15.121	-21.335	19.540
Partially purified BII			
5	-8.507	-18.746	36.830
20	-8.507	-19.290	36.802
37	-8.507	-19.904	36.764
45	-8.507	-20.199	36.767

4.4.2.2. Thermodynamic Parameters of Transition State

According to the transition state theory, the interaction of CA125 to CA125 antibody to form the final product `proceeds through the formation of an activated complex (transition state).

CA125+CA125 antibody → [CA125…CA125antibody] → CA125-CA125antibody

An activated complex   Final product
(Transition state)

Arrhenius equation and the kinetic constants have been used to determine thermodynamic parameters of the transition state (Ea, ΔH^*, ΔS^* and ΔG^*).

Figure (4-7) and (4-8 A&B) shows Arrhenius plots of ln k+1 against 1/T values. The slope of the straight line represents the activation energy Ea. Tables (4-9) and (4-10) show the values of thermodynamic parameters of the transition state of all studied groups (OI, OII, OIII, BI and BII). OIII group showed the highest Ea value, which reflects the high energy required to overcome the energy barrier of transition state for the formation of (125I-antiCA125 antibody-CA125) complex in comparison to the rest groups. On the other hand the value of activation energy is in accordance with the high positive values of ΔG^*, which indicates that the formation of an activated complex (125I-antiCA125 antibody…CA125) is a non spontaneous process and required a lot of energy (equal to Ea) to overcome the transition state energy barrier and giving the final product .Also the positive values of ΔG^* is mainly attributed to the decrease in entropy of the transition state ($\Delta S^* < 0$) in addition, the positive value of ΔH^* in all groups shows that the heat content of the activated complex is more than that of isolated species.(169)

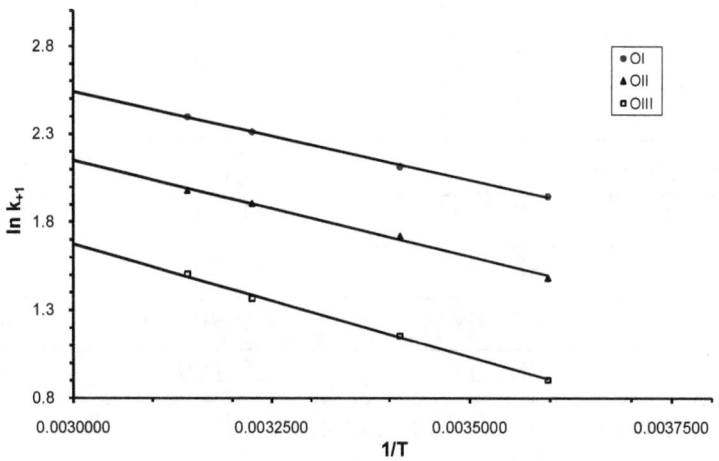

Figure (4-7): Arrhenius plot of the binding of 125I-antiCA125 antibody with its CA125 in ovarian tumor homogenates for OI, OII and OIII. (All other details are explained in the text).

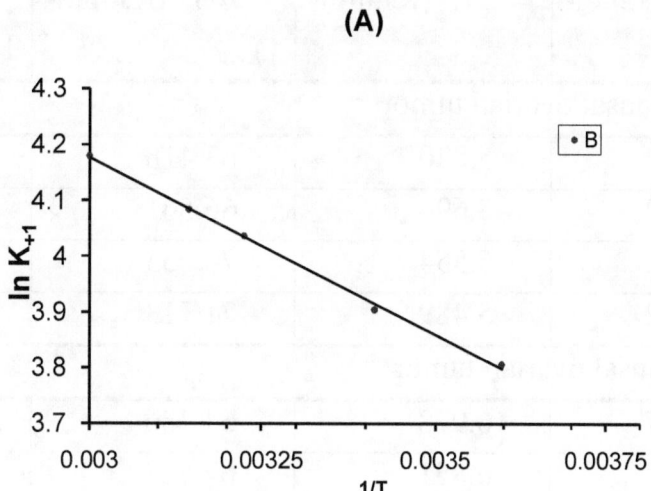

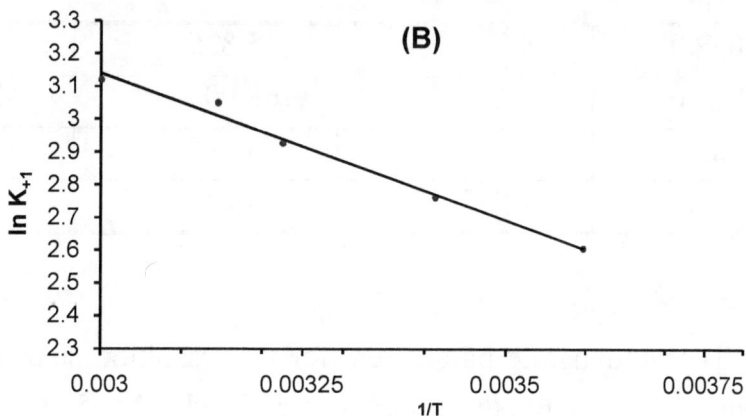

Figure (4-8): Arrhenius plot for the binding of 125I-antiCA125 antibody with partially purified CA125 A) BI, B) BII. (All other details are explained in the text).

Table (4-9):Thermodynamic parameters for the transition state for the binding of 125I-antiCA125 antibody to CA125 in ovarian tumor homogenates at different temperatures. (All details are explained in the text).

Temperature °C	Ea(KJ.mol-1)	ΔH*(KJ.mol-1)	ΔG* (KJ.mol-1)	ΔS*(J.mol-1.K-1)
Malignant post – menopausal ovarian tumor				
5	8.132	5.820	63.418	-207.187
20	8.132	5.696	66.561	-207.730
37	8.132	5.554	70.053	-208.061
45	8.132	5.489	71.713	-208.251
Malignant pre – menopausal ovarian tumor				
5	9.287	6.978	64.486	-206.863
20	9.287	6.851	67.528	-207.088
37	9.287	6.710	71.113	-207.751
45	9.287	6.644	72.790	-208.006
Benign				
5	10.640	8.325	65.825	-206.820
20	10.640	8.204	68.903	-207.163
37	10.640	8.063	73.498	-207.854
45	10.640	7.997	75.044	-207.777

Table (4-10): Thermodynamic parameters for the transition state for the binding of 125I-antiCA125 antibody to partially purified CA125 at different temperatures. (All other details are explained in the text).

Temperature °C	Ea(KJ.mol-1)	ΔH*(KJ.mol-1)	ΔG* (KJ.mol-1)	ΔS*(J.mol-1.K-1)
Partially purified BI				
5	5.430	3.119	59.118	-201.435

20	5.430	2.994	62.220	-202.136
37	5.430	2.853	65.640	-202.538
45	5.430	2.787	67.255	-202.729
Partially purified BII				
5	7.156	4.845	61.890	-205.197
20	7.156	4.720	65.004	-205.747
37	7.156	4.579	68.482	-206.138
45	7.156	4.513	69.802	-205.311

The values of thermodynamic parameters of the binding reaction gave an overall idea about the nature of forces that regulate the formation of complex. Comparisons of the values of transition state with those of standard state led us to choose a thermodynamic model shown in figure (4-9).

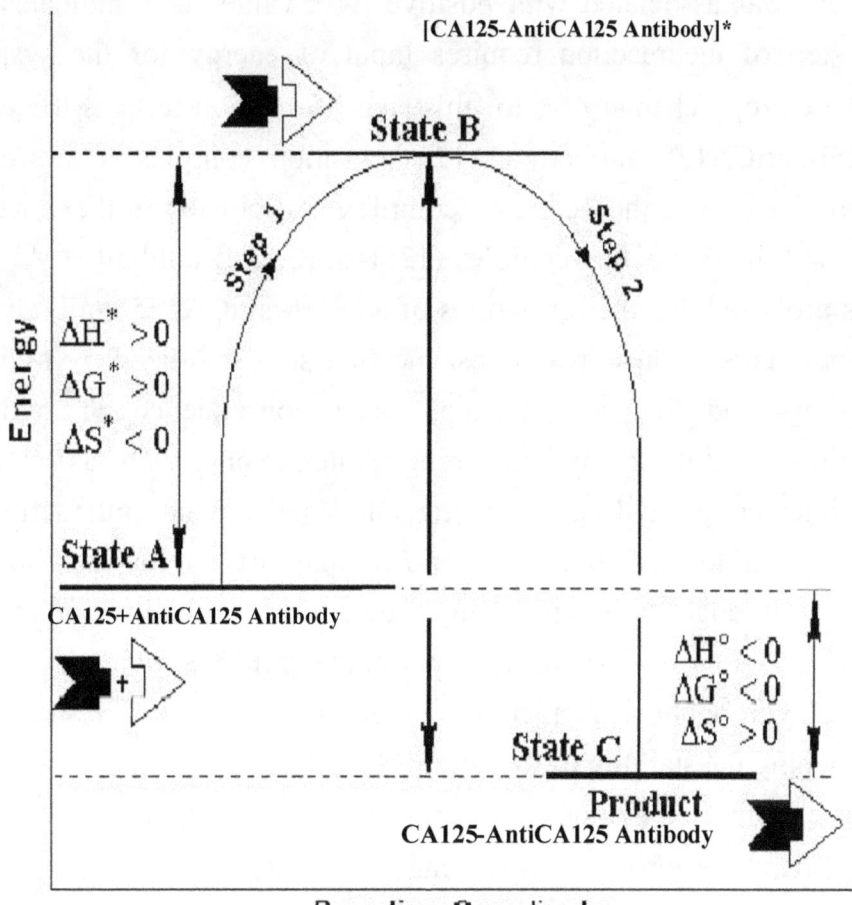

Figure (4-9): General energy diagram and thermodynamic Model applied to the interaction of 125I-anti antibody to CA125 of ovarian human homogenates.

This model proposes that the formation of the (125I-antiCA125 antibody/CA125) complex undergoes three thermodynamic state (170). The thermodynamic state A represents the initial energy level of 125I-AntiCA125Antibody and its CA125. In the thermodynamic state B, the two species had come together and mutually penetrated their hydration sphere to form a partially immobilized hydrophobically associated species. Thermodynamic state C represents the fully interacting complex (125I-antiCA125 antibody/CA125).

In step 1 of the reaction, the binding of 125I-AntiCA125Antibody to CA125 was associated with positive ΔG^* value. This indicates that the initial step of the reaction requires input of energy for the system. The negative entropy change ΔS^* for this step of reaction reflects the change of the 125I-antiCA125 antibody/CA125 transition complex to more ordered structure. In step 2, the activated complex participates further interactions, giving the fully interacting complex (125I-antiCA125 antibody/CA125).

It is proposed that the formations of a (125I-antiCA125 antibody/CA125) complex occurs in these two steps, the first step stabilized by hydrophobic interactions and the second step, as a consequence of hydrophobic interactions, stabilized by short-range interactions such as electrostatic (ionic) interactions, hydrogen bonding, and Vander Waals' interactions which become possible due to the juxtapositioning of appropriate amino acid residues. Although these short-range interactions probably cannot maintain the integrity of the 125I-antiCA125 antibody/CA125 complex in the absence of the hydrophobic interactions, they are probably responsible for strengthening the stability of the complex. (171)

Hydrophobic interactions contribute to the stability of the complex via high positive excited entropy change ($\Delta S^* > 0$), while electrostatic interactions , hydrogen bonding and Vander Waals' interactions contribute to the stability of the complex via high negative change in entropy ($\Delta S^* < 0$) (171,172) .

The thermodynamic data from this study indicates that the binding of 125I-antiCA125 antibody to its CA125 are mainly entropically driven and come in agreement with the concept that hydrophobic and short-range interactions have an important role in the binding of 125I-antiCA125 antibody to its CA125antigen.

Chapter Five
Spectroscopic Studies
On Isolated (125I-anti CA125 antibody/CA125) Complex

Abstract

Spectroscopic studies in the ultraviolet region were carried out to characterize the (125I-antiCA125 antibody/CA125) complex of partially purified CA125 antigen (BI and BII) forms which are partially purified from malignant ovarian tumor homogenates.

Gel filtration technique was used to separate 125I-anti CA125 antibody bound to partially purified CA125 (BI and BII) from unbound (free) 125I-antiCA125 antibody. Factors affecting the absorption properties of the two types of complexes such as pH, solvent polarity (solvent perturbation technique), spectrophotometeric pH titration and thermal stability in the presence of different concentration of sodium chloride have been studied.

The spectroscopic pH titration curves for complex of partially purified CA125 (BI) and (BII) for histidine residue gave pka of 6.5 and 7.2 respectively, while 11.4 and 11.2 for tyrosine residue respectively. Also, it was showed that 60% of histidine and 36.8% of tyrosine residues are located on the surface of complex of (BII) antigen while these residues were 80% and 25% on the surface of complex of (BI).

5.1 Introduction

Spectrophotometry is one of the most valuable analytical techniques available to biochemists. Unknown compounds may be identified by their characteristic absorption spectra in the ultraviolet, visible or infrared. The wave length that is absorbed and efficiency of absorption depend on both the structure and environment of the molecule.

The most uses of spectroscopic technique in biochemistry employ UV region spectrum. Proteins absorb U.V light at approximately 280 nm due to the presence of tryptophane, tyrosine and (to a lesser extent) phenylalanine residues within their structure, while the absorption of UV light at (215-230) is due to the presence of the polypeptide chain backbone and histidyl residues (173).

The electronic transitions for these chromophors come from n $\longrightarrow \pi^*$ and $\pi \longrightarrow \pi^*$. Change in the charge and the environment of these chromophors can lead to alteration in the absorption spectrum, and the conformational changes of a protein may also involve environmental change in its chromophoric groups.(174) A large number of environmental factors produce detectable changes in λmax. Among these factors is the pHs of the solvent which determines the ionization state of ionizable chromophore. Also the solvent polarity affects the chromophore electronic transition where the λmax for n- π^* transition occurs at shorter wavelength in polar solvents (H_2O, Alcohol) than in longer wavelength. The shift may or may not be accompanied by a change in intensity of spectrum. (175, 176) Thus absorbance measurements can give an idea of location of particular amino acid in protein structure.

Although several new Immunochemical techniques were developed to study antigen/antibody interactions (173, 177), U.V spectra remain as one of the most important methods in immunology because it provides a sensitive and quantitative measurements for the study of antibody structure and its specific ligand binding. (178)

Very limited work concerning physical properties of CA125 specially those related to U.V spectroscopy has been done, such as the studies on CA125 in breast cancer by Haider (179) and In colorectal cancer by Al-Jobory (180). Also the U.V studies on interaction of CA125 with its specific antibody are not wide spread. Hence, the goal of this chapter is to study the spectroscopic behaviour at the region of U.V of the partially purified CA125 and its complex formed with   125I-antiCA125 antibody at different conditions.

Material and Methods

5.2 Materials

5.2.1 Chemicals

All chemicals and reagents mentioned in section (2.2.1) have been used in the experiments of this chapter.

5.2.2. Instruments

All instruments mentioned in section (2.2.2) have been used in the experiments of this chapter.

5.2.3. Buffers and Reagents

Buffers and reagents mentioned in section (2.3.4) are used in this chapter. Other additional solutions are indicated in each experiment.

5.3 Methods

5.3.1. Gel filtration technique for separation of free and bound   125I-antiCA125 antibody.

5.3.1.1. Preparation of the column.

The dimensions of the column were (1x27cm) chosen according to the equation in section (3.3.1.1).

5.3.1.2. Preparation of the Gel and determination of void volume.

The sepharose CL-6B was used to separate free and bound 125I-antiCA125 antibody,(157) and was prepared as mentioned in section (3.3.1.3) the void volume was determined and found to be 10.ml.

5.3.1.3. Separation procedure of (125I-anti CA125 antibody / CA125) complex.

A. Partially purified CA125 (BI) form with 125I-anti CA125 antibody.

6. Two hundred micro liter from partially purified CA125(BI) antigen in section (3.3.1.5) (360 µg.ml-1) was incubated with 80 µl of

125I-anti CA125 antibody (1440 µg.ml-1), and the reaction was completed to final volume of 600 µl with Tris-buffer (0.05 M, pH 6.8). The tubes were incubated for 180 min at 5°C.

7. At the end of the incubation, the mixture was applied to the surface of a sepharose CL-6B column equilibrated with Tris-buffer 0.05M, pH 6.8.Elution was carried out using the same buffer to separate CA125 bound to 125I-anti CA125 antibody from unbound antigen with flow rate 12ml.hr-1.

8. The radioactivity of each fraction was counted in gamma counter for 1min.

Calculations

Radioactivity (c.p.m) for each fraction was plotted against the fraction number.

B. Partially Purified CA125 (BII) form with 125I-antiCA125 antibody.

1. One hundred and eighty micro liter (440 µg.ml-1) from partially purified CA125 antigen (BII form) in section (3.3.1.5) was incubated with 100 µl of 125I-antiCA125 antibody (1800 µg.ml-1) and the reaction was completed to final volume of 600 µl with Tris-buffer (0.05M pH 7.2). The tubes were incubated for 210 min. at 5°C.

2. At the end of the incubation, the mixture was applied to the surface of a sepharose CL-6B column equilibrated with Tris-buffer 0.05M pH 7.2. The elution was carried out using the same buffer to separate CA125 bound to 125I-antiCA125 antibody from unbound antigen with flow rate 12 ml.hr-1.

3. The radioactivity for each fraction was counted in gamma counter for 1 min.

4. 80 µl of 125I-antiCA125 antibody was completed to 600 µl with Tris-buffer (0.05M pH 7.2), then this volume was applied to the surface of the column in step 2, and step 2 and 3 were repeated.

Calculations

Radioactivity (c.p.m) for each fraction was plotted against the fraction number.

5.3.2. The U.V Spectrum of (125I-anti CA125 antibody/ CA125) Complex, 125I-antiCA25 antibody and Partially Purified CA125.

5.3.2.1. The U.V Spectrum of (125I-anti CA125 antibody / CA125) Complex

The gel filtration profile in section (5.3.1.3 A & B) gave two peaks. The fractions under each peak were pooled and the absorption spectrum was scanned in U.V region against the appropriate blank in reference beam.

5.3.2.2. The UV Spectrum of 125I- anti CA125 antibody.

Twenty five micro litter of 125I-anti CA125 antibody was mixed with 475 µl of Tris (0.05M pH 7.2) and placed in 0.5 cm3 cuvette. The absorption spectrum was scanned in the UV region against appropriate blank in the reference beam.

5.3.2.3. The UV Spectrum of partially Purified CA125

Two hundred micro litter from partially purified CA125 antigen (BI) was mixed with 300µl of Tris pH 6.8 and placed in 0.5cm3 cuvette. The absorption spectrum was scanned in UV region against appropriate blank in the reference beam. The same procedure was repeated for partially purified CA125 antigen (BII) using 100 micro liter of (BII) and 400µl Tris-buffer pH7.2 for dilution.

5.3.3. Factors Affecting the Absorption Properties of (125I-anti CA125antibody / CA125) Complex.

5.3.3.1. The pH Effect on the Complex

Reagents

1. KCl-HCl buffer (pH) was prepared as follows

Solution A: Potassium chloride (0.1M), 0.788 gm was dissolved in a final volume of 100ml deionized distilled water.

Solution B: Hydrochloric acid (0.1 N)

The required pH (3.0) was prepared by mixing 50ml of solution A with an appropriate amount of solution B to obtain the required pH, and then the volume was made up to 100ml with deionized distilled water.

2. Citrate-phosphate buffer at different pH was prepared as follows.

Solution A: citric acid (0.05M): 0.9605 gm of citric acid dissolved in 100ml deionizer distilled water.

Solution B: Dibasic sodium phosphate (0.1M): 1.4198gm of $Na_2HPO_4$was dissolved in a final volume of 100ml deionized destilled water.

Working buffer pH (4 and 6) was prepared by mixing a volume of solution A with appropriate amount of solution B to obtain the required pH in a final volume of 100ml.

3. Tris buffer at different pH values was prepared as follows:

Solution A: Tris (hydroxyl methyl amino methan) (0.1M): 1.215gm was dissolved in a final volume of 100ml of deionized distilled water.

Solution B: Hydrochloric acid (0.1N)

The required pH (7 and 8) was prepared by mixing 50ml of solution A with appropriate amount of solution B to obtain the required pH, and then the volume was made up to 100ml with deionzied distilled water.

4. Glycine – NaOH buffer was prepared as follows:

Solution A: Glycine (0.1M): 0.7505gm $C_2H_5NO_2$ was dissolved in a final volume of 100ml deionized distilled water.

Solution B: Sodium hydroxide (0.1M):0.4gm NaOH was dissolved in a final volume of 100ml deionized distilled water.

Working buffer pH (9 – 12) was prepared by mixing 50ml of solution A with appropriate amount of solution B to obtain the required pH, then the volume was made up to 100ml with deionized distilled water.

Procedure

One hundred micro liter of pooled fractions under the first peak in (Fig 5-1A) and Fig (5-1 B) which represent (125I-antiCA125 antibody / CA125) complex of BI and BII respectively were completed to 500 μl with different buffers at different pH values (3, 4, 9 and 12) individually then each sample tube was scanned in UV region against a buffer blank at each pH.

5.3.3.2. Effect of Solvent Polarity on UV Spectra of Complex.

The effect of 20% ethanol, and the same amount of ethylene glycol, glycerol and DMSO on the complex was studied.

One hundred micro liter of (125I-antiCA125 antibody/CA125) complex of BI and BII [pooled fractions under the first peak in figure (5–1–A) and (5–1–B)] were mixed with 100 μl of either ethanol, ethylene glycol, glycerol and DMSO) separately. The volume was completed to 500 μl with Tris pH 6.8 and pH 7.2 for complex of BI and BII respectively. The absorbance of each sample was scanned immediately in the UV region (200–350 nm) against blank reference contains 20% appropriate solvent.

5.3.3.3. Spectrophotometric pH Titration of complex

A Series of complexes from of BI and BII (100µl) were completed to 500µl with buffer at pH ranging from 8 to 12. The absorbance of each sample was measured at 295 nm and the absorbance of λmax at each pH value was plotted versus the corresponding pH. Other series of the same complex (100µl) were completed to 500 µl with buffers ranging from 4 to 8. The maximum absorbance of each sample was measured at 211nm and the absorbance of λmax at each pH values was plotted against the corresponding pH.

5.3.3.4. The Effect of NaCl Concentration on the thermal Stability of the complex by UV spectral studies.

Reagents

Buffers used in thermal stability studies of complex of BI and BII were prepared as follows:-

Twenty percent ethylene glycol buffer was prepared by mixing 20ml of ethylene glycol and 80ml of Tris-buffer pH 6.8. NaCl (0.01M) in 20% ethylene glycol buffer was prepared by dissolving 0.05844 gm of NaCl in 100 ml of 20% ethylene glycol buffer, while NaCl (0.1M) in 20% ethylene glycol buffer was prepared by dissolving 0.5844 gm of NaCl in 100ml of 20% ethylene glycol buffer.

20% Ethylene glycol buffer in Tris buffer pH 7.2 was also prepared and used to prepare (0.01M) NaCl and (0.1M) NaCl solution.

Procedure

One hundred micro litter of complex of BI and BII were completed to final volume 500µl with (0.01M) NaCl in 20% ethylene glycol buffers pH 6.8 and pH 7.2 for complex of BI and BII respectively. Each mixture was placed in 0.5cm cuvette in the sample beam and the buffer at the adjusted pH in the reference beam. The absorption was measured at the wavelength of (292 and 295 nm) at different temperatures 20, 30, 40, 50, 60, 70, 80. The experiment was repeated for each complex with another solution (0.1M NaCl in 20% ethylene glycol) at 292 and 295 nm.

5.3.3.5. The Effect of Urea, KCl and Urea - KCl mixture on the spectrum of the complex.

Reagent

1. Eight molar urea was prepared by dissolving 24.02 gram of urea in the final volume of 50 ml of Tris pH 6.8

2. KCl (0.03M) was prepared by dissolving 0.2737 gram of the salt in the final volume of 50 ml of corresponding buffer.

3. 8M urea and 0.03 M KCl solutions were also prepared using Tris pH 7.2 buffers.

Procedure

One hundred micro liters of complex of BI and BII were pipetted in a set of three tubes. The volume was completed to 500 µl with Tris buffer pH 6.8 for complex of BI and Tris pH 7.2 for complex of BII contains either 0.03M KCl, 8M Urea or mixture 1:1 of both 0.03M KCl and 8M urea respectively. Then each Sample was placed in 0.5cm cuvette in the sample beam and the buffer at the same pH in the presence of the same salt in the reference beam.

The absorption of each sample was scanned immediately in the area of (200 – 350 nm).

5.4. Results and Discussion

5.4.1.Gel Filtration Technique for Separation of Free and Bound 125I-anti CA125 antibody

Figures (5-1 A & B) show the results of gel filtration technique to separate 125I-anti CA125 antibody bound to partially purified CA125 (BI) and (BII) forms respectively. The elution profile in figure (5-1A) revealed two peaks: the first peak with low retention time at fraction number 10 (high molecular weight) represent the complex of partial purified CA125 (BI) with 125I-anti CA125 antibody bound to 125I-antiCA125 antibody, while the second peak at fraction number 19 represents the unbound (free) 125I-anti CA125 antibody. The elution profile in figure (5-1B) also revealed two peaks: the first peak at fraction number 15 represent the complex of partial purified CA125 (BII) bound to 125I-anti CA125 antibody, while the second peak at fraction number 19 represents the unbound (free) 125I-anti CA125 antibody. The elution profile for the label antiCA125antibody is shown in Figure (5-2) in which one peak appeared in the same position of second peak of Figure (5-1A&B) which represents the unbound 125I-antiCA125 antibody. The resultant fractions under the first peak in figures (5-1A) or (5-1B) were collected and pooled.

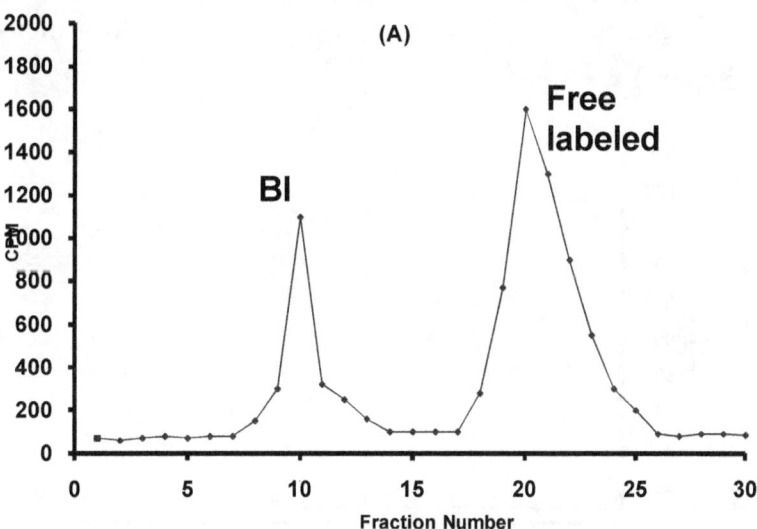

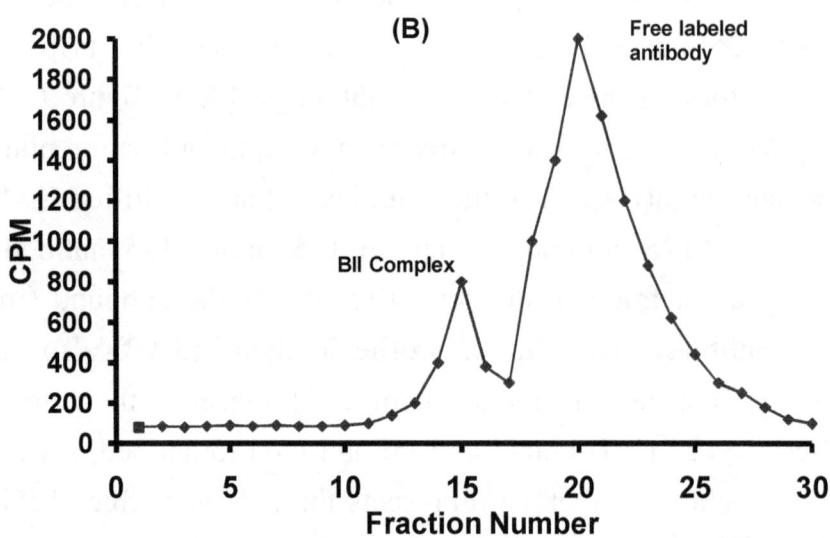

Figure(5-1) The elution profile of the isolated complex (125I-antiCA125 antibody/CA125) and free antibody in

(A) Partially purified CA125 antigen (BI)

(B) Partially purified CA125 antigen (BII)　　　　　　using sepharose CL-6B gel.　　　　　　(All other details are explained in the text)

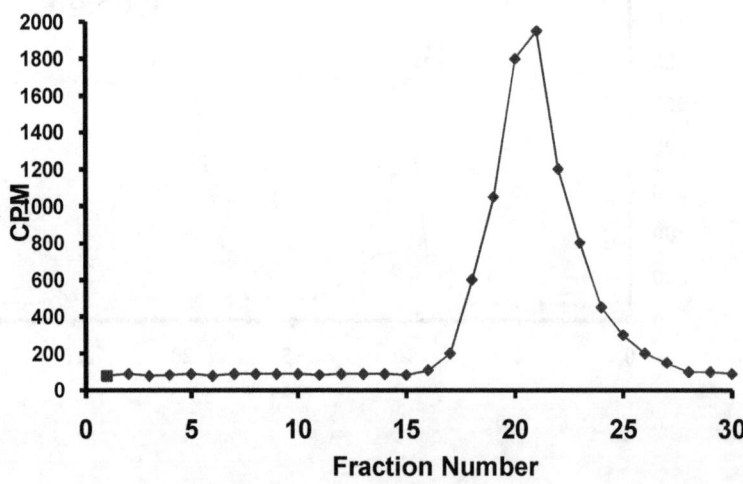

Figure(5-2): The elution profile of free 125I-antiCA125 antibody/ using sepharose CL-6B gel.(All other details are explained in the text).

5.4.2. The UV Spectra of Partially purified CA125, anti CA125 antibody and (125I- antiCA125 antibody/CA125) complex molecules.

The ultraviolet absorption spectra of protein in the regions 250 to 300 nm are contributed from tyrosyl, tryptophan and (to a less extent) phenylalanine residues, but at shorter wavelengths; the contributions come from other groups such as histidyl residues and the peptide bond. The absorbance at lower wave lengths is directly related to the amount of polypeptide material and is usually considerably more sensitive than at 280nm. Absorbance at 215-230nm is useful for monitoring peptides may not contain tryptophan or tyrosine (173).

The UV spectra of partially purified CA125 (BI) and (BII), 125I-antiCA125 antibody and (125I-antiCA125 antibody/CA125) complex were scanned from 200-350nm to determine the absorption spectra and the alteration in the UV spectra as a result of their interaction.

5.4.2.1. The UV Spectrum of Partially Purified CA125.

Figure (5-3) and (5-4) shows the UV spectra of partially purified CA125 (BI) and (BII) respectively. The spectrum of (BI) antigen consisted of two peaks; a large one at 220 nm and smaller at 278nm, while the UV spectrum of BI antigen shows two peaks at 212 and 270nm as shown in table 5-1.

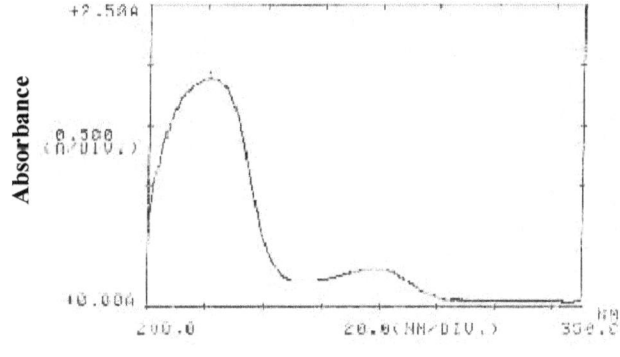

wavelength nm

Figure (5-3): UV Spectrum of partially purified CA125 (BI) (All other details are explained in the text).

313

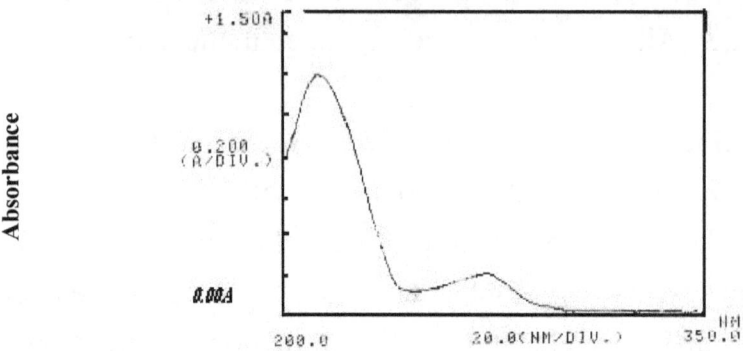

Figure (5-4): UV Spectrum of partially purified CA125 (BII) (All other
wavelength nm
details are explained in the text).

As a result it seemed that each form of CA125 antigen (BI and BII) has a
characteristic spectrum and can be identified by its peaks, the first peak at
(220 or 212 nm) could be due to the amide group in polypeptide bond of
CA125 molecule with contribution of the histidyl residues. While the second
peak (at 278 or 270) is assigned to tyrosyl residue.

5.4.2.2. The UV spectrum of 125I- anti CA125 antibody.

The UV spectrum of 125I-anti CA125 antibody has shown in figure (5-5).
The spectrum consisted of two obvious peaks. The first peak at 225nm is
assigned to the amide groups in the poly peptide bond with contribution of
histidyl residues(173) while the small peak at 278nm is assigned to tyrosyl
residue.

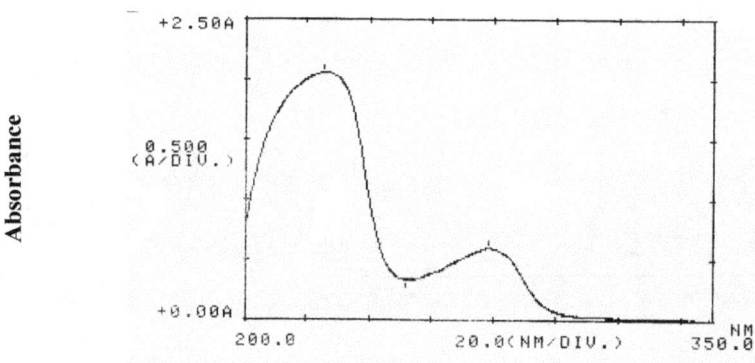

wavelength nm

314

Figure (5-5): UV spectrum of 125I-antiCA125 antibody (All other details are explained in the test).

5.4.2.3. The UV spectrum of (125I-anti CA125 antibody / CA125) complex.

Figure (5-6 and 5-7) shows the spectra of partially purified CA125 antigen (BI) and (BII) bound to 125I-antiCA125 antibody respectively. The spectra of both complexes consisted of one peak at (214 or 208 nm) for the complex of BI and BII of CA125 antigen respectively shown as shown is table (5-1).

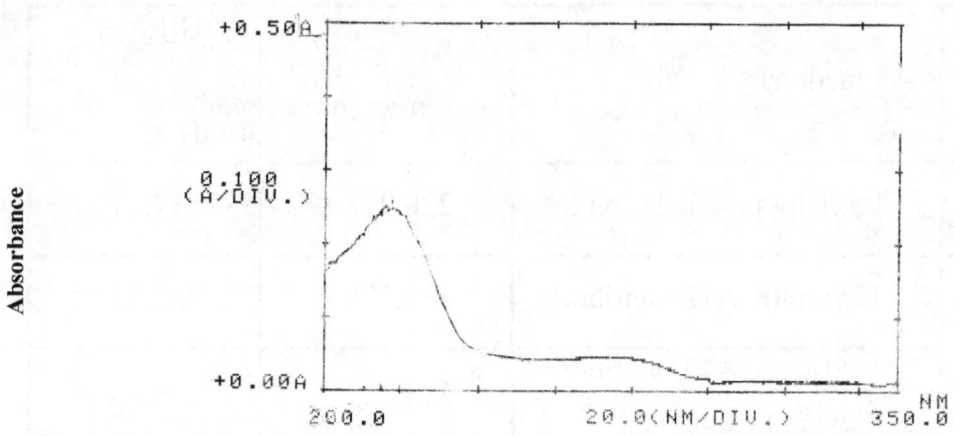

Figure (5-6): UV spectrum of CA125 (BI)/ 125I-antiCA125 antibody complex. (All details are explained in the text).

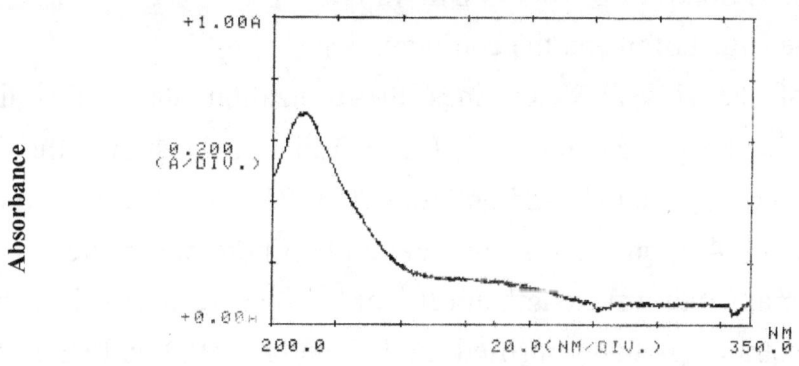

Figure (5-7): UV spectrum of CA125 (BII)/ 125I-antiCA125 antibody complex (All details are explained in the text)
wavelength nm

The strong absorption of these peaks (214 or 208 nm) arises from electronic transition in the peptide backbone itself and is therefore sensitive to backbone conformation (181). There was disappearance of tyrosine peaks in both complexes. These changes are due to fitting of antibody to its antigen to form (125I-Anti CA125 Antibody/CA125) complex. This result is in agreement with Seinerman etal observation who found that the surface of protein interactions was polar as well and the complex formation lead to the burial of charged and polar residues. (182)

Table (5-1): The λ max of (125I-antiCA125 antibody/CA125) Complex, partially purified CA125 and unbound (free) 125I-anti CA125 antibody. (ALL other details are explained in the text).

N o.	Fractions	BI λ max (nm)	BII λ max (nm)
1	Partially purified CA125	220,278	212,270
2	125I-antiCA125 antibody	225,278	225,278
3	125I-antiCA125 antibody /CA125) complex	214	208

5.4.3. Factors Affecting the Absorption Properties of (125I-antiCA125 antibody/CA125) Complex of BI and BII Antigen.

5.4.3.1. The Effect of pH on the complex.

The pH of the solvent determines the ionization state of ionizable chromophore in the protein molecule.(181) Table (5-2) shows the λmax values of isolated (125I-antiCA125 antibody /CA125) complex of BI and BII at different pH (3, 4, 9 and 12). At an acidic pH 3 both complexes of BI or BII have one maximum wavelength at (205 or 202 nm) respectively compare to the UV spactra of partially purified CA125 antigen (BI) and (BII) or the spectra of   125I-anti CA125 antibody.

It seems that in acid region there was a blue shift in λmax from (214 or 2 08 nm) in neutral pH to (205 or 202) in acidic pH for both complexes of (BI) and (BII) respectively. The blue shift is due to the increasing of hydrogen bond formed in the presence of highly positively charged state (183).

When the pH value was increased from neutral to pH 9, there was also only one maximum wavelength found in the spectra of both complexes with the increase in λmax value from (214 or 208) to (223 or 220) for complex of BI and BII respectively. At pH 12 two λmax were obtained for each complex. λmax1 and λmax2 of complex of (BI) were at (225, 284nm) respectively whereas λmax1 and λmax2 of complex of BII were (223, 282nm) respectively.

These results indicate that tyrosine residue in both complexes molecules at neutral pH are located in a way that a small part of it is on the surface of the protein molecule while a large part of these residues is buried but at high pH = 12 the protein becomes denatured (unfolded) and the internal tyrosine has become exposed to the solvent and absorb light. A red shift observed in absorption of these tyrosine residues is certainly related to the ionization of side chain of the tyrosine and this led to the availability of the lone pair on the oxygen atom to happen easier and at lower energy level (red shift).

Table (5-2): The effect of different pH on λ max value of (125I-anti CA125 antibody/CA125) complex. (All details are explained in the text).

| pH | λ max | |
	(125I-antiCA125 antibody / CA125) (BI complex)	(125I-antiCA125 antibody / CA125) (BII complex)
3	205	202
4	212	207
7	214	208
9	224	221
12	225, 284	223, 282

5.4.3.2. The Effect of solvent polarity on the UV spectrum of the complex

The determination of whether an amino acid is internal or external by measuring the spectra of a protein in polar and non- polar solvent is called the solvent perturbation method. In fact, proteins are rarely studied in completely non- polar solvents. However, significant solvent effects can be induced by the use of a mixture of water and substance of a reduced polarity such as ethanol, ethylene glycol, glycerol and dimethylsulfoxide (144).

317

Several spectral changes were obtained in the presence of these perturbants, like the alteration of the peak position and intensities of protein spectrum, and the appearance of new chromophores on the surface of protein molecule. These chromophores were embedded in an interior region of the protein in the absence of the solvent. One of the main assumptions of the solvent perturbation technique is that solvents alter the peak position and intensities by altering the energy and probability of electronic transitions.(184-185) In reality the preferential solvation is caused not only by the perturbant interaction with chromophor itself, but also with the group adjacent to the chromophor in the protein.

Table (5-3) shows the effect of different solvents on the (125I-antiCA125 antibody/CA125) complex of (BI) and (BII) form. It was found that (λmax 214 or 208 nm) shown in previous experiments for complex of BI or BII respectively, was shifted to longer wavelength (red sheft) in the presence of ethanol, ethylene glycol and glycerol at a concentration of (20%). These shifts are attributed to the amide group in polypeptide bond with contribution of histidyl residues inter molecular hydrogen bonding between amide group of polypeptide bond in the complex molecule and the solvent may cause these shifts the intermolecular hydrogen bonding increase as the concentration of the solution increase and additional bands start to appear at longer or shorter wavelength (186). The contribution of histidyl residues in the observed spectra λmax1 is difficult to detect because of the overlapping of its absorbance with that of peptide bond.(176) Table (5-3) shows that the spectrum of both protein complexes are is sensitive to change in the polarity of the solvent which may indicate that high percent of histidine residues is located on the surface of the protein molecule.

In the presence of DMSO (20%) there was an increase in λmax1 from (214 or 208) to 242 nm for both complexes and new λmax at (284, 282 nm) appeared which belongs to complexes of BI and BII respectively. The new peaks are related to tyrosyl residues. The appearance of λmax of tyrosine residue is related to the perturbing solvent which makes the possibility for the presence of this residue to the surface of the protein structure.

Table 5-3: The effect of solvent polarity on λ max of (125I-antiCA125 antibody / CA125) complex

(All other details are explained in the text)

Solvent 20% of	(125I-antiCA125 antibody/CA125) (BI)		(125I-antiCA125 antibody/CA125) (BII)	
	λ max1	λ max2	λ max1	λ max2
Ethanol	222	-	219	-
Ethylen glycol	217	-	215	-
Glycerol	223	-	221	-
DMSO	242	284	242	282

5.4.3.3. Spectrophotometric pH Titration of the Complex.

Spectrophotometric pH titration is the following of the changes in absorbance of the chromofor with increasing pH (144). Many studies of protein structure require the determination of Pka values for protein dissociation from ionizable amino acid side chains, because these values give an indication of the location of the amino acid in the protein. This can often be done spectrophotometricaly because dissociation often changes the spectrum of one of the chromophores, the observation of tyrosine dissociation was performed by measuring the absorption at 295 nm (λmax for the ionized form of tyrosine), and the observation of histidine dissociation was carried out by measuring the absorption at 211 nm

The titration curve of (125I-antiCA125 antibody/CA125) complex of (BI) and (BII) for both tyrosyl and histidyl residues are illustrated in figure (5-8 A&B) respectively. Figure (5-8A) shows that the Pka for tyrosine is 11.4 for (125I-Anti CA125 Antibody / CA125) complex of (BI), while the Pka for tyrosine is 11.2 for (125I-antiCA125 antibody / CA125) complex of (BII) form. From the same curves it could be concluded that about (36.8%) and (25%) of tyrosyl residues are located on the surface of protein complex of BI and BII respectively. The other residues are buried interiorly in a polar environment of protein complex of both forms of CA125 antigen. A large arise in the absorbance was observed at high pH because protein complexes become denatured.

Figure (5-8B) shows that Pka values of histidine residues in complex from BI and BII antigen are (6.5) and (7.2) respectively. Also from these curves it was found that (80%) histidyl residues are located on the surface of the complex of BI antigen, while (60%) located on the surface of the complex of BII antigen. the other histidine residues are buried interior the protein complex of both antigens.

These results are in agreement with those found in solvent perturbation experiment in section (5.4.3.2.) for the percent of histidine residue on the surface of protein complex molecule.

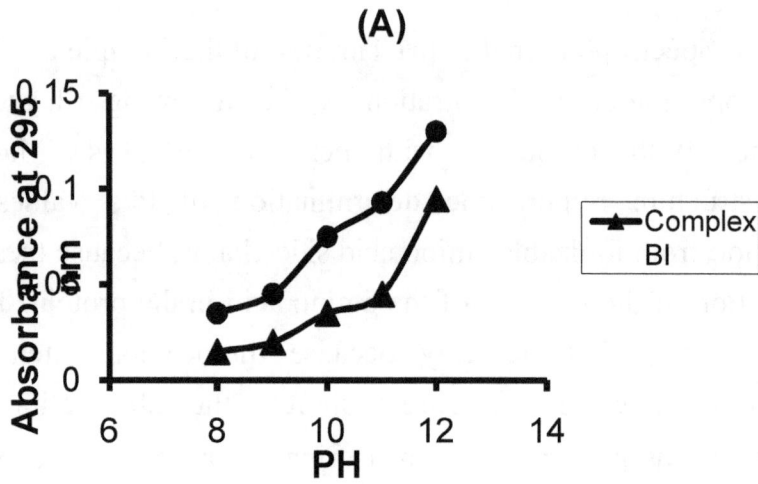

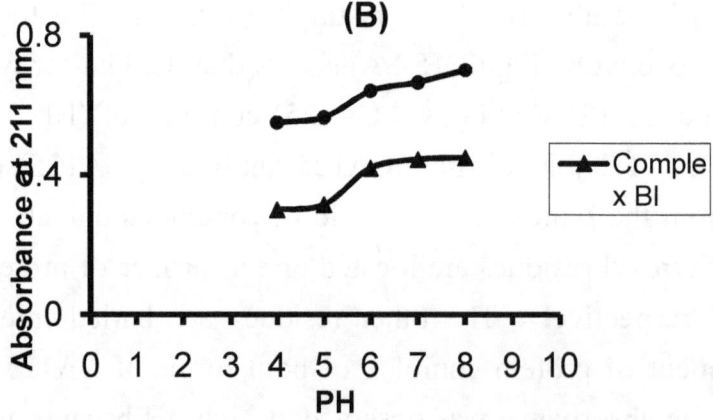

Figure (5-8): Spectrophotometric pH titration of (125I-antiCA125 antibody/CA125) complex from BI and BII antigen.

A=for tyrosine, (B) for Histidine.

(All other details are explained in the text).

5.4.3.4. The effect of NaCl concentration on the thermal stability of the complex by UV spectral studies.

The effect of the different concentration of NaCl on the thermal stability of (125I-antiCA125 antibody/CA125) complex of BI and BII of partially purified CA125 antigen was examined in this experiment. The values of absorbance at λmax (292, 295 nm) for tryptophyl and tyrosyl residues respectively, in two different concentrations of NaCl 0.01 M and 0.1 M in 20% ethylene glycol buffer are shown in figure (5-9A&B) and (5-10A&B).

As shown in figure (5-9A&B) the internal tryptophane and tyrosine are completely exposed to the solvent at 60°C in the presence of 0.01 M NaCl in both complexes of BI and BII. The increment in the absorbance of both tryptophyl and tyrosine residues with increasing temperature could be due to those buried chromophores becomes exposed to the solvent during thermal denaturation (187).

Figure (5-10 A&B) shows that in presence of 0.1 M NaCl, the absorbance of both tryptophan and tyrosine reach higher value at 70°C for both complexes of (BI) and (BI), therefore higher concentration of NaCl causes more stabilization for protein complex .

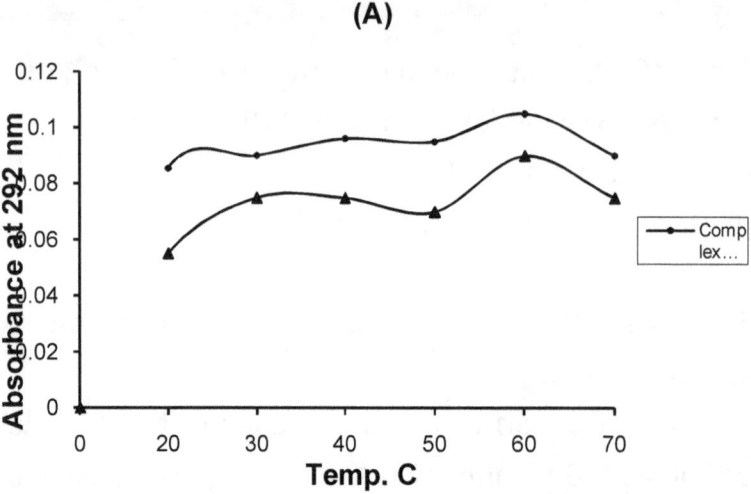

(A)

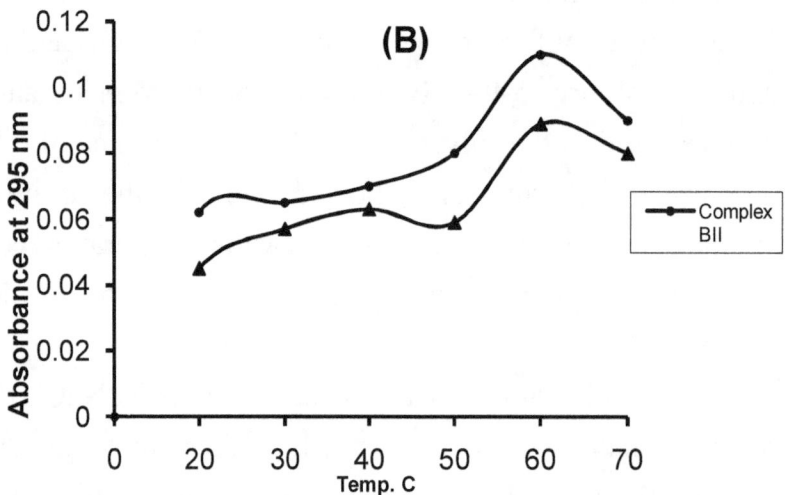

(B)

Figure (5-9): Thermal stability curve for complex of BI and BII

(A) at λmax 292 in presence of 0.01M NaCl,

(B) at λmax 295 in the presence of 0.01M NaCl.

(All other details are explained in the text).

The decrease of the absorbance in presence of 0.1M NaCl as compared with that in 0.01M NaCl could be due to salt concentration. Each protein in solution containing salts will collect around it a counter ion atmosphere enriched in oppositely charged small ion, (chloride ion and sodium ion), and such a cloud of ions will tend to screen the protein, the larger the

322

concentration of small ion present, the more effective this electrostatic screening will be, and decrement in the absorption intensity will be observed (181).

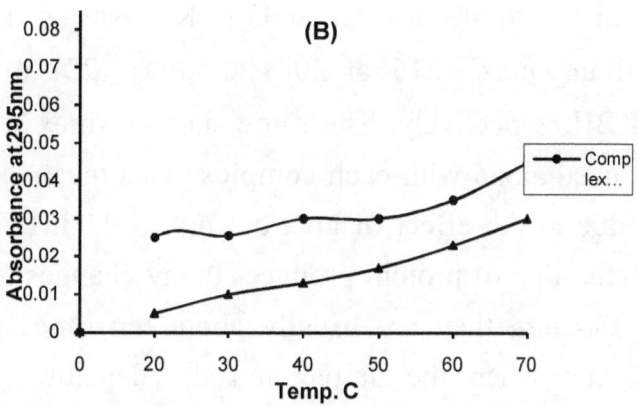

Figure (5-10 A&B): Thermal stability curve for complex of BI and BII:

(A) at λmax 292 in presence of 0.1M NaCl,

(B) at λmax 295 in presence of 0.1M NaCl.

(All other details are explained in the text).

5.4.3.5. Effect of Urea, KCl and (Urea- KCl) Mixture on the Spectrum of the Complex

Table (5-4) shows the effect of 8M urea, 0.03M KCl and a mixture of 1:1 of 8 M urea and 0.03 M KCl on λmax of the complexes of both forms of partially purified CA125 antigen. Comparing the values of λmax of these molecules obtained in the absence of urea or KCl (table 5-1) with those obtained in the presence of 8M urea in table (5-4), it seems that there was a significant red shift in λmax1 of poly peptide bond from (215 or 208nm) to λmax (223 or 221 nm) for complex from BI and BII antigen respectively. While there is no λmax2 peak assign for aromatic amino acid, i.e. tyrosine residue in both complexes. These results indicate that the molecule solvated with urea (dipole –dipole interaction) and produce a red - shift and new chromofore come to the surface .The red shift is due to the intermolecular hydrogen bonding between the oxygen of the amide group and the solvent (176). When 0.03M KCl was used, there was a slight blue shift (3-1nm) in λmax1 of polypeptide bond in the complex of BI and BII antigen respectively such blue shift can arise by introducing positive (K^+) or negative (Cl^-) charges near the chromophore (the amide group, which might interact with π – electron system of the amide group (174).

When a mixture of 1: 1 of 8M urea and 0.03 M KCl was used, there was a significant red shift in λmax, (215 or 208) to λmax (221 or 218nm) in complex of BI and BII respectively. The same shift in λmax was observed when 8M urea was used alone with each complex. This means that the shift caused by mixture due to the effect of urea but not to 0.03M KCl. Solvent perturbation or denaturation of protein produces many changes in absorption near 230 nm and 280 nm, they are usually about ten times greater near 230nm than at 280nm when the native and the denatured protein are compared. (2) Some of these changes in absorption may be produced by the change in $n – \pi^*$ absorption of poly peptide bond in protein either because of a change in their geometrical arrangement or because of environment changes (181).

Table (5-4): The effect of 8M Urea, 0.03M KCl and mixture (Urea-KCl) on the λ max of complex UV spectrum (All other details are explained in the text).

Solvent	λmax (nm)	
	complex of BI	complex of BII
Urea 8M	223	221
KCl 0.03M	211	207
Urea-KCl Mixture 1:1	221	218

Conclusions

Out of the results obtained in this work we can conclude the following:

1. CA125 is more specific tumor marker for ovarian malignancy than CEA. A higher ratio of CA125 to CEA could be used to differentiate ovarian from non ovarian malignant diseases when both sera contain increased CA125 concentration.

2. The modified protocol for the assay of CA125 is suitable for the assessment of CA125 in the tissues of ovarian tumor homogenates.

3. Partial purification of CA125 showed two forms (BI) with 670 kDa molecular weight and (BII) with 100 kDa molecular weight.

4. The kinetic studies of 125I-antiCA125 antibody with CA125 of benign and malignant ovarian tumor tissues and with partially purified CA125 of malignant post-menopausal ovarian tumor tissues revealed that the binding reactions are time and temperature dependent. The binding data fits the second order reaction kinetics at (5, 20, 37 and 45 °C) in all cases.

5. Thermodynamic studies for the binding reaction of 125I-antiCA125 antibody with CA125 in benign and malignant ovarian tumor tissues and with partially purified CA125 of malignant post-menopausal ovarian tumor tissues, revealed that the binding reactions were exothermic ($\Delta H° < 0$) and spontaneous ($\Delta G° < 0$) and the binding reactions were entropically and enthalipically driven ($\Delta S° > 0$) and ($\Delta H° < 0$).

6. The spectroscopic studies revealed that partially purified forms of CA125 and their complexes with 125I-antiCA125 antibody have characteristic spectra and give an idea of the location of particular amino acids in (125I-antiCA125 antibody/CA125) complex molecules.

Future work

According to the results obtained in this work, the following works are suggested for the future:

1.   Manufacturing of IRMA kit, using the optimum conditions concluded out of this study's results, to determine CA125 in ovarian tumor tissues.

2.   Application of the modified IRMA method for the assessment of CA125 in other tissues such as lung and pancreas.

3.   Assessment of new markers adjuvant to CA125 to be used for early diagnosis and follow up of the patients with ovarian cancer.

4.   Additional works are needed for farther purification of partially purified CA125 from ovarian tissues using high performance liquid chromatography (HPLC) based on affinity chromatography or ion-exchange technique. Then using the purified CA125 antigen to produce specific antiCA125 antibody and   125I-CA125 tracer.

5.   Development of radioreceptor-assay protocol to determine the receptors of CA125 in ovarian tissues, then molecular characterization of these receptors.

References

1. White A, Handler PH, and Smith E. Principles of Biochemistry; 5th Ed; Mc Gray-Hill. 1972; pp.812.

2. Ablev GI. Alpha-feto protein in ontogenesis and its association with malignant tumors. Adv Cancer Res 1971; 14:292.

3. Gold P, and Freeman SO .Demonstration of tumor –specific antigen in human colonic carcinoma by immunological tolerance absorption technique J Exp Med 1965; 121:439-450.

4. Kohler G, and Milstein. Continuous cultures of fused cells secreting antibody of predefined specificity Nature 1975; 257(5517):495-497.

5. Kreuzer H and Massay A. Recombinant DNA and Biotechnology; ASM press comp, USA, 1996, chapter 24, pp. 190-198.

6. Hayes DF, Bast R, Desch CE, Fritsche H, Kemeny NE, et al . A tumor marker utility grading system (TMUGS). A framework to evaluate clinical utility of tumor markers. Nati Cancer Inst 1996; 88:1456.

7. Bates S E and Longo D L .Use of serum tumor markers in cancer diagnosis and management. Semin Oncol. 1987(2)102.

8. Stearns V, Yamauchi H, and Hayes DF. Circulating tumor markers in breast cancer: Accepted utility and novel prospects. Breast Cancer Research and treatment. 1998; 52:239-259.

9. Costa J, and Cordon CC. Cancer Diagnosis: Molecular Pathology; in: cancer principles and practice of oncology; 6th ed.; De Vita V.T., Hellman S., Rosenberg Eds. Lippincott Williams and Wilkins. 2001; pp.641-657.

10.Anderson SC, and Cockayne S. Clinical Chemistry; concepts and applications; An HB. Jint .ed; Philadelphia; W.B. Saunders company; 1993; chapter 16, pp.322-330.

11.Moossa AR, Schempff SC, and Robson MC. Comprehensive Textbook of Oncology; 2nd ed.; Eds. Baltimopre, Williams & Wilkins, 1991; pp.225-238.

12.Haber D and Fearon E. The promise of cancer genetics. Lancet, 1998; 351:SII1.

13.Orr-weaver TL and Weinberg RA. A checkpoint on the road to cancer. Nature 1998; 392:223-224.

14.Brown JM, and Wouters BG. Apoptosis, p53 and tumor cell sensitivity to anticancer antigen. Cancer Res 1999; 59: 1391-1399.

15.Kastan MB, Onyekwere O, Sidransky D, Vogelstein B, and Graig RW. Participation of p53 in the cellular response to DNA damage. Cancer Res.; 1991; 51: 6304.

16.Wu J. Diagnosis and management of cancer using serologic tumor markers. In; Clinical Diagnosis and Management by Laboratory Methods; 20th ed.; J.B. Henry Ed. W.B. Saunders Company; 2001; pp.1028-1042.

17.David W. Immunoassay Hand Book; 2nd ed.; U.K. Nature Publishing Group, 2001; chapter 63, pp.635-662.

18.Zurawski VR, Broderick SF, Pickens P, et al. CA125 levels in group of non hosptalised women: relevance for the early detection of ovarian cancer. Obstet Gynecol 1987; 69:606-611.

19.European Group of Tumor Markers (EGTM). http://www.med.uni.muenchen.de/egtm/detail/4.htm .

20.Thomas j, Nowak A, and Gordon H. Essential of Pathophysiology; 2nd ed. WcB Mc Graw-Hill; 1999; pp. 501-504.

21.Eric V Mackay, Norman A Beischer, Lloyd W Cox, and Carl wood. Illustrated text book of Gynecology; W.B. Saunders Company 1983, p. 282.

22. Cotran RC, Kumor V, and Collins T. Robbins Pathologic Basis of Disease; 6th ed.; WB Saunders Company; 1999; pp.1068-1069.

23. Carol Mattson Porth; Pathophysiology; 4th ed.; J. B. Lippincott company Philadelphia; 1994, p.749.

24.Fuys Woodruff J D; Pathology: Practical Gynecologic Oncology; 2nd ed.; Williams and Wilkins Company; 1995; p.1079.

25.Kristensen GB and Trope C. Epithelial ovarian carcinoma. Lancet 1997; 349:113-117.

26. Scott JR, Disaia PJ, Hammond CB, and Spellacy WN. Danforth's Obstetrics and Gynecology; 8th ed.,; Lippincott Williams & Willkins ; 1999; pp 678-695.

27.Rosa J. Ackerman's Surgical Pathology; 8th ed. Atimes Mirror Company; 1996; p1474.

28.Caroline Van Haaften and Cinda M Boyer. Epithelial ovarian tumors in the reproductive age group: Age is not an independent prognostic factore. Cancer 1996; 77: 1131.

29.Karlan BY and Platt LD. The current status of ultrasound and color Doppler imaging in screening for ovarian cancer .Gynecol Oncol. 1994;

55:528

30. Charles R Whitefield; Dewhurst's text Book of Obstetrics and Gynecology; 5th ed.; Black well science; 1995; PP.759-774.

31. Tiernery JR, Mcphee SJ, and Oapadakis Mia.; Current Medical Diagnosis & Treatment; 38th ed.; Appelton & Lange; 1999; P. 718.

32. Parkin DM, Whelan SL, Ferlay J, Raymond L, and Young J. Cancer incidence in five continents; vol VII Lyon: International Agency for Research on cancer 1997 (IARC scientific Publication No. 143).

33. Greenlee RT, Hill-Harmon MB, Murray T, and Thun M. Cancer statistics. CA Cancer J. Clin 2001; 51:15.

34. Iraqi cancer registry 1995-1997.

35. Piver MS, Baker TR, Piedmote M, and Sandecki AM .Epidemiology and etiology of ovarian cancer. Seminars in Oncology 1991; 18 (3): 177-185.

36. Kerlikowske K, Brown JS, and Grady DG. Should women with familial ovarian cancer undergo prophylactic oophorectomy? Obstet Gynecol; 1992; 80:700.

37. Serova O, Montagna M, Torchard D, et al. A high incidence of BRAC1 mutations in 20 breast-ovarian cancer families. Am J. Hum. Genet; 1996; 58:42

38. Wooster R, Bignell G, Lancaster J et al. Identification of breast cancer susceptibility gene BRAC2. Nature 1995; 378: 789.

39. Gillis CR, Hole DJ, still RM, Davis J, and Kaye SB. Medical audit, cancer registration and survival in ovarian cancar. Lancet 991; 337: 611-612.

40. Yancik R, Ries LG, and Yates JW. An analysis of surveillance, epidemiology, and end results program data. Is J Obstet Gynecol 1966; 154:636-47?

41. Whittermore AS, Harris R, and Itnyre J. Characteristics relating to ovarian cancer risk: Collaborative analysis of twelveU.S.case-controlstudics .II Invasive epithelial ovarian cancers in white women. Am. J. Epidemiol 1992; 136: 1184.

42. Gross TP and Schlesselman JJ. The estimated effect of oral contraceptive use on the cumulative risk of epithelial ovarian cancer. Obstet Gynecl 1994; 83:419.

43. Risch HA, Marrett LD, and Howe GR. Parity, contraception, infertility and risk of epithelial ovarian cancer. Am. J Epidemiol 1994; 140: 585-97.

44.Daniel L, Clarke-Pearson M, and Yousif D. Green's Gynecology: Essentials of Clinical Practice; 4th ed., Little, Brown Company; 1990; pp. 531-541.

45.Wong C, Hempling RE, Piver MS, et al. Perineal Talc exposure and subsequent epithelial ovarian cancer: A case control study. Obstet Gynecol 1999; 93:372.

46.Bristow RE and karlan BY. Ovulation induction, infertility, and ovarian cancer risk. Fertil steril 1996; 66:499.

47.Rodrigue ZC, Tatham LM, Calle EE, et al. Infertility and risk of fetal ovarien cancer in a prospective cohort of U.S. women Cancer control .Cancer Causes Control ; 1998 ;9 :645.

48.Rossing MA, Daling JR, Weiss NS, et al .Ovarian tumor in a cohort of inferite women. N Engl J Med. 1994; 331: 771.

49."General Information about Ovarian Epithelial Cancer" NCl Cancer. Gov. web site (Http://www.cancer.gov.).

50.Smith LH and Oi RH. Detection of malignant ovarian neoplasm's: A review of the literature I. Detection of the patient at risk, clinical, radiological and cytological detection. Obstet Gynecol Surv.; 1984; 39:313.

51.Pollock RE.   Manual of Clinical Oncology; 7th ed.; Wiley. Liss, Inc.; 1999; p.542.

52.Campbell S, Bhan V, Royston P, et al. Transabdominal ultrasound screening for early ovarian cancer. BNJ 1989; 299:1363.

53.Bast RC, Klug TL, St John E, Jenison E, Niloff JM, Lazarus H, Berkowitz RS, Leavitt T, Griffiths CT, parker L, zurawski VR, and knapp RC . A radioimmunoassay using a monoclonal antibody to monitor the course of epithelial ovarian cancer.   N Eng J Med 1983; 309:883-887.

54.Schwartz PE, and Taylor Kjw. Ovarian Cancer: Epidemiological perspectives with Developments in Early Diagnosis; the Parthenon publishing group New York; 1994, p. 257.

55.James B, Wyngaarden Lloyd H, and smith JR, Claude Bennett Cecil: textbook of Medicine. 20th ed.; W.B. Saunders Company; 1996; pp. 1021-1022.

56.Celluzzi CM, Mayordomo CI, Storkns WJ, Lotze MT, and Falo LD. Peptide-pulsed dentritic cells induce antigen-specific CTL-mediated protective tumor immunity. J Exp Med 1996; 183:283.

57.Kawashima I, Hudson SJ, Tsai V, Southwood S, Takesako K, Appella E, Sette A, and Celis E. The multiepitope approach for immunotherapy for cancer: identification of several ETL epitopes from various tumor associated antigens expressed on solid epithelial tumors. Hum Immunol 1998; 59:1.

58.Vogle FD, Strickeler E, Weyermann M, Kohler T, Gill H, Negri G, kreienberg R, and Runnebaum IB . p53 auto antibodies in patients with primary ovarian cancer are associated with higher age, advanced stage and higher proportion of a p53-posative tumor cell. Oncology; 1999; 57:324.

59.Vikhanskaya F, D'Incalci, and Broggini M. p73 competes with p53 and attenuates its response in a human ovarian cancer cell line. Nucleic Acid Res 2000; 28: 513.

60.Werness BA, Freedman A, Piver MS, Romero-Gutierrez M, and petrow E. Prognostic significance of p53 and p21 (waf1/cip1) immunoreactivity in epithelial cancer of the ovary. Gynecol Oncol 1999; 75:413.

61.Presneau N, Laplace-Marieze V, sylvain V, Lortholary A, Hardouin A, Bernard- Gallon D, and Bignon Y. New mechanism of BRAC1 mutation by deletion / insertion at the same nucleotide position in three unrelated fresh breast cancer. Hum. Genet 1998; 103:334.

62.Lancaster JM, Garney M, and Futreal PA. BRAC1 and 2: A genetic like to familial beast and ovarian cancer. Medscape women's Health 1997; 2:7.

63.Woolas RP, xu FG, Jacobs IJ, Yu YH, Daly L, Berchuck A, Soper JT, Clarke- pearson DL Oram DH, and Bast RC. Elevation of multiple serum markers in patients with stage I ovarian cancer. J Natl Cancer Inst 1993; 85:1748.

64.kufe D, Inghirami G, Abe M, Hayes D, Justi-wheeler H, and schlom J. Differential reactivity of a novel monoclonal antibody (DF3) with human malignant versus benign breast tumors . Hybridoma 1984; 3:223.

65.Mckenzie SJ, Desombre KA, Bast BS, Hollis DR, Whitaker RS, Berchuck A, Boyer C M, and Bast RC. Serum levels of HER-2 neu(C-erbB-2) correlate with over expression of p158 neu in human ovarian cancer. Cancer 1993; 71:3942.

66.Hancock MC, langton BC, Chan T, Toy P Monahan JJ, Mischak RP, and Shawver L K. A monoclonal antibody against the c-erbB-2 portion enhances the cytotoxicity of cis-diaminedichloro-platinum against human breast and ovarian tumor cell lines. Cancer Res 1991; 51:4575.

67.Alexander WK and William RH. Ovarian papillary serous tumors of low malignant potential (serous borderline tumors). A long term follow-up study, including patients with micro invasion, lymph node metastatasis, and transformation to invasive serous carcinoma. Cancer 1996; 78:278.

68. Thigpen JT, Lambuth BW, and Vance RB. Management of stage I and II ovarian cancer. Semin Oncol 1991; 18:596.

69.Kristensen GB and Trope C. Epithelial ovarian carcinoma. Lancet 1997; 349:113-117.

70.Kumar P, Rehani MM, Kumar L, Sharma R, Bhatla N, Chaudharg R, Thulkar S, Sunderam KR, and Kumar N. Tumor marker CA125 as an evaluator and response indicator in ovarian cancer : its quantitative correlation with tumor volume. Med Sci Monit 2005; 11: CR 84.

71.Colakovic S, Lukic V, Mitrovic L, Jelic S, Susnjer S, ,and Marinkovic J. Prognostic value of CA125 kinetics and half time in advanced ovarian cancer . Int J Biol. Marker 2000; 15:147-152.

72.Hempling RE, Piver MS, Natarajan N, Baker TR, Thompson JM, Hicks ML, and Metlin CJ. Predictive value of serum CA125 following optimal cytoreductive surgery during weekly cisplatin induction therapy for advanced ovarian cancer.   J of Surg Onco 1993; 54:38-44.

73.Jacobs IJ and Bast RC. The CA125 tumor –associated antigen: a review of the literature. Human Reproduction; 1989; 4:pp.1-12.

74.Backston T, Mahlck CA, and Kjellgrea O. Progesterone as a possible tumor marker for nonendocrine ovarian malignant tumors. Gynecol Oncol 1983; 16:129.

75.Heinnon PK, Tuimala R, Pyy KK, and Pystyam P. Human placental alkaline phosphatase in benign and malignant ovarian neoplasia. Br J Obstst & Gynecol 1982; 89:84.

76.Tholander B, Taube A, Lingew A, sjoberg O, Stendahi U, and Tamsen L. Pretreatment serum level of CA125, CEA, tissue polypeptide antigen and placental alkaline phosphatase in patient with ovarian carcinoma. Gynecol Oncol 190; 39:26-33.

77.Shabana A, Onsrud M. Tissue polypeptide-specific antigen and CA125 as serum tumor markers in ovarian carcinoma. Tumor Biol 1994; 15:361.

78.John R, Van Nagell JR, Pletsch A, and Goldenberg M. A study of cyst fluid and plasma carcinoembrionic antigen in patients with cystic ovarian neoplasm's. Cancer Res 1975; 35:1433-1437.

79.Negishi Y, Iwabuchi H, Sakunaga H, et al. Serum and tissue measurement of CA72-4 in ovarian cancer patients. Gyncol Oncol 1993; 48:149-54.

80.Berek JS and Martinez-Maza O. Molecular and biological factors in the pathogenesis of ovarian cancer. J Reprod Med 1994; 39:241-248.

81.Schwartz FE, Chambers SK, Chambers JT, Gutman J, Katopodis N, and   Foemmel R. Circulating tumor markers in the monitoring of gynecological malignancies Cancer 1987; 60:353-61.

82.Berek JS, and Bust RC. Ovarian cancer screening "the use of serial complementary tumor markers to improve sensitivity and specificity for early detection" Cancer 1995; 76:2092-96.

83. Hanisch FG, and Dienst C. CA125 and CA19-9: two cancer associated sialylsaccharide antigens on a mucus glycoprotein from human milk. Eur J Biochem 1985; 149:323-330.

84.Sekine H, Ohno Tand Kufe DW. Purification and characterization of a high molecular weight glycoprotein detected in human milk and breast carcinomas. J Immunol 1985; 135:3610-3615.

85. Shimizu M, and Yamauchi K. Isolation and characterization of mucn like glycoprotein in human milk fat globule membrane. J Biochem 1982; 91: 515-524.

86.Tsubura A, Morii S, Vdea S, Sasaki M, Zother S , Waltzing V, Mooi W, Hageman PC, Hilkens J, and Tweel JV. Immunohistochemical demonstration of MAM-3 and MAM-6 antigen in normal human skin and their tumors. Arch Dermatol Res. 1987; 279:550-557.

87. Sekin H, Hayes DF, Ohno T, et al. Circulating DF3 and CA125 antigen levels from patients with epithelial ovarian carcinoma. J Clin Oncol 1985; 3:1355-63.

88.Harbest AL. The epidemiology of ovarian carcinoma and the current status of tumor markers to detect disease. J Obstet Gynecol 1994; 170:1099-107.

89.Berek JS, Chung C, kaldi K, Watson JM, Knox RM, and Martinez Maza O. Serum interleukin-6 levels correlate with disease status in patients with epithelial ovarian cancer. J Obstet Gynecol 1991; 164:1038-43.

90.Gotlib WH, Abrams JS, Watson JM, Velu T, Martine Z, Mazo O, and Berek JS. Presence of interleukin 10 (IL 10) in the ascites of patients with ovarian and other intra abdominal cancer. Cytokine 1992; 4:385-90.

91. Ramakrishhan S, Xu FJ, Brandt SJ, Niedel JF, Bast RC, and Brown EL .Constitutive production of macrophage colony-stimulating factor by human ovarian and breast cancer cell lines. J Clin invest 1989;83:921-926.

92.Xu FJ, Ramakrishhan S, Daly L, Soper JT, Berchuck A, Clarke PD, et al. Increased serum levels of macrophage colony stimulating factor in ovarian cancer. Is J Obstet Gynecol 1991; 165:1356-62?

93.Xu FJ, Yu YH, Daly L, Desombre K, Anselmino L, Hass GM, et al. The OVX1 radioimmunoassay complements CA125 for predicting the presence of residual carcinoma at second-look surgical surveillance procedures. J Clin Oncol 1993; 11:1506-11.

94.Knauf S, Anderson DJ, Knapp RC, and Bast RC. A study of NB/70K and CA125 monoclonal antibody radioimmunoassay for measuring serum. Am J Obstet Gynecol 1985; 152(7):911-913.

95.Schwartz PE, Chaambers JT, Taylor KJ, et al. Early detection of ovarian cancer: preliminary results of the Yale Early Detection Program Yale. J Biol Med 1991; 64:573-82.

96. Soper JT, Hunter VJ. Daly L, Tanner M, Creasman W, and Bast RC. Preoperative serum tumor-associated antigen levels in women with pelvic masses. Obstet Gynecol 1990; 75:249.

97.Davis HM, Zurawski VR, Bast RC, and Klug TE. Characterization of the CA125 antigen associated with human epithelial ovarian carcinomas. Cancer Res 1986; 46:6143-6148.

98.Nagata A, Hirota N, Sakai T, Fujimoto M, and Komoda T. Molecular nature and possible presence of a membranous glycophosphatidylinositol anchor of CA125 antigen. Tumor Biol 1991; 12:279.

99. Bast RC, Boyer JI, Xuf J, Wiener J, Kohler M, and Berckuck A. Cell growth regulation in epithelial ovarian cancer. Cancer 1993; 71:1597-1601.

100. O'Brien TJ, Beard JB, Underwood LJ, and Shigemasa K. The CA125 gene: A new discovered extension of the glycosylated N-terminal domine doubles to size of this extracellular superstructure. Tumor Biol 2002;

23: 154-169.

101.   O'Brien TJ, Beard JB, Underwood LJ, Dennis RA, Santin AD, and York L. The CA125 gene: an extacllular superstructure dominated by erepear sequences. Tumor Biol 2001; 22:348-366.

102.   Kui Wong N, Easton RL, Panico M, Sutton Smith M, Morrison JC, Lattanzio FA, Morris HR, Clark GF, Dell A, and Patankar MS. Characterization of the oligosaccharides associated with the human ovarian tumor marker CA125.   J Biol Chem 2003; 278: 28619-28634.

103.   Yin BW and Lloyd KO. Molecular cloning of the CA125 ovarian cancer antigen identification as a new mucin, MUC16.   J Biol Chem 2001; 276, 27371-27375.

104.   Wreschner DH, McGuckin MA, Williams SJ, Baruch A, Yoeli M, Ziv R, Okun L, ZareTsky J, Smorodinsky N, Keydar I, Neophytou P, Stacey M, Lin HH, and Gordon S. Generation of ligand-receptor alliances by "SEA" model-mediated cleavage of membrane-associated mucin proteins. Protein Sci 2002; 11:698-706.

105.   Hardardottir H, Parmely TH, Quirk JG, Sanders MM, Miller FC, and   O' Brien TJ. Distribution of CA125 in embryonic tissue and adult derivation of the fetal periderm.   J Obstet Gynecol 1990; 163:1925-1931.

106.   Fukuda M, Roles of mucin-type O-glycans in cell adhesion. Biochim Biophys Acta 2002; 1573:394-405.

107.   Bresalier RS, Byrd J, Wang L, and Raz A. Colon cancer mucin: A new ligand for the beta-galactoside binding protein galactin-3. Cancer Res 1996; 56: 4354-4357.

108.   Seelenmeyer C, Wegehingel S, Lechner J, and Nickel W. The cancer antigen CA125 represents a novel counter receptor for galactine-1. J Cell Science 2003; 116:1305-1318.

109.   Perillo NL, Marcus ME and Baum LG. Galectins: versatile modulators of cell adhesion, cell proliferation, and cell death. J Mol Med 1998; 76: 402-412.

110.   Gaetje R, Winnekendonk DW, Scharl A, and Kaufmann M. Ovarian cancer antigen CA125 enhances the invasiveness of the endometriotic cell line EEC145. J Soc Gynecol Investig 1999; 6: 278-281.

111.   Rump A, Morikawa Y, Tanaka M, Minami S, Umesaki N,

Takeuchi M, and Miyajima A. Binding of ovarian cancer antigen CA125/MUC16 to mesothelin mediates cell adhesion. J Biol Chem 2004; 279(10): 9190-9198.

112. Hassan R, Bera T, and Pastan I. Mesothelin: A new target for immunotherapy. Clin cancer Res 2004; 3937-3942.

113. Bast RC, Siegal FP, Runowiecz C, Klug TL, and Knapp RC. Elevation of serum CA125 prior to diagnosing of an epithelial ovarian carcinoma. Gynecol Oncol 1985; 22:115-120.

114. Bon GG, Kenemans P, Verstraeten R, Van kamp GJ and Hilgers J. Serum tumor marker immunoassay in gynecologic oncology : establishment of reference values. J Obstet Gynecol 1996 174:107-114.

115. Lloyd KO and Yin BW. Synthesis and secretion of the ovarian cancer antigen CA125 by the human cancer cell line NIH: OVCAR-3. Tumor Biol 2001; 22: 77-82

116. Meyer T, and Rustin GJ. Role of tumor markers in monitoring epithelial ovarian cancer. Br J Cancer 2000; 82:1535-1538.

117. Bast RC, Feeney M, Lazarus H, Nadler LM, Colvin RB, and Knapp RC. Reactivity of monoclonal antibody with human ovarian carcinoma. J Clin Invest 1981; 68: 1331-1337.

118. Nustad, et al. Specificity and affinity of 26 monoclonal antibodies against the CA125 antigen: first report from the ISOBM TD-1 workshop. Tumer Biol 1996; 17:196-219.

119. Lehtovirta P, Apter D, and Stenman VH. Serum CA125 levels during the menstrual cycle. Br J Obstet Gynecol. 1999; 97: 930-933.

120. Bonfrer JMG, Korse CM, Verstraeten RA, Van Kamp GJ, Hart AAM, and Kenemans. Clinical evaluation of the BYK LIA-mat CA125 II assay: Discussion of a reference value. Clin Chem 1997; 43: 491-497.

121. Guadagni F, Marth CH, Zeimet AG, Ferroni F, Spila A, Abbolito R, Roselli M, Greiner JW, and Schlom J. Evaluation of markers in patients with gynecologic diseases. AMJ Obstet Gynecol 1994; 171:1183-91.

122. Austoker J. Screening for ovarian, prostatic and testicular cancer. Br Med J 1994; 309:315-320.

123. Monagham JM. Malignant diseases of ovary. Dewhursts text book of Obstetrics and Gynecology for postgraduates, 6 editions; Blackwell

science Ltd. 1999; PP.590-592.

124.   Zurawski VR, Orjaseter H, Andersen A, et al. Elevated serum CA125 levels prior to diagnosis of ovarian neoplasia: relevance for early detection ovarian cancer   Int J Cancer 1988; 42:677.

125.   Roupaz FE, Raftopoulos V, Tzavelas G, Kotrotsiou E, Sotiropoulou P, Karanikola E, Skifla, and Ardavanis A. Serum CA125 combined with transvaginal (TSV) ultrasonography for ovarian cancer screening. Invivo 2004;18(6):831-836

126.   Bast RC, Xu F, Woolas RF, Yu Y, Conaway M., O' Briant K, et al. complementary and coordinate markers for detection of epithelial ovarian cancers, In: sharp F., Mason P, Blackett T, and Berek JS, editors. Covarian Cancers 3; Chapman and Hill; London; 1995; P.P. 189-192.

127.   Schutter EMJ, Kenemans P, Sohn C, Kristen P, Crombach G, Westermann R et al. Diagnostic value of pelvic examination, ultrasound and serum CA125 in post-menopausal women with pelvic mass. Cancer 1994; 74:1398-1406.

128.   Rustin GJS. The clinical value of tumer markers in the malignant of ovarian cancer. Ann Clin Biochem 1996;33:284-289.

129.   Wagner U, Kohler S, Prietl G, Giffels P, Schmidt-Nicolai S, Schlebusch H, et al. Monoclonal antiidiotypic antibodies in immunotherapy of ovarian carcinoma (MAB CA125) and breast carcinoma .Zentrabl Gynakol 1999; 121:190.

130.   Wagner U, Schlebusch H, Kohler S, Schmolling J, Grunn U, and Krebs D. Immunological responses to the tumor associated antigen CA125 in patient with advanced ovarian cancer induced by the murin monoclonal anti-idiotypic vaccine A CA125. Hybridoma 1997; 16:33-40.

131.   Nusted K, Lloyd KO, Nilsson O, and O'Brient TJ. Epitopes on CA125 from cervical mucus and ascites fluid and characterization   Tumer Biol 2002; 23:303-314.

132.   Einhorn N, Sjovall K, Knapp RC, Hall P, Scully RE, Bast RC, and Zurawski VR. Prospective evaluation of serum CA125 levels for the early detection of ovarian cancer. Obstet Gynecol 1992; 80: 14-18.

133.   Boerman OC, Thomas GMG, Segers MFG, Kenemans P, Lovgren, Zurawski VR, Haisma HJ, and Poels LG. Time-resolved immunoflurometric assay for the ovarian carcinoma-associated antigenic determinant CA125 in serum. Clin Chem 1987; 33(12): 2191-

134.   Schollerr N, Crawford M, Sato A, Drasche CW, O'Biant KC, Kiviat N, Andrson GL, and Urban N. Bead-based ELISA for valedation of ovarian cancer : Erley detection   markers . Clin Cancer Res 2006 ;12:2117-2124.ancer

135.   Bast RC and Knapp CC. CA125: History, current status, and future prospects. MJM, 1997; 3:67-71.

136.   Lowry OH, Rosenrough NJ, Farr AL, and Randel RJ. Protein measurement with folin phenol reagent. J Biol Chem 1951; 193: 365-375.

137.   Fleuren GJ, NAP M, Aalders JG, Trimbos JB, and DE Bruijn NWA. Explanation of the limited correlation between tumor CA125 content and serum CA125 antigen levels in patients with ovarian tumors. Cancer 1987; 60: 2437-2442.

138.   Al-Barazanji AK. (2002) "The accuracy of malignant risk index based onCa125, ultrasound and menopausal state". Thesis, supervised by Kais Kubba and Suhail Najim Al-Salam, submitted for the degree of fellowship of Arab Board of Obstetrics and Gynecology.

139.   Malkasion G.D. Jr., Knapp R.C., Lavin ph. T., Zurawski V.R. Jr., Podratz K.C., Stonhope CR, Mortel R, Berck JS, Bast RC, and Ritts RE. Preoperative evaluation of serum CA125 levels in pre-menopausal and post-menopausal patients with pelvic masses: Discrimination of benign form malignant disease.   J Obestet Gynecol 1988; 159:341-6.

140.   James T Wu, Terry M, Joseph AK, and David PK. Improved specificity of the CA125 Enzymeimmunoassay for ovarian carcinomas by use of the ratio of CA125 to carcinoembryonic antigen. Clin Chem 1988; 34/9: 1853-1857.

141.   Nagell JR, Meeker WR, Parker J., and Harraison JD. Carcinoembryonic antigen in patients with gynecologic malignancy. Cancer 1975; 35: 1372-1376.

142.   Nagell JR, Donaldson ES, Gay EC, Sharkey RM, Rayburn P, and Goldenberg DM. carcinoembryonic   antigen   in ovarian epithelial cystadenocarcinomas. Cancer 1978; 41: 2335-2340.

143.   Donaldson ES, Nagell JR, Pursell S, Gay EC, Meeker WR, Kashmiri R, and Voorde J. Multiple biochemical marker in patients with gynecologic malignancies. Cancer 1980; 45: 948-953.

144.   Freifrlder   D.   "Physical   Biochemistry: Application   to

Biochemistry and Molecular Biology"; 2nd ed.; San Francisco: W.H. Freeman & Company. 1982; Chapter 14; pp. 494-591.

145.   Changux JP. Responses of actylcholinesterase from torepedo marmorata to salts and curarizing drugs. Mol. Pharmacol 1966, 2:369.

146.   Helen CH, Mansel H, Siraj M, and Niel S. Essential of Clinical Immunology; 4th ed.; London Blackwell Science Ltd; 1999; Chapter 19:pp.314-321.

147.   Clackson T, Hoogenboon HR, Griffiths AD, and Winter G. Marking antibody fragments using phage display libraries. Nature 1991; 352:624-628.

148.   Dixon M, and Webb E, Enzymes; 3rd ed.; London; Longman Group Limited; 1979; pp.273.

149.   Devlin TM. Text Book of Biochemistry with Clinical Correlation; 2nd Ed; John Wiley and Sons Inc.; New York; 1986; pp.125-66.

150.   Melander W and Horvath C. Salt effect on hydrophobic interactions in precipitation and chromatography of proteins: an interpretation of the lyotropic series. Arch Biochem Biophys 1977; 183: 200-215.

151.   Collins KD. Charge density-dependent strength of hydration and biological structure. Biophys J.; 1997; 72: 65-76.

152.   Evans JS and Levine BA. Protein–protein interaction sites in the calcium modulated skeletal muscle troponin complex. J Inorg Biochem 1980; 12:695.

153.   Jones S, and Thornton JM. Principles of protein –protein interactions. Proc Natl Acad Sci 1996; 93:13-20.

154.   O'Brien TJ, Hardin JW, Bannon GA, Norris JS, and Quirk JG. CA125 antigen in human amniotic fluid and fetal membranes. Am J Obstet Gynecol 1986; 155(1): 50-55.

155.   Scopes RK, Protein Purification Principles and Practice; New York; Springer Verlag. 1982; pp. 162-197.

156.   Price NC, and Stevens L. Fundamentals of Enzymology; 2nd ed.; Newyork, Oxford University Press; 1986; pp. 125.

157.   Ormerod MG, Steel K, Westwood JH, and Mazzini MN. Epithelial membrane antigen: partial purification, assay and properties. Br J Cancer 1983; 48:533-541.

158.   Segal I.H.; Biochemical Calculations; 2nd ed.; John Wiley and Sons; 1976; pp. 278-373.

159.   Haisma HJ, Battaile A, Stradtman EW, Knapp RC, and Zurawski VR. Antibody antigen complex formation following injection of CA125 monoclonal antibody in patients with ovarian cancer. Int J Cancer 1987; 40: 758-762.

160.   Wiseman T, Williston S, Randts J, and Lnng-Nam Lin. Rapid measurement of binding constants and heats of binding using a new titration calorimeter. Anal Biochem 1989; 179:131-137.

161.   Rosier JS, Gokulrangan G, Girault H, Sovojanovsky S, and Wilson GS. Characterization of protein adsorption and immunosorption kinetic in photoabelated polymer microchanals. Langmuir 2000; 16: 8489-8494.

162.   Weiland GA, Minneman KP, and Molinoff PB. Thermodynamic of agonist and antagonist interactions with mammalian β adrenergic receptors. Mol. Pharmacol 1980; 18: 341.

163.   Camacho Cj, Weng Z, Vajda S, and Delisi C. Free energy landscapes of encounter complexes in protein-protein association. Biophys J 1999; 76:1166-1178.

164.   Seeley DH, Wang WY, and Salhanick HA. Temperature dependence of kinetic interactions between progesterone and uterine cytoplasmic receptor. Biochem Biophy Acta 1980; 632: 536-543.

165. Forde A, and Coley J. Choosing and characterizing antibodies. In: Goaling JP. Editor. Immunoassays A practical approach ; Oxford university press London; p.p.62-63

166.   Weiland GA and Molinoff PB. Qutitative analysis of drug-receptor interaction I. Determination of kinetic and equilibrium properties. Life Science; 1981; 29: 314.

167.   Nemethy G and Scherag AJ. The structure of water and hydrophobic bonding in proteins: III the thermodynamic properties of hydrophobic bond in protein. Phys Chem 1962; 66:1775.

168.   Waelbroeck M, Van Obberghen E, and De Meyts p. Thermodynamics of the interaction of insulin with its receptor. J Biol Chem 1979; 259:7736.

169.   Haro LS, and Talamantes FJ. Thermodynamics and kinetics of mouse prolactin-hepatic receptor interaction. Mol Cell Endocrinol 1985; 43:199

170.   Ross PD and Subramanian S. Thermodynamics of protein association reaction: Forces contributing to stability. Biochemistry 1981; 20:3096.

171.   Blumenthal DK and Stull JT. Effect of pH, ionic strength, and temperature

on activation by calmodulin and catalytic activity of myosin light chain kinase. Biochemistry 1982; 21:2386-2391.

172.   Laport DC, Wireman EM, and Storm DI. Calcium-induced exposure of a hydrophobic surface on calmodulin. Biochemistry 1980; 19: 3814.

173.   Johnstone A and Thorpe R. Immunochemistry in Practice; 3rd ed.; Blackwell Science Ltd.; 1996; p.p. 1-4, 292-311.

174.   Bujalowski W and Jezewska MJ. Quantitative determination of equilibrium binding isotherms for multiple ligand-macromolecule interactions using spectroscopic methods. In: Michael G. Spectrophotometry and spectrofluorimetry: a practical approach .New York: Oxford; 2000; pp. 141.

175.   Nolta K and Steck. Isolation and initial characterization of the bipartite contractile vacuole complex from dictyostelium discoideum. J Biol Chem 1994; 269:2225.

176.   Scheraga HA. Protein Structure; New York: Academic Press; 1961; pp. 365-571.

177.   Kiernan JA. Histological and Histochemical Methods Theory and Practice; 3rd ed., Reed Educational and Professional Publishing Ltd.; 1999; Chapter 19: pp. 391-398.

178.   Williams CA and Chanse MW.   Methods in immunology and immunochemistry; New York., Academic Press; 1968; vol II; Chapter10: pp 163-174.

179.   Haider TM. (2004) "Development of Radio Receptor Technique for Measurement of CA125 in Malignant and Benign Breast Tumors". Thesis, supervised by Al-Mudhaffar S.A., College of Science, Baghdad University.

180.   Al-Jobory E. (2004) "Biochemical Characterization of CA125 in Sera and Tissue of Some Colorectal Tumors". Thesis, supervised by Al-Mudhaffar S.A., College of Science, Baghdad University.

181.   Mathews Ch k, and Holde KE. "Biochemistry" California the Benjamin /Cummings Publishing Co.; 1990; Chapter 6: pp. 191.

182.   Sheinerman FB, Norel L, and Honig B. Electrostatic aspects of protein-protein interaction. Curr Opin Struct Biol 2000; 10:153-159.

183.   Nils H Axelsen. "Hand book of immuno precipitation"-in Gel Techniques; 3rd ed.; WA. Benjamin Inc. London; 1983.

184.   Nagacura S, and Baba H. Dipole moment and near ultraviolet absorption of some monosubstituted benzenes: The effect of solvent and hydrogen bonding. Am Chem. Soc 1952; 74:5693.

185.   Pimentel GC. Hydrogen bonding and electronic transitions: The role of the Franck-Condon principle. J Am Chem   Soc 1957; 79:3323.

186.   Silvestien. RM, Bassalar GC, and Marril. TC. "Spectrophotometric identification of organic compounds"; New York: John Wiley and Sons; 1981; pp.181.

Leach SJ. physical principles and techniques of protein chemistry; New York: Academic Press;

Part c
Biochemical Characterization
Of CA125 in colorectal tumors
Sami A .AL-Mudhaffar
Enas Ghazi Shakir AL-Joboury

List of Contents

343

Chapter one
Introduction

1 – 1 Historical Background of Tumor Markers:

The first tumor marker reported was the Bence – Jones protein. Since its discovery in 1847 by precipitation of a protein in acidified boiled urine, the measurement of Bence – Jones protein has been a diagnostic test for multiple myeloma (a tumor of plasma cells). More than one hundred years after its discovery, Edelman and Poulik identified the Bence–Jones protein as the monoclonal light chain of immunoglobulin secreted by tumor plasma cells. Monoclonal paraproteins appear as sharp bands in the globulin area in electrophoretic patterns of serum. Diagnosis of multiple myeloma is often made based on this finding or on the presence of an elevated level of monoclonal immunoglobulin in the serum (1).

1 – 2 Definition of Tumor Marker:

A tumor marker is a substance present in or produced by a tumor itself or by the host in response to a tumor that can be used to differentiate a tumor from normal tissue or to determine the presence of a tumor based on measurement in the blood or secretions. Such a substance can be found in cells, tissue or body fluids. It can be measured qualitatively or quantitatively by chemical, Immunological, or molecular biological methods to identify the presence of a cancer.

Morphologically, cancer tissue has been recognized by pathologists as resembling fetal tissue more than normal adult differentiated tissue. Tumors are graded according to their degree of differentiation as being (1) well differentiated (2) poorly differentiated, or (3) an plastic (without forms). Tumor markers are the biochemical or immunological counterparts of the differentiation state of the tumor. In general, tumor markers represent re–

expression of substances produced normally by embryogenically closely related tissues (1).

Few markers are specific for a single individual tumor (tumor – specific markers); most are found with different tumors of the same tissue type (tumor – associated markers). They are present in higher quantities in cancer tissue or in blood from cancer patients than in benign tumors or in the blood of normal subjects (1).

1 – 3 Classification of Tumor Markers:

Tumor markers may be classified to chemical and genetic tumor markers.

Chemical Tumor Markers:

Markers produced by cancers include enzymes and isoenzymes, hormones, oncofetal antigens, carbohydrate epitopes recognized by monoclonal antibodies, receptors, and oncogene products.

Enzymes were of the first groups of tumor markers identified. Their elevated activities were used to indicate the presence of cancer.

Hormones as tumor markers were used for the detection and monitoring of cancer.

Oncofetal antigens were discovered using conventional antisera produced against fluids from cancer – bearing animals or extracts of cancer tissues (1).

The development of monoclonal antibody techniques allowed more sensitive and specific measurements of tumor antigens. More importantly, new antigens were discovered by developing monoclonal antibodies against tumor cell preparations. They appear to have better clinical sensitivity and specificity than do the oncofetal antigens (1).

Table (1– 1) summary of the chemical tumor markers.:

Marker type	Associated malignancy	Example
Enzyme	Liver	Alcohol dehydrogenase
	Bone, Liver, Leukemia, Sarcoma	Alkaline phosphatase
	Ovarian, Lung, Trophoplastic, Gastrointestinal, Seminoma, Hodgkin's	Alkaline phosphatase placental

	Pancreas,	Amylase
	Colon, Breast	Aryl Sulfatase B
	Colon, Bladder, Gastrointestinal, Vanous	Galactosyl Transferase
	Lung (small– cell) neuroblastoma, carcinoid, melanoma, Pancreatic	Neuron – Specific enolase
	Prostate, Vanouse (large bowel, lung, ovarian)	Prostate – Specific Antigen (PSA) Ribonuclease
	Colorectal, Breast, etc.	Telomerase
	Colon, Breast, Lung	Sialyl Transferenase
Hormone	cushing s syndrome, Lung (small cell)	ACTH
	Lung (small cell) adrenal cortex, duodenal	Antidiuretic hormone
	Modularl thyroid	Calcitonin
	Pituitary adenoma, Renal, Lung, Embryonal, choriocarcinoma, Testicular (non seminomatous)	Growth hormone hCG
	Torophoblastic, Gonads, Lung, Breast	Human placental lactogen
	Liver, Renal, Breast, Lung, Various	Parathyroid hormone
	Pitutary adenoma, Renal, Lung	Prolactin
	Pancreas, Bronchognic	Vasoactive intestinal
	Pheochromocytoma neuroblastoma	Peptide
Oncofetal Antigen	Hepato cellular, germline (non seminoma)	(α– feto protein)
	Colon	Beta– Oncofetal Antigen (β– oncofetal Antigen)
	Liver	Carcino fetal ferritin
	Colorectal, Gastrointestinal, Pancreatic, Lung, Breast	CEB (Carinoembryonic Antigen)
	Pancreatic	Pancreatic oncofetal

	Cervical, Lung, Skin, Head and neck (Squamous)	Squamous cell Antigen
	Colon, Gastrointestinal, Bladder	Tennessee Antigen
Mucin	Breast, Ovarian	CA 15–3
Mucin	Breast	CA 27–29
Mucin	Breast, Ovarian	MCA
Mucin	Pancreatic, Ovarian, Gastrointestinal, Lung	Du–PAN–2
Protein	Multiple Myeloma, β– –cell lymphoma chronic lymphocytic leukemia, Waldenstrom's macroglubulinnemia	β2 Macroglobulin
Protein	Insulinoma	C– Peptide
Protein	Liver, Lung, , Leukemia	Ferritin
Protein	Multiple myeloma, Lymphomas	Immunoglobulin
Protein	Pancreatic, Stomach	Pancreas associated Antigen
Protein	Trophoplastic, Germ cell	Pregnancy specific protein [2]
Protein	Hepatocellular	Prothrombin precursor
Protein	Ovarian	Tumor associated trypsin inhibitor
Blood group related Antigen	Pancreatic, Hepatic, Gastrointestinal	CA 19–9
Blood group related Antigen	Gastrointestinal, Pancreatic, Ovarian	CA 19–5
Blood group related Antigen	Colon, Gastrointestinal, Pancreatic	CA 50
Blood group related Antigen	Ovarian, Colon, Breast, Gastrointestinal	CA 27,4, CA242
Others	Breast	Estrogen and Progesterone receptors
Others	Brain, Various	Polyamine
Others	Bone metastasis, Breast, (multiple myeloma)	Hydroxy Proline

	Neuroblastoma, Pheochromocytoma	Catecholamine metabolites
	Gastrointestinal, Lung, Rheumatoid	Lipid– associated sialic acid

Genetic Tumor Markers:

Two classes of genes are implicated in the development of cancer, oncogenes ((cell activation genes and suppressor genes)) involved in the recognition and repair of damaged DNA.

Oncogenes are derived from proto–oncogenes, which may be activated by dominant mutations. The type of mutation could be point mutation, insertion, deletion, translocation, or inversion. Most oncogenes code for proteins that function at same stage of activation of cells for proliferation, and their activation leads to cell division. Most oncogenes are associated with hematological malignancies, such as leukemia and to a lesser extent, solid tumors (1).

The other class of tumor genes, the suppressor genes, has been isolated from mostly solid tumors. The oncogenicity of suppressor genes is derived from the loss of the gene rather than their activation, as with oncogenes. The major tumor suppressor gene, P53, functions to repair damaged DNA by apoptosis (programmed cell death). Repair is mediated by activation of the production of P21, which blocks the cell cycle in late G1 to allow repair to take place. The loss of function of this gene due to loss or mutation may result in the inability of the DNA repair process and lead to the development of tumorogensis (2).

The exciting promise of using detection of oncogenes and suppressor genes for the diagnosis, determining the prognosis, and predicting the response to the chemotherapy remains to be realized. Oncogene detection remains an experimental approach to human cancer, with great expectation not yet fulfilled. The ability to predict susceptibility to develop cancer by the detection of mutations in tumor suppressor genes raises ethical questions that remain to be resolved (2).

1 – 4 Ideal Tumor Markers:

The ideal tumor markers have the following properties (3):–

* High clinical sensitivity.

* High clinical specificity.
* Tumor markers levels proportional to tumor volume.
* Reflect tumor heterogeneity.
* Low levels in healthy population.
* Low levels in benign diseases.
* Discriminatory to identify tumor and metastasis from benign to healthy states.
* Provide adequate times lead for early diagnosis and early treatment.
* Assay sensitivity to detect stage I cancer.

1 – 5 Clinical Applications of Tumor Markers:

The potential clinical applications of tumor marker assay are listed below.

Screening:

Some tumor markers have been used in mass screening programs of asymptomatic individuals, with limited success, in high – risk sectors of the population. However, it is to be emphasized that no biochemical tumor marker is yet specific and sensitive enough to be recommended as a definitive screening test for cancer (3).

Diagnosis:

Almost every tumor marker has been investigated for its suitability as a primary diagnostic test for cancer in symptomatic individuals. However, sufficient false – positive and false – negatives have been encountered with every marker so far discovered to preclude their use in distinguishing malignant and nonmalignant conditions. The ultimate goal of identifying tumor – specific antigens has so far eluded oncologists because most tumor markers have been found in some normal tissue and the serum of some non – cancerous individuals and in many benign diseases. For this reason, these antigens are often referred to as tumor associated antigens. Nevertheless, a number of tumor markers have proved to be useful in confirming diagnosis, often in conjunction with a battery of other clinical methods. Another approach attempts to use multiple tumor markers to diagnose tumors and to identify the primary origin of metastic disease (3).

Differential Diagnosis and Classification:

Immunoassay for some tumor markers are used in clinics to distinguish between clinical conditions with similar symptoms , where one or both could be cancerous, For example, the measurement of neuron– specific enolase levels allows differentiation between neuroblastoma and Wilm's tumor when a child present with a palpable abdominal mass (3).

Staging and Grading:

The degree of elevation in the concentration of several tumor markers can help to stage tumors. In general the mean circulating levels of these tumor markers increase with the stage of the cancer. In contrast, placental alkaline phosphatase is a tumor marker related to the grade of cancer, and serum levels of this anylate are higher in grade 1and 2 tumors than in grade 3 ovarian carcinomas (3).

Prognosis:

Prognosis is the probability of cure of a cancer patient. Positive lymph node detection is a classical method of determining prognosis invasively. The magnitude of tumor marker levels in several cancers corresponds to the mass of tumor. Moderate elevations are suggestive of better prognosis than persistent high levels. Tumor aggressiveness resulting in widespread metastasis; precipitates very high serum tumor marker levels indicating poor prognosis. Generally, well– differentiated tumors tend to be less aggressive than undifferentiated or anaplastic tumors. Whereas most tumor marker over expression indicates poor prognosis, the increased levels of progesterone and estrogen receptors in breast cancers determine the type of treatment (hormone) as well as good prognosis (3).

Monitoring and Recurrence:

The profile of tumor marker concentration against time can mirror the condition of patients diagnosed to have cancer (3).

Tumor markers profiles usually reflect one of the following classical patterns:–

* A rapid decline in tumor marker level to normal concentrations following surgery or other forms of first– line therapy suggests that treatment has been successful.

* The lack of a decline to basal levels following first– line therapy may indicate that treatment has been only partially successful.

* Continued low levels of the tumor marker indicate that remission has been maintained as a result of treatment.

* A subsequent rise in the concentration of the tumor marker (from the basal level) suggests a recurrence of the disease. Tumor markers can warn of renewed tumor growth or recurrence 3 – 12 months before other methods provide confirmation.

* Decline of the marker levels after an increase has been associated with a recurrence, is suggestive of the responsiveness of a tumor to second– line or subsequent treatment.

* If tumor marker concentrations remain elevated after treatment, the tumor may be resistant to the therapeutic method employed and prognosis of the patient is poor unless alternative therapeutic modalities are available.

Table (1–2) Refers to the up to date clinical usefulness of tumor markers (4):

Type of cancer	Tumor Marker	Clinical use
GI (colorectal, pancreas, stomach)	CEA CA19–9, CA195, CA72.4 CA50	Prognosis and Monitoring therapy.
Liver	AFP	Screening, diagnosis, Prognosis, Monitoring therapy.
	CEA	Monitoring therapy.
Breast	CEA, CA15–3, CA549, CAM2, M29, CA27, 29 MCA	Monitoring therapy.
Prostate	Estrogen /progesterone receptors PSA–total, Free, Complexes	Screening, Prognosis,
Ovarian	CA125	Prognosis, therapy.
Lung (small cell carcinoma)	NSE, CK–ββ	Monitoring therapy
Neuroblastoma	VMA, Catecholamine	Screening, diagnosis, Prognosis, Monitoring therapy.
	NSE	Monitoring therapy.
Testicular (gem cell tumors)	AFP, β–hCG	Diagnosis, Prognosis and Monitoring therapy.
Myeloma	Immunoglobulin	Diagnosis, Prognosis.
Thyroid	Thyroglobulin	Screening, Monitoring

		therapy.
	Calcitonin	Diagnosis, Monitoring therapy.
Neuron endocrine	variety of hormones	Diagnosis.
Bone	ALP, 5–NT	Diagnosis, Monitoring therapy.
Bladder	BTA, NMP22	Recurrence Detection.
Liver metastases	ALP	Diagnosis, Prognosis, Monitoring therapy.
Trophoblastic diseases	hCG	Diagnosis, Prognosis, Monitoring therapy.

1 – 6 Tumor Marker in Colorectal Cancer:

There are several tumor markers correlated with the incidence of CRC, but the most important markers are:

* CA 19 – 9:

It is a monoclonal antibody raised against colon carcinoma cells(5).The carbohydrate antigen is a glycolipid(1), it is shown to react against a monosialoganglioside antigen(5).The Antibody did not react against a panel of other ganglioside, but it did react to elements in human meconium(6).

In colon cancer patients with the elevated value had a four folds which increase in death compared to patients with lower values (p<0.001)(7).

* CA – 50:

It is a monoclonal antibody developed against the human adenocarcinoma cell line. CA – 50 was a marker for colorectal cancer and pancreatic .The clinical use of CA–50 is in the prognosis and monitoring therapy (1).

* CA – 242:

Studies of cancer antigen CA – 242 have been described (8) .It has a little advantage over CEA alone. But when it is used in panel of multiple markers, it may provide an enhanced sensitivity and specificity to serve as a monitoring tool (8).

* CEA:

It is an oncofetal antigen, CEA is currently in wide spread use as a marker for colorectal cancer.

Elevation can be observed in a variety of benign gastrointestinal disease (9, 10), in smokers (11), and other malignancies including breast (12), lung (13), gastric (14), pancreatic (15), and gynecologic cancers (16). Because of the lack of specificity for colon cancer and resulting false–positive results, CEA cannot be recommended for use in cancer screening.

The major clinical role for CEA is in monitoring response to surgery and detecting recurrence. The most effective indicator of recurrent disease is a progressive increase in serial CEA levels (17). CEA may provide additional prognostic information at the time of staging (18).

* CA 72 – 4:

It is a monoclonal antibody purified from human colon carcinoma xemograft. CA72–4 and CEA value may be complementary. The clinical use of CA72–4 is in prognosis and monitoring therapy (1).

* Cathepsin B:

It is a lysosomal cystein protease that can degrade matrix components, and result in a higher metastatic potential and a worse prognosis (19, 20). It was found that Cathepsin B in colon cancer correlated with the stage, that it had less elevated in stage I/II than in stage III/IV.

In addition there are several tumor markers for colorectal cancer are under study. Walach et al.(21) found that leukocyte alkaline phosphatase was more sensitive for detecting metastases than CEA. Verazin et. al. (22) compared total sialic acid (TSA)/total proteins (TP) ratio to CEA in 146 consecutive patients undergoing colorectal resections. TSA/TP was more frequently elevated than CEA levels in cancers in earlier stages (A, B2) (22). In a study comparing TPA and CA19 – 9 to CEA, the combination of markers was more sensitive for detecting recurrence than CEA alone (23).

1 – 7 Developing the CA125 Assay:

The development of an assay for the CA125 as a tumor marker grew out of attempts to obtain monoclonal reagents for serotherapy of patients with ovarian cancer .In the early 1970s, it was discovered in an animal model that the intraperitoneal injection of a heteroantiserum developed in rabbits against a partially purified tumor – associated antigen could inhibit the intraperitoneal growth of syngeneic murine ovarian cancer transplants (24, 25). Soon after, it was found that the anti tumor activity of hetroantiserum could be augmented by coinjection of the immunostimulant Corynebacterium parvum (26), which was shown to attract and activate inflammatory cells capable of mediating antibody – dependent cell – mediated cytotoxicity (27) .By the early 1980s, clinical studies using intraperitoneal injection of Corynebacterium parvum as a single agent demonstrated the objective regression of small amounts of ovarian cancer in patients with persistent or recurrent disease(28).

With the discovery of the monoclonal technology by Kohler and Milstein in 1975(29), the present authors attempted to develop antibodies reactive with ovarian cancer that might be administered in combination with Corynebacterium parvum. Mice were repeatedly injected with a human ovarian cancer cell line and hybridomas were prepared from immune spleen cells and the P3NS–1 plasmacytoma. From these hybridomas, clones were isolated based on the production of antibodies that bound to the ovarian cancer cell line used for immunization, but not to a B lymphocyte cell line developed from the tumor cell donor. The one hundred twenty – fifth promising clone produced an IgG1 antibody of the desired specificity and was designated OC (ovarian cancer) 125(30).

Characterization of CA125:

It was originally described for serous cystadenocarcinoma of ovary. Its half – life in the body is 20 days or more (31).

Chemical study has revealed sensitivity of CA125 to proteases, low pH, and high temperature, and high ionic strength, properties consistent with a conformational peptide determinant. However, CA125 activity can also be destroyed with relatively high concentrations of periodate and blocked with different lectins, suggesting a close association with carbohydrate. Despite these observations, the chemical composition of the CA125 determinant is still not completely defined.

Further more, despite repeated attempts to clone the CA125 associated protein, the isolation of an appropriate gene has not yet been reported. Using polyclonal heteroantiserum, a gene was isolated from bacterial expression library that mapped to the region of this bacteria. The product of this gene does not, however, appear to react with OC125(32).

Biochemistry of CA125:

CA 125 is a marker for ovarian and endometrial carcinoma. CA125 is actually a heterogeneous mixture of glycoprotein with a molecular weight range of 200–1000KD ,which is different from classical mucines by means of carbohydrate conversion (less than 50%) and the presence of both N and O–linked carbohydrate residues(34), but lower molecular weight species have also been reported(33). Much of the heterogeneity of the CA125 antigen is most likely related to differences in glycosylation. The antigenic domains reactive with the monoclonal antibodies appear to be located on the protein part of the CA125.

CA125 is a Tumor–derived Mucin:

Tumor–derived mucins are high molecular weight glycoproteins; carbohydrate–rich cell surface components of epithelial tissues. They have a polypeptide backbone with numerous O–linked oligosaccharide chains attached to the backbone. Monoclonal antibodies generated against tissue mucins usually recognize epitopes on the carbohydrate portions of the molecules. It was found that some monoclonal antibodies recognize carbohydrate epitopes somewhat selectively on cancer cells despite the fact that most of these epitopes are also expressed on some normal tissues. Changes in cell surface carbohydrate of cancer cells are often not clear, however, alternations in the cell surface carbohydrate of cancer cells are caused by a shift to high molecular weight glycans. These changes in carbohydrate have been associated with reduced cellular adhesion to extracellular matrix and increased invasiveness and metastatic potential of tumor cells (35, 36).

Function of CA125:

CA125 is an antigen expressed by fetal amniotic and celomic epithelium. In the adult, it is found in tissue derived from celomic epithelium (mesothelial cells of the pleura, pericardium and peritoneum) and müllerin epithelium (tubal , endometrial , and endocervical). The surface epithelium of normal fetal and adult ovaries does not express the determinant, except in inclusion cysts, areas of metaplasia, and papillary excrescences (37, 38). The antigen is not present in the normal serum, or in adult or fetal ovaries. The antigen is also found in the chorionic membrane, extracts of maternal decidua.

The function of CA125 antigen is largely unknown and one hypothesis associates the antigen with müllerian differentiation (3).

Purification of CA125:

Several methods have been reported for the purification of CA125 antigen. Caristedt et. al(39). ,were isolate CA125 by using perichloric acid from patients with cervical tumors then the acidified solution was centrifuged, and the supernatant was then used as a source of CA125 antigen. Another method was reported by Schneider et. al(40). who describe a method by which an immuno affinity matrix was constructed by binding antibody directly or indirectly to protein A–Sepharose 4B followed by cross linking of the complex with dimethyl pimelimidate and SDS–poly acrylamid gel electrophoresis.

By using gel filtration technique, pools of sera from normal healthy control and ovarian cancer patients were purified separately on columns containing Sephacryl S–200 and Sephadex G–200(41).

Binding of CA125:

Using immunohistochemical analysis, the CA125 antibody was found to bind antigen expressed by approximately 80% of epithelial ovarian cancer, as well as by other gynecologic, breast, lung, and colon carcinomas (42). The murine monoclonal antibody (OC125), which is used to detect the CA125 antigen, was obtained after immunization with OVCA433 cell line(37). The original CA125 test uses the OC125 antibody as both the capture and indicator antibody in a RadioImmunometric Assay (43). More recently, the CA125 II test has been developed, which use the M11 monoclonal antibody as the capture antibody for CA125.A recent epitop – mapping workshop has defined the binding characteristics of monoclonal antibodies reactive with

CA125 and has identified two major regions on the antigen, which are called OC125–like (OC125) and M11 (OC 133) –like epitopes (44 – 46).

Clinical Application of CA25:

The CA125 was originally developed to monitor the course of patients with epithelial ovarian cancer. After cytoreductive surgery, small, non–palpable nodules of residual disease below the limits of resolution for computerized tomography and magnetic resonance imaging often remain within the peritoneal cavity. Cytotoxic chemotherapy is often administered for many months without a clear indication of weather the disease is responding to treatment .If a cut of 35 U/ml is chosen, which excludes 95% of apparently healthy individuals, more than 80% of patients with clinically evident ovarian cancer will have elevated CA125(47).

It has been shown that CA125 is not a specific marker for ovarian cancer in that it can be elevated in sera from patients with other gynecological adenocarcinomas, as well as lymphomas, malignant mesotheliomas, immature teratomas, and carcinomas of the pancreas, colon, breast, and lung (48, 49) CA125 is a marker of the clinical and homodynamic status and the course of patients with heart failure before and after heart transplantation (50).

CA125 is a valuable marker for both short and long – term monitoring of treatment effectiveness. Post operative serum level is related to the extent of tumor resection. After complete removal of the tumor, elevated CA125concentrations to normal with a half – life of about 5 days (51, 52). However, CA125 values may still be increased up to 300 U/ml 2 – 3 weeks after surgery due to the pathological (53).

CA125 in Colorectal Cancer:

An investigation has revealed that CA125 has been shown to be present in the sera of 32% of patients with carcinoma of the colon and 30% of patients with miscellaneous gastrointestinal tract tumor (54). In the search for a method to facilitate the preoperative discrimination of ovarian carcinoma from colorectal carcinomas, CA125 level was measured and found to be a helpful marker in the differentiation between the two cancers(55).

Subsequent researches have been performed for measuring the level of CA125 in the serum of advanced colorectal cancer, it has been found to be a good indicator in the diagnosis of advanced colorectal adenocarcinoma (56, 57)

1 – 8 Colorectal Tumors:

A – Benign Tumors (polyps):

A polyp is a growth extending into the lumen of the gastrointestinal tract, and is defined as a visible protrusion above the surface of the surrounding normal large bowel mucosa in the colon. Although polyps occur in all sections of the gastrointestinal tract, but are most common in the colon. Polyps may be detected endoscopically by sigmoidscope or radiographically by bariumenema. Colorectal polyps can be classified either according to their shape or according to their histology; table (1 – 3) shows the classification of colorectal polyps histological as either neoplastic (adenomatous polyps) or non–neoplastic. Although all adenomatous polyps have malignant potential, the majorities are benign when detected. In contrast, hyperplastic, mucosal, inflammatory and hamaratomatous polyps are non – neoplastic and thus have no malignant potential .Lastly, sub mucosal polyps include lymphoid polyps , lipomas ,and less common histological types (58).

Table (1–3) Histological Classification Of Colorectal Polyps

Neolpastic Adenomatous (polyps)	Non–Neoplastic polyps	Sub mucosal polyps
1–Benign (Adenomatous)	Hyperplastic	Lymphoid
A–Tubular	Mucosal	Lipoma
B–Tubulovillous	Inflammatory	Other
C–Villous	Hamartomatous	
D–Malignant(carcinomatous)	Juvenile	
	Peutz–Jeghers	
2 – Other benign colon carcinoma(59)		
A–Leiomyoma		
B–Pnuo omatosis cystoides intestinalis		
C–Colitis cystica profunda		
D–Polyposis Syndrome 1–Familial adenomatous Polyposis (FAP) 2–Gardner's adenomatous Polyposis		

3–Turcot's adenomatous Polyposis
4–Familial Juvenile Polyposis Coli (FPC)
E–Cowden's Disease
F–Muri – Torre Syndrome
G–Cronkhite – Canada Syndrome

Neoplastic Polyps (Adenomatous Polyps):

Adenomatous polyps, or adenomas, are attached to the bowel wall by a stalk "pedunculated" or by a broad, flat base "sesile". The clinical significance of identifying adenomas is that it has malignant potential and many develop into a cancer (50). It is generally accepted that all colorectal cancers originate from a precursor adenoma.

The National polyp study has demonstrated that colonscopic removal of adenomatous polyps significantly reduce the risk of developing colorectal cancer(50).

Adenomatous polyps occur more frequently in men than in

 women (60, 61). Older patients have an increased risk of having adenomas. Although adenomas vary greatly in size, most are small, measuring less than 1.0 cm in diameter. In the national polyp study of the 3.371 colonoscopically removed adenomas, 38% were only 0.5 cm or less, 36% were 0.6 to 1.0 cm, and 26% were larger than 1.0 cm (62). In those found to have adenomatous polyps at colonscopy, about 60% have a single adenoma and 40% have multiple adenomas (63). Increased age was associated with increased rate of multiple adenomas (61). Adenomatous polyps exhibit the same predominantly left – sided colonic distribution that is found with colorectal cancers. Several clinical studies have reported that more than 60% of colonscopically removed adenomas are located distal to the splenic of flexure (62, 64)

1 – 9 Epidemiology of Colorectal Cancer:

Colorectal cancer encompasses carcinoma of both colon and rectum (65). Colorectal cancer is fourth most common incident cancer (after breast, lung and prostate) and the second most common cause of cancer death (after lung) (66) in the United State, with 111,000 new cases per year and 51,000 deaths. Rates vary approximately 20 – fold   around the world .The highest rates are seen largely in the developed world, North America, western Europe, and Australia, with age – adjusted (world standard) incidence rates of 25 to 35 per 100,000 in the late 1980s.It is notable that rates in northern Italy (>30 per 100,000 for males) now higher than in England and Wales (<20 per 100,000).The formerly lower rates in Japan have now risen to a level comparable to those in England and Wales. The lowest rate is seen in India (1 to 3 per 100,000).

In the 1960s and 1970s, colorectal cancer was essentially the only cancer that occurred approximately equal frequency in men and women. in North America and Australia (high rates) and Japan and Italy (rapidly rising rates) in particular, the male age adjusted rates now appear to exceed those of females, sometimes by more than 20% .The difference are less marked in England and Wales .The male and female rates in New Zealand non – Maoris (around 30 per 100,000) are equal (65) .There is a tendency for the rates to be similar between the sexes or to show a female excess before the age of 50 and, regularly, to shown a male excess after that age. The risk of cancer varies by subsite within the colon and rectum. The subsite risk varies between the sexes and further by age, women have higher rates of rightsided neoplasms than men and tend to develop cancer at an earlier age (67). The American Cancer Society estimates that 133,500 person in the United State will develop colorectal cancer in 1996 with 54,900 deaths. Approximately 6% of the American populations will eventually develop colorectal cancer. Studies of migrant population in the USA have shown the risks for colorectal cancer approach those of United States – born whites in the first generation or after >20 years of residence (68). Data from surveillance, Epidemiology and End Results Program of the National Cancer Institute indicate that over the past decades there have been proximal shifts in the sites of the colorectal cancer development: an increase in the cecal and ascending colon tumors and decrease in the rectal lesions (69).

More than half of all colonic cancers now develop either in the sigmoid (35%) or the cecum (22%).The distribution throughout the remaining colon is as follows: ascending colon (12 %) transverse colon (10 %) and descending colon (7%).

The incidence of colonic cancer (36.2 per 100,000 in the United States is about 2.5 times that reported for rectal cancer (14.6) per 100,000)).Within the large intestine,69% of cancers are in the colon and 31% in the rectum or at rectosigmoid junction(70).

The population of colorectal cancer in Iraq(71-75), like other Asian and Middle East countries were lower than that in the North America and Western countries, however it was witnessed an increasing in an alarming way in the percentage at the last ten years. It was also showed that colorectal cancer when combined colon and rectal cancer was among the commonest ten cancers in Iraq for the last ten years .Fig (1 – 1) shows the population of colorectal cancers in Iraq for the last ten years. From the figure there are two fold increasing in the population of colorectal through the last ten years.

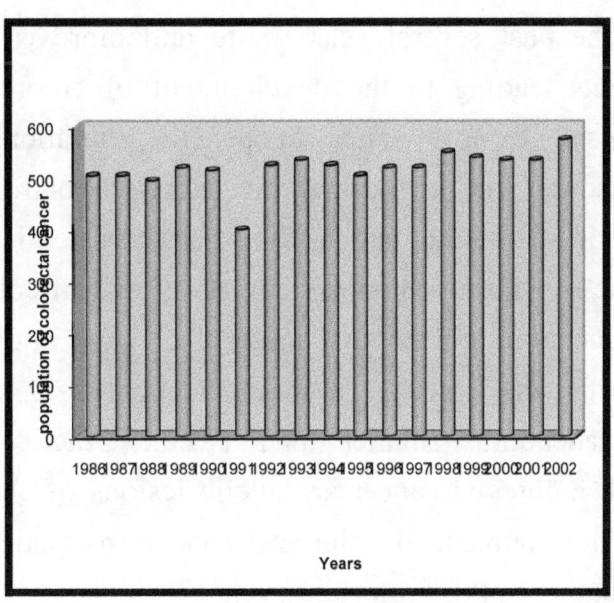

Figure (1–1): The population of colorectal cancer in Iraq through (1986 – 2002)

1 – 10 Etiology for Colorectal Cancer:

In contrast to pancreatic cancer, smoking does not play an etiologic role. Dietary factors however may play important causative and protective role. Fat intake has been the most consistently positive association and fiber intake the most consistantly inverse association. Comparing the incidence in different countries, the rates of colon cancer are strongly associated with the intake of animal fat and meat.

Carcinogenesis in the colon and rectum has been described in terms of an initiation – promotion model based on observation in laboratory animals. The first step involves initiating factors that directly interact with cellular DNA to induce mutations in genome. After wards the process is driven by promotional factors, which are not mutagenic by, themselves but enhance cellular proliferation of previously mutated cells. The human diet contains a lot of naturally occurring mutagens or substances that can be metabolized into mutagens.

During the past several years more and more is known about the molecular events leading to the development of colorectal cancer. It is believed to result from a series of genetic alterations leading to the progressive disorder of the normal mechanisms controlling growth. An important genetic alternation that has been demonstrated is a mutation within codon 12 of the K – ras – protooncogen. About half of colorectal carcinoma and similar percentage of adenomas larger than 1 cm in diameter have been found to have the ras – gene – mutation compared to less than 10 % of patients with adenomas smaller than 1 cm. Other genetic alterations associated with colorectal cancer are allelic lesions of chromosomes 5,17p and 18q .The development of colorectal cancer from adenomas appears to reflect accumulation of this molecular event (76 – 78).

Harden (79), implicated that in all cancers; their importance would vary depending on environmental effect strength. The current etiologies of colorectal cancer are:

1 – Genetics (80 – 83).

2 – Environmental factors (Diet including fat, fibers, and meat).

3 – Biological factors (84).

4 – Pathological disorders (84).

5 – Family History (84).

6 – Viruses (85 – 87).

1 – 11 Screening of Colorectal Cancer:

Screening procedures for colon cancer can be divided into two categories (88, 89). First are the procedures for patients who fall into high–risk group, and second are for those with no known risk factor other than age.

☐Screening High–Risk Individuals:

Patients with prior colon cancer, patients who have already colon or rectal cancer carry as significantly increased risk of a metachronous lesion (90). Often, these lesions are not cancer but are pre–malignant polyps.

Removal can preempt cancer and often can be done endoscopically, obviating further abdominal surgery.

First Degree Relatives of Patients:

A family history remains the primary starting point for identifying individuals who are at risk.

Individuals with first degree relative who have colorectal cancer are at significantly greater risk RR = (1.72) for developing colorectal cancer than the population at large (91, 92). This relative risk is most pronounced in those under 45 years at age RR = (5.37) (92).

The following family history diseases could be developed to colorectal tumors.

I – Crohn's Disease:

Patients with Crohn's disease also fall into the high–risk category(93). The clinical implications for Crohn's disease are complex. Because the segment of bowel involved is not predicable, removal of involved bowel "large or small" does not prevent the reoccurrence of Crohn's disease, thus, the surgical opportunity for preempting GI epithelial transformation in these patients is not available.

II – Ulcerative Colitis (U.C.)

At present, a lack of defined criteria for morphologic assessment of the conversion risk of ulcerative colitis mucosa from severe dysphasia to cancer creates a dilemma for pathologists.

Individual advice usually is based on population statistic .The empiric rule is to consider proctocolectomy after ten years of active ulcerative colitis; up to 50% of patients with a history of continuing ulcerative colitis(92,94).

III – Familial Polyposis Coli (FPC)

Patients with familial polyposis coli (FPC) and their first degree relative should be screened by colonscopy .New molecular biologic techniques can define whether young relatives of patients with FPC have a genetic constitution responsible for FPC, the absence of or mutation of the FAP locus on chromosome 5(95,96).

Screening in Asymptomatic Populations at Standard Risk:

Data accumulated over the last twenty years by the Strange Clinic Study support rectal examination and testing stool for occult blood as an essential part of every complete physical examination (97). Patients who have appropriate diagnostic work–ups after finding occult blood on systematic stool sampling are apt to have early bowel cancer or pre–cancer. (i.e., polyps)(89, 98). Systematic testing "fecal occult blood testing "can be recommended for appropriate age patients.

:Person at Increased Risk

The recommendations of patients with a family history of CRC are a colonoscopy within one year of initial resection. If the exam produces normal findings, follow up evaluations should be offered at three and five years (99).

1 – 12 Staging System of Colorectal Cancer (100):

A – Dukes Classification and its Modifications:

The first practical staging was the classification outlined initially in 1930 by Cuthbert Dukes, based on an earlier clinical categorization of rectal cancer by the surgeon, Lockhart – Mummery. Dukes classified rectal tumors from A to C:

* Stage A– penetration into but not through the bowel wall.
* Stage B– penetration through the bowel wall.

* Stage C– involvement of lymph nodes, regardless of the extent of the bowel wall penetration.

Subsequently, many modification, were made by Dukes, as well as by others (100).

Dukes, stage C was further subdivided into C1 (closely positive nodes) and C2 (positive nodes at the point of ligature).

A fourth stage, D, was added to indicate disease beyond the limit of surgical resection. Duke's classification is still widely used in staging colorectal cancer because of its simplicity and ease of use particularly by the surgeon and oncologist. However, the TNM system is increasingly being applied internationally.

B – TNM Classification:

The TNM classification for colorectal cancer is shown in table (1– 4) of the American Joint Committee on cancer and the Union International Control Cancer (AJCC/UICC) is compatible with the Dukes classification in that each of the three subsets of tumoral, nodal and metastatic involvement makes no assumption about the status in another part of the system that is, it allows for the exceptions to the general role of orderly progression of tumor spread.

The different Dukes classifications do not encompass all three prognostic factors in one staging system.

Table (1–4): TNM clinical classification system for staging colorectal cancer

Primary tumor (T)		
Tx	Primary tumor cannot be assessed.	
To	No evidence of primary tumor.	
Tis	Carcinoma in stiu confined within the glandular basement membrane (intra epithelial) or lamina propria (intramucosal) Tumor invades the sub mucosa.	
T1	Tumor invades the muscular is propria.	
T2	Tumor invades through the muscularis propria into the serosa or	
T3	into the non–peritonealized pericolic or perirectal tissue. Tumor directly invades other organs or structures and/or pre forates the visceral peritoneum tissues.	
T4		
Regional Lymph nodes (N)		
NX	Regional lymph nodes cannot be assessed.	
No	No regional lymph nodes metastasis.	
N1	Metastasis in 1–3 pericolic or perirectal lymph nodes.	
N2	Metastasis in >4 pericolic or perirectal lymph nodes.	
Distant Metastasis (M)		
M1	Presence of distant metastasis cannot be assessed.	
x	No distant metastasis.	
Mo	Distant metastasis.	
M1		
Stage Grouping		
	AJCC/VICC	Dukesa

Sta ge O	Tis	N0	M0	–
	T1	N0	M0	A
Sta ge I	T2	N0	M0	–
	T3	N0	M0	B
	T4	N0	M0	–
Sta ge II	Any T	N1	M0	C
	Any T	N2	M0	–
	Any T	Any N	M1	–
Sta ge III				
Sta ge IV				

aDukes B is composite of better (T3, N0, M0) and worse (T1, N0, M0) prognostic groups as in Dukes C (any T, N, M0 and any T, N2, M0).

1 – 13 Symptoms of Colorectal Cancer:

Clinical Picture:

Adenocarcinoma of the colon and rectum may be present as long as five years before symptoms appear; however, persons with symptomatic disease often have occult blood loss from their tumors, and the bleeding rate increase with tumors size and degree of ulceration.

Symptoms depend to some extent on the site of the primary tumor. Cancers of the proximal colon usually grow longer before they produce symptoms than those of the left colon and rectum. Constitutional symptoms "fatigue, shortness of breath, angina"secondary to microcytic hypochromic anemia may be the principle manner of presentation of right colon tumors. Less often, blood from right colon cancers is admixed with stool and appears as "mahagany feces" .As the tumor grows, it produce vague abdominal discomfort or presents as a palpable mass. Obstruction is uncommon because of the large diameters of the cecum and ascending colon, although rectal cancers may block the ileocecal valve and cause distal small bowel obstruction (58).

The left colon has a narrower lumen than the proximal colon, and cancers of the descending and sigmoid colon often involve the bowel circumferentially and cause obstructive symptoms. Patients may present with colicky abdominal pain, particularly after meals, and a changes in bowel habits. Constipation may alternate with increased frequency of detection, as small amounts of retained stool moved beyond the obstructing lesion. Hematochezia is present more often with distal lesions than with proximal ones, and bright red blood passed per rectum or coating the surface of the stool is common with cancers of the left colon and rectum. Rectal cancers also cause obstruction and changes in bowel habits, including constipation, diarrhea, and tenesmus .Rectal cancer may invade locally to involve the bladder, Vaginal wall, or surrounding nerves, resulting in perineal or sacral pain, but this is a late occurrence.

Symptomatic patients with colorectal cancer are often misdiagnosed. Symptoms are ascribed to benign conditions such as diverticular disease (abdominal pain, bleeding, change in stool caliber) ,irritable bowel syndrome (abdominal pain, change in bowel habits) ,or hemorrhoids (rectal bleeding).

Colorectal carcinoma should be considered when a patient, especially older than 40 years presents with hypochromic microcytic anemia or frank hematochezia and rectal bleeding. Too often, anemia in the elderly is ascribed to "chronic disease", only to be diagnosed later as a sign of colorectal cancer (101).

Abdominal pain – in any form–and bleeding also merit evaluation cancer in this age group. Large bowel cancer affects younger patients. Particularly those with inflammatory bowel disease or strong family history for colorectal and other cancers.

Judicious evaluation of younger patients for CRC is therefore warranted when suggested by history and clinical presentation.

1 – 14 Diagnosis of Colorectal Cancer:
   Diagnosis of colorectal cancer is first accomplished by (66):
1. Immunodiagnosis:
A.Immunohistochemistry:
   Several procedures are available but the most commonly used at present being peroxidase–antiperoxidase immune complex method and biotin - avidin immunoenzymatic technique.

Since immunoperoxidase – staining is directly applicable to electron microcopy, this added feature allows expanded ultrastructural studies with only slight modification of the same method used at the light microscope level (102).

B.Immunotargeting:

In this approach antibodies can be used in diagnostic clinical applications. Thus antibodies against pathology – specific markers such as carcinoembryonic antigen (CEA) can be used for targeting purposes.

During the last years a pioneer work has performed in the field of tumor targeting, such as the used of radiolabeled MAbs for detection of CRC by immunoscintigraphy (103,104), or the coupling of photoreactive substances to antitumor antibody (103,104). Other means are the use of dimeric mouse – human chimeric anti–IgA, which has the property to translocate the pseudo lumen of carcinomas glands, were the target CEA, is accumulating and the development of high activity molecule called peptabody (107).

2. Cytogenetic Diagnosis:

In colorectal cancer, there appears to be a relationship between the frequency of DNA aneuploidy and stage of the disease. There is also a correlation between histologic grade and aneuploidy. The significance of S–phase fraction measurement in colorectal cancer relative to that of DNA ploidy is not certain (108). Fischbach, Wet. al, have found significant difference in tissue concentration of CEA. Using FCM technique, DNA aneuploidy was present in 31.6%, 10.5% and 51.6% of chronic inflammatory bowel disease, CR–adenoma and CR–carcinoma respectively. This agrees with data in the literatures indicating DNA aneuploidy in 55% to 60% of CRC(109).

3. Flow Cytometry (FCM):

The rapidly expanding field of FCM consist of simultaneous measurement of several parameters (cell size, cytoplasmic granularity, cell viability, cell cycle time, DNA content, surface marker photype and enzyme content)(110). Jonssen AM et .al., (1999) studied the change of the activity levels of the antioxidant enzymes manganese and copper / zinc superoxidase disutase and found that the development of neoplasia in the human colorectal was accompanied by a major changes in the level activity of manganese superoxide dismutase (Mn–SOD) which illustrates that Mn–SOD might have a functional role in human CR carcinogenesis(111).

4. Imaging Techniques:

In vivo immunotargeting of specific antigens with radiolabeled monoclonal antibodies is a new method of diagnosis, which has greatly improved (112).

The most commonly used radionuclides in radioimmunodetection (RAID) are iodine–131, indium–111, and iodine–123 and technetium–99 m (113). An increasing number of different monoclonal antibodies, development against tumor–associated markers (114), are currently used for tumor targeting in cancer imaging.99mTc–labeled CEA and alpha – fetoprotein antibody fragments are used in combination with tomographic methods to increase target–to–background contrast. These techniques are used successfully for imaging small tumors (<0.5 cm), which can sometimes be missed by other radiologic methods, including computed tomography (CT) scans and magnetic resonance (MRI) imaging (115). With refinement of the technique, an increasing number of antibody–based imaging agents have become available in rapid, single step labeling kits that permit imaging within a few hours after injection (113), giving RAID many clinical applications. Other imaging techniques are:

1 – Whole–body positron emition tomography (PET), with flourine–18–2–Fluro–2–deoxy–D–glucose (116).

2 – Positron emission tomography (PET) joint to computed tomography (CT) (117).

3 – Computed tomography with arterial photography (CTAP).

4 – Trans abdominal ultrasonography (TUS).

5 – Hydrocolonic ultrasonography (HUS).

6 – Endosonography (Endoscopic Ultrasonography).

1 – 15 Treatment of Colorectal Cancer:
Surgery:

Surgical resection is the treatment of choice for most colorectal cancer. Preoperative colons copy should be performed, if possible, to rule out synchronous lesions and serum CEA should be measured to inform staging and post follow – up.

The goal of surgery is wide resection of the involved segment of bowel together with removal of its lymphatic drainage vessels. The resection should include a segment of colon at least 5 cm on either side of the tumor.

In patients, with colorectal cancer the primary tumor should be resected, even in the presence of distant metastasis to prevent obstruction or bleeding. In patients with advanced disease and multiple medical problems, repeated palliative fulguration or rectal tumors may be preferable to surgery. Newer modalitres, such as laser photoablations are being tested as alternative means of palliation in these patients (118,119).

Radiation Therapy

Radiation therapy is used preoperatively or post – operatively to decrease local recurrence in those with high–risk rectal and rectosigmoid cancers (Dukes' B2 and C lesions), or in a combined pre–operative and post operative "sandwich approach". Given the rectal demonstration of decreased recurrence and increased survival in patients with rectal cancer receiving combined post operative radiation and chemotherapy, this would appear to be the treatment of choice for high risk patients with transmural tumor extension or lymph node metastases (120).

Endoscopic Therapy:

Endoscopic therapy using the neodymium– yttrium–aluminum garnet (Nd:YAG) laser has been used to recanalize the rectum as palliative therapy in patients with obstructing rectal cancers who are poor surgical risks or who have advanced stages of malignant disease(119).

Photodynamic Therapy (PDT):

PDT has also been used to treat patients who are poor surgical risks. Patients are sensitized with a hematoporphyrin derivative, which is taken up by the tumor. Phototheraphy is then performed using a tunable dye laser and a flexible optical fiber, which can be inserted into the tumor (118).

Chemotherapy:

The mainstay of chemotherapeutic palliation is 5–fluorouracil (5–Fu). 5–Fu is a pyrimidine antimetabolite action in the "S" phase of the cell cycle (121). The cytotoxic effects of 5–FU are mediated by active metabolites, which inhibit the synthesis of thymidine, DNA and proteins (122). The clinical effectiveness of 5–FU is schedule dependent. Bolus regimens give consistently poor results with response rates of 5–25 %(123–127). Response rates improve markedly when 5–FU is administered by i.v. Infusion over 5 days or by protracted i.v. infusion over a period of many months (128,129). Several studies have demonstrated that in vitro 5–FU cytotoxic activity may be enhanced significantly by many drugs such as interferon, folates, and other antineoplastic drugs. In particular it has been shown that folinic acid strengths the binding of the 5–FU active metabolite, 5–FdUMP, to its target enzyme thymidylate synthase, forming a stable ternary complex that dissociates very slowly, increasing the fluoropyrimidine cytotoxic activity (130). The ability of folinic acid (FA) to enhance 5–FU antineoplastic activity has been confirmed in some prospective randomized trials in colorectal carcinoma patients (131,132). Other drugs for chemotherapy are: Methortrexate (MTX)(133),PALA [N–phosphonoacety ,L–aspartic acid](134) ,Hydroxy urea(135), Cisplatin(136), Dipyridanol(137),Tomudex,Oxalipaltin(137), Doxifluridine(137), Taxotere(135).

Immune Therapy:

A – Monoclonal Antibody (MAb):

Recent advance in immunology, molecular biology had let the development of radiolabeled antibodies that can be used in the detection of metastases lesions from CRC (radioimmuno detection).

These same antibodies can be linked to cytoxic agent such as the A subunit of the plant toxin ricin, the toxin A chain killer cells or chemotherapeutic agents for immunotargeted therapy (138–140)

Liposomes containing chemotherapeutic agents can be linked to monoclonal antibodies (MAbs) and delivered in a similar fashion (141). But in clinical application it was found that the major limitations of monoclonal conjugates as therapeutic agents have been their poor tumor targeting, in adequate tumor penetration and immunogenicity. More even and deeper tissue penetration has been demonstrated with smaller Antibody (Ab) fragments. The smaller size and absence of an FC segment may contribute to a lowered immunogenicity (142).

B – Cytokine Therapy:

The isolation and cloning of various cytokine gene has facilitated their large scale production. Among the cytokines that have been valuated in cancer immunotherapy are IFN–α, β and γ; IL–1, IL–2, IL–4, IL–5 and IL–12, GM–CSF, and INF. Although these trails have produced occasional hopeful results, many obstacles remain to the successful use of this type of cancer immunotherapy (142).

1 – Interferons (IFNs):

Use of interferons (IFNs) is based on in vitro data showing synergism with 5 – Fu in a dose–and schedule dependent manner. When combination with (FA) and 5–FU, IFN– α continues to produce clinically significant and probably prohibitive toxicity (143).

2 – Interleukin–2 (IL–2):

Early studies have established the effective doses of recombinant IL–2 (144–146) with 5–FU or with MAbs which have been synergistically interactive with IL–2 in vitro (147).

Gene Therapy:

Future novel approaches include use of gene therapy or gene engineering to exploit differences between normal and neoplastic cells. An artificial chimera is created that is composed of a tumor marker gene and a non mammalian enzyme. This is introduced and selectively expressed by the tumor cells bearing the marker (148). The non mammalian enzyme that slips along with the marker is a "Trojan horse" that can then be used to convert a pro drug harmless to normal tissue into a compound that is toxic to the chimera bearing cells.

Huber and Colleagues (148), created a chimera consisting of the CEA gene and cytosine deaminase gene; this made the tumor cells express cytosine deaminase and therefore become susceptible to toxicity from 5–Flurocytosine, which is harmless to the other cells. In chimera bearing cells, the pro drug is converted to 5 – FU (145). Transfect ion of the genes for IL–2 or GM – CSF (149) by a retroviral vector has evoked immunologic response against the inoculated cytokine secreting cells as well as recently injected parental cells. Efforts to transfer this approach to human investigation are in progress (149,150)

In order to find a suitable method for CA125 detection in colorectal tumors, the following ideas could be followed.

The Aim of the Work:

1 – Determination of CA125 Antigen level in sera of patients with benign and malignant colorectal tumors, pre and post–surgical resection the tumor.

2 – Development of IRAM method for cytosolic CA125 in benign and malignant colorectal tumors by using labeled Antibody (125 I–anti CA125 Antibody).

3 – Molecular characterization and determination of the optimum conditions for the binding of 125I – anti CA125 Antibody with CA125 in crude and partially purified from colorectal tissues homogenates and studying the effect of various factors affecting the binding   (temperature, time, pH, halides salts).

4 – Determination of the kinetic and thermodynamic parameters of the binding reaction of CA125 with its specific Antibody.

5 – Isolation of (anti CA125/CA125) isoforms in patients with colon cancer.

6 – SpectroscAbstract:

In this chapter we tried to find the optimum conditions of the binding of 125I – anti CA125 Antibody with A125 in nuclear and cytosolic fractions in the groups of colorectal tissue homogenate. The results obtained revealed a higher incidence of CA125 in two groups of malignant tumors than those in benign colorectal tumors (U.C) and in the cytosolic fractions more than the nuclear fractions.

The level of CA125 in serum of patients with benign and malignant colorectal tumors (preoperative) was measured by ImmunoRadiometricAssay (IRMA). The results obtained from this method showed that there was a highly significant differences between serum CA125 levels in colon and rectum tumors (P <0.001) as compared with benign tumors and significantly lower in benign colorectal tumors as compared with healthy subjects.

The binding of 125I–anti CA125 Antibody with CA125 was studied in three groups: benign colorectal tumors (U.C), malignant colon tumors (Colon Cancer Stage B) and malignant rectal cancer (rectum cancer Stage C).

The optimum conditions for the binding were as follows:

CA125 concentrations in tissue homogenate: $100\mu g$ .mL–1 for (U.C),

$400\mu g$ .mL–1 for Colon Cancer Stage B (CCB) and 200 μg .mL–1 for rectum cancer Stage C (RCC) .125I – anti CA125 Antibody concentration were: 1.44 mg.mL–1 for (U.C), 2.88 mg.mL–1 for (CCB) and 2.16 mg.mL–1 for (RCC). The optimum pH was 7.2 for (U.C), 7.8 for (C.CB) and (RCC). The optimum time and temperature were: three hours at 5oC for (U.C), seven hours at 25 oC for (CCB) and three hours at 5oC for (RCC).

The uses of different halides were shown to cause inhibitary effects on the binding of 125I –anti CA 125 Antibody to CA125 in all groups.

The use of different divalent cations was shown to increase the binding of CA125 to its Antibody (125I – anti CA125 Antibody) in all groups ,while the use of monovalent cations was shown to inhibit the binding of 125I – anti CA125 Antibody to CA125 in all groups studied

.Chapter Two

Introduction:

CA125 is a tumor – associated Antigen which was identified by a monoclonal antibody raised in mice against cell line (152), although increased serum concentrations are most commonly found in epithelial ovarian cancer (153,154), increases have also been described in patients with other gynecological malignancies (155,156).

Recently a murine monoclonal Antibody , was produced and designated 130 – 22 by fusing myeloma cells and spleen 130 – 22 recognized CA125 Antigen bound to aseparate antigenic determinant from that recognized by OC125(157) . Some patients with adenocarcinoma of lung also showed elevated levels of serum CA125 (157) .Indicating that CA125 was shared by ovarian and lung adenocarcinoma cells. Elevated CA125 level in serum was found in many cases including normal bronchial mucus(158) , firstimester of pregnancy(159) , during menstruation(160,161) ,endometriosis(162) , and also liver diseases associated with ascites(163) .

Serum CA125 level was determined by several methods including Enzyme Immunoassay (EIA) (164), ImmunoRadiometric Assay (IRMA) (165), and ImmunoFluoroMetric Assay (IFMA) (166).

There were no references to evaluate CA125 in colorectal tumors tissues by ImmunoRadiometric Assay, therefore the goal of this chapter is to develop a diagnostic utility of serum CA125 level in patients with colorectal tumors and demonstrate the optimum conditions of 125I –anti CA125 Antibody binding with CA125 in colorectal tissue homogenate.

2–1 Chemicals, Instruments and Samples:

All chemicals and reagents used in this study were of analar grade

Table (2–1): Chemicals used and companies provided with

Chemical.	Company.
1– ImmunoRadiometric kit for CA125 Antigen level	Immunotech (Beckman coulter) (France)
2–Tris (hydroxy methyl amino methane , Bovine Serum Albumin (BSA) ,Tris (hydroxy methyl amino methane) hydrochloride ,MgCl2, ZnCl2, and CaCl2 ,EDTA ,Sucrose	Fluka (Switzerland)
3– CuSO4.5H2O, Na,K–tarterate ,NaOH , HCl , Na2CO3 ,NaF ,NaCl ,NaBr ,NiCl2.6H2O ,and MnCl2 , Folin – ciocalteaue	BDH ,Limited pool (UK)
4– Blue dextran (2000) , Sepharose Cl– 6B	Pharmacia Fine Chemicals (Sweden)

2–2 Instruments:

Table (2–2): Instruments used and companies provided with:

Instruments	Company
1 – Gamma counter Type 1270–rack GammII	LKB
2 – Cintra 5 UV/visible Spectrophotometer, SM–Shaker	England
3 – PH M62 Standard pH meter	Denmark
4 – Sartorius analytical balance BL 210 S	Germ

	any
5 – Cooling centrifuge type 202– ; with maximum Speed 13500 r.p.m.	Sigma

2–3 Patients:

A total of 95 colorectal patients involved in this study with benign and malignant tumors (50 male), (45 female) subjected to curative surgery. Their mean age was 49 year ranges (16–88 years).

Two groups of CRC patients and one group with benign colorectal tumors were involved in this study.

According to the histopathological examination of the resected pieces, the patients were grouped into the following:

Group (1): Consisted of 15 patients with benign colorectal tumors (Ulcerative Colitis).

Group (2): Consisted of 39 patients with Colon Cancer Stage B.

Group (3): Consisted of 41 patients with rectal cancer Stage C.

Blood samples were also collected from all patients involved in this study, and also from normal donors with age range between (15–75)

Years .The patients were admitted for treatment and diagnosis to the following hospitals in Baghdad:

*Kadumia Teaching Hospital.

*AL–Yarmook Teaching Hospital

*AL–Kindy Teaching Hospital

*Baghdad Teaching Hospital.

*Nursing Home Private Hospital.

*AL–Najat Private Hospital.

*AL–Mustaunsiryah Private Hospital.

*AL–Zahra 'a Private Hospital .

Patients with diseases that may interfere with this study were excluded. All surgical operations of malignant and benign tumors were done under the supervision of surgeons:

Dr. Zuhair AL–Bahraini, Dr.Saaeb Sedeq, Dr.Faleh AL–Aubaidy, Dr.Abd AL–Salam AL–Tai, Dr. Azam Qanber Aga, Dr.Maa'd Medhat and Dr. Nazar Taha Maky .

2–4 Blood Sampling:

Blood samples (3–5) mL were obtained from patients of groups mentioned above , by vein puncture before surgical operation .The whole blood was left for (10–20) min. at room temperature . After coagulation, the serum was separated by centrifugation at 3000 r.p.m. for 10 min. Serum specimens were then frozen at –20oC until assayed.

Table (2–3): The host information of patients and healthy which are used in this study

Patients	Number	Type of Tumor	Age Range Year
Group I	15	Benign tumor (Ulcerative Colitis)	16–38
Group II	39	Colon Cancer Stage B	41–75
Group III	41	Rectal cancer Stage C	50–88
Group IV	30	Control	30–65

The weight of resected tissue samples range between (1.5–25) gm.

2–5 Specimens Collection:

The tumors were surgically removed from patients of colon and rectum (CR). They were immediately rinsed with ice–cold saline solution, and immersed in the same solution. They were collected and stored at –20oC until homogenization.

2 – 6 Preparation of Tissue Homogenate:

The frozen tissues were washed with ice cold normal saline and then weighed. They were minced, pulverized, with a scalpel scissors in the Petri dish placed on ice bath, and then homogenized at 4oC in tris buffer (0.05M , pH 7.4) with a ratio of 1 : 3 (weight : volume) using normal homogenizer .

The homogenates were filtered through a nylon mesh sieve in order to eliminate fiber connective tissue, and then centrifuged at 9000 r.p.m. for 30 min. in cooling centrifuge at 4oC. The supernatants and pellets were considered cytosolic and nuclear fractions respectively. The pellet (sediment)

was discarded and the cytosolic (supernatant) was used in experiments involved cytosolic cancer Antigen CA125 (125) source.

Solutions:

TES Buffer solution (0.05M, pH 7.4) was prepared as follows : (3.0285gm) of tris (hydroxy methyl amino methane), 0.93060 of Ethylene di amine tetra acetate di sodium salt (EDTA) and (42.7875gm) of sucrose was dissolved in 400 mL of deionized distilled water , and the pH was adjusted with HCl (1M) at 7.4 then the solution was completed to 500 mL with deionized distilled water

2 – 7 Protein Determinations:

The method of Lowry et. al. (151) was used to determine total proteins in tissue and sera, using Bovine Serum Albumin (BSA) as standard protein.

Solutions:

1– Standard Bovine Serum Albumin (BSA) (1mg/mL).

2– Solution A, Alkaline Sodium carbonate solution (2% Na_2CO_3 in 0.1N NaOH).

3–Solution B (Copper Sulphate –Sodium Potassium tartrate solution (0.5 % $CuSO_4$.$5H_2O$ in 1% Na–K tartrate.

4– Solution C, Alkaline copper solution, 50 mL of solution A was mixed with 1mL of solution B discards after one day.

5– Solution D, Folin ciocalteaue solution, prepared by the dilution of the commercial solution with an equal volume of distilled water on the day of use.

Procedure:

1- One milliliter of standard Bovine Serum Albumin (BSA) containing (0, 25, 50, 75, 100, 150, 175, 200) µg /mL protein was pipetted in a set of duplicate tubes.

2- A set of duplicate tubes containing 150 µL of cytosolic fraction of tissue specimens, and the volume were made to one mL with deionized distilled water.

3- Five milliliter of solution C was added to all tubes. Then the contents were mixed by vortexing, and allowed to stand for 10 min. at room temperature.

4- Half milliliter of solution D was added drop by drop with mixing. The mixture was left to stand for 30 min. at room temperature.

5- The absorbance of the developing color was read at 600 nm. against the blank.

6- The standard curve was obtained by plotting the absorbance against the corresponding concentrations of standard protein and used to determine the unknown protein concentration of tissue homogenate specimens and serum as shown in Fig. (2–1).

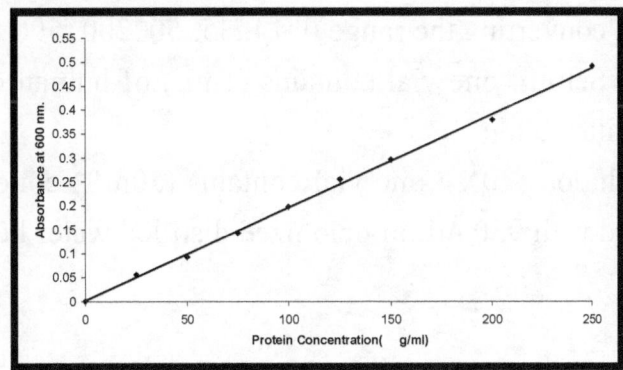

Figure: (2–1) Standard curve of protein determination (All other details are explained in the text).

2–8 Determination of Cancer Antigen CA125 Level in Sera of Patients with Benign and Malignant Colorectal Tumors:

Serum CA125 levels were measured by ImmunoRadiometric Assay (IRMA). The assay is a two site "Sandwich" assay in which two mouse monoclonal antibodies directed against two different epitopes of the molecule, are used.

Samples or standards were incubated in tubes, coated with the first monoclonal Antibody, in the presence of the second, 125Iodine – labeled monoclonal Antibody. Following incubation the liquid contents of the tubes are aspirated and the excess unbound, labeled Antibody is removed by washing.

Solutions:

The solutions used in this assay were provided with the kit described as follows:

1- Monoclonal 125I– labeled anti CA125 tracer Antibody, one vial contains 33 mL (13μci) (480KBq) of 125I–labeled in buffer, BSA, Sodium azide (<0.1%) and dye.

2- Anti– CA125 monoclonal Antibody coated tubes.

3- CA125 Serum Standard: six vials, four vials contain (2 mL) and two zero vials contain (5 mL). The six standard vials contain human CA125 in liquid form with BSA and sodium azide (< 0.1%) for a construction of a standard curve, converting the range 0, 14, 35, 50, 200, 500 IU/mL.

4- Controls Serum: one vial contains (1mL) of human CA125 in human serum with sodium azide.

5- Wash solution (20X): one vial contains (50mL) concentrated solution has to be diluted with 950 mL of deionized distilled water before use.

Procedure:

The assay details in the following procedure described in the leaflet provided from Immunotech Company are:

1- Number a duplicate series of 125I – anti CA125 Antibody coated tubes.

2- Add sequentially either 100 μL of standard control or samples to the bottom of tube, followed by 300μL of tracer, vortex gently.

3- To two additional tubes add 300 μL of tracer in order to obtain total c.p.m (T).

4- Incubate all tubes for four hours at room temperature (18–25oC) with moderate horizontal shaking (4000r.p.m)

5- Aspirate contents of all tubes carefully, except of those for total c.p.m.

6- Add 2 mL of wash solution to each tube (except tubes for total c.p.m) and immediately aspirate contents of the tubes. Repeat this operation twice. No trace of dye should remain.

7- Measure radioactivity of tubes for counts bound (B) and total (c.p.m) (T).

Calculations:

1– The mean net count c.p.m for each group after subtracting the background of each pair of duplicate tubes were counted in gamma counter for one minute.

2– The (B/T %) ratio was computed for each standard and unknown samples as follows :

$$(B/T\%) = \frac{\text{Standard or sample mean count}}{\text{Total activity mean count}} \times 100$$

3– The standard curve was drawn by plotting the percent value for each standard (vertical axis) versus CA125 concentration (horizontal axis) on semi – logarithmic graph paper. As shown in fig. (2–2)

4–CA125 concentration of unknown was calculated from the standard curve using their duplicate counts.

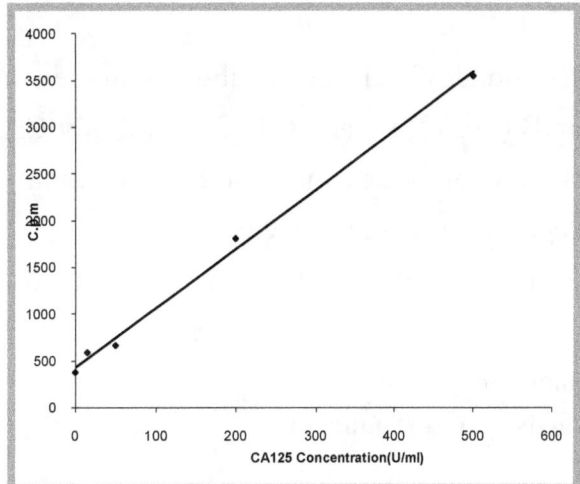

Figure (2–2) : Standard curve of CA125 determination in human sera by IRMA method (All other details are explained in the text) .

2–9: Binding Studies of Cancer Antigen CA125 in Colorectal Tumors Homogenate with 125I–Anti CA125 Antibody:

The detection of cytosolic and nuclear CA125 was carried out using ordinary tubes (not coated with MAb.)

393

1- 100ml of crude colorectal cytosolic homogenate (i.e. Ulcerative Colitis (U.C), Colon Cancer Stage B. and Rectal cancer Stage C having (1300,1100 and 1000) µg protein was incubated with 50µl of 125I–anti CA125 Antibody, the volume of mixture was completed to 250µl with tris buffer (0.05M, pH7.4).

2- All tubes were incubated at 25 oC for four hours.

3- After incubation, the tubes were centrifuged at 4000 r.p.m for one hour at 4oC by using cooling centrifuge.

4- The supernatant was discarded and the complex formed was counted in gamma counter for one minute.

5- Nuclear CA125 was estimated by dissolving the sediment of nuclei in tris buffer (pH7.4) with a ratio 1:10 (weight: volume) with shaking.

6- In order to detect the nuclear CA125, 100µl of colorectal homogenate i.e. (U.C, Colon Cancer Stage B and rectal cancer Stage C having (216,183,167µg) protein were incubated with 50ml of 125I–anti CA125 Antibody and volume the was completed to 250µl with tris buffer (0.05M , pH7.4).

7- Steps 2, 3, 4 for cytosolic fractions were repeated.

Calculations:

1- The count radioactivity in each tube (expressed in c.p.m) represents the bound fraction B (i.e. 125I – anti CA125 Antibody/CA125) complex.

2- The count ratio activities in the tubes containing 125I–anti CA125 Antibody alone represent the total activity.

3- The ratio of (B/T)% for each tube was count as follows:

$$(B/T) = \frac{\text{Sample mean count (B)}}{\text{Total activity mean count (T)}} \times 100$$

Solution:

Tris buffer (0.05M, pH7.4) was prepared by dissolving (0.6057gm of tris (hydroxy methyl amino methane in 50 ml of deionized distilled water and the pH was adjusted with HCl (1M) at pH7.4, the volume was completed to 100ml with deionized distilled water.

2–10: Factors Effecting 125I–Anti CA125 Antibody Binding to CA125 in Colorectal Tissue Homogenate:

2–10–1: The Effect of Different Protein Concentrations of the Homogenate on the Binding:

1- Fifty milliliter of 125I–anti CA125 Antibody were added to 100µl of crude cytosolic homogenate (U.C, Colon Cancer Stage B and Rectal cancer Stage C) containing increasing amounts of protein concentration (50,100,200,300,400,500) µg. ml – 1 completed to a final volume of 250µl with tris buffer (0.05M,pH7.4).

2- The tubes were incubated for four hours at 25 oC.

3- Two additional tubes containing 50µl of 125I–anti CA125 Antibody only, for total activity computation, were set aside until counting.

4- After incubation, the tubes were centrifuged at 4000r.p.m for one hour at 4oC by using cooling centrifuge.

5- The supernatant was decanted and the radioactivity of the complex formed was count.

Solutions:

Tris buffer (0.05, pH7.4) prepared as described in the experiment of (Binding studies of Cancer Antigen in colorectal tumors homogenate with 125I – anti CA125 Antibody.

Calculations:

1 – The B/T percent were determined according to the experiment of (Binding studies of Cancer Antigen CA125 in colorectal tumors homogenate with 125I – anti CA125 Antibody).

2 – The percent of binding values B/T were plotted versus increasing amount of protein of the colorectal tissue homogenate.

2–10–2: The Effect of 125I–Anti CA125 Antibody Concentration on the Binding:

1– Increasing amounts of 125I–anti CA125 Antibody (10, 20, 30, 40, 50) µl were added to 100µl colorectal tissue homogenate (100) µg.ml – 1 for U.C, 400µg.ml – 1 for Colon Cancer Stage B and 200µg.ml – 1 for Rectum cancer C).

2– The volume was made up to 250µl with tris buffer pH7.4.

3 – Steps 2,3,4,5 in the experiment of (The effect of different protein concentration of homogenate on the binding) were repeated

Calculations:

Values (B/T) % was calculated as described in the experiment of (Binding studies of Cancer Antigen CA125 in colorectal tumors homogenate with 125I – anti CA125 Antibody).

1- Values of (B/T)% were plotted versus concentration of labeled Antibody (125I–anti CA125 Antibody).

2–10–3: The Effect of pH on Binding:

1- One hundred µl of human colorectal homogenate (U.C, CC Stage B and RC Stage C containing (100,400,200µg.ml– 1) respectively were added to (20, 40 and 30µl) respectively i.e. (1.44, 2.88 and 2.16mg.ml– 1 of 125I–anti CA125 Antibody.

2- For each tube in step1 were completed to 250µl with tris buffer (0.05M) with different pH (6.8 – 8).

3- Steps 2,3,4,5 the experiment of (The effect of different protein concentration of homogenate on the binding) were repeated.

Calculations:

1- Values (B/T) % was calculated as described in the experiment of (Binding studies of Cancer Antigen CA125 in colorectal tumors homogenate with 125I – anti CA125 Antibody).

2- Values of (B/T) % were plotted versus different pH.

Solutions:

        Tris Buffer used as described in the experiment of (Binding studies of Cancer Antigen CA125 in colorectal tumors homogenate with 125I – anti CA125 Antibody).

2–10–4: Time Course of CA125 Binding in Colorectal Tissue Homogenate:

1-   One hundred µl of colorectal tissue homogenate (U.C, CC Stage B and RC Stage C) containing (100, 400, and 200 µg .ml – 1) protein were added to (1.44, 2.88, and 2.16 mg.ml– 1) of 125I – anti CA125 Antibody.

2-   The volume was completed to 250 µl with tris buffer (0.05 M , pH 7.2 , 7.8 , and 7.8) respectively

3- All tubes were incubated at 25oC at different time intervals (1, 2, 3, 4, 5, 6, 7, and 8) hours.

4- To determine the time course of CA125 binding to 125I – anti CA125 Antibody at different temperatures. Steps 1, 2 in the same experiment were repeated at different temperature (5, 37 and 45) oC.

5- Steps 3, 4, 5 in experiment of (The effect of different protein concentration of homogenate on the binding) were repeated.

Calculations:

1 – (B/T) % was calculated as described in the experiment of (Binding studies of Cancer Antigen CA125 in colorectal tumors homogenate with 125I – anti CA125 Antibody) at each time and temperature.

2 – The values of (B/T) % were plotted versus the time at different temperatures.

Solutions:

Tris buffer was used as described in the experiment of (Binding studies of Cancer Antigen CA125 in colorectal tumors homogenate with 125I – anti CA125 Antibody).

2–10–5: The Effect of Different Halides on Binding:

1- At the optimum conditions of colorectal tissue homogenate for the three groups (i.e. U.C, CC Stage B and RC Stage C) by incubation 100µl of each group of homogenate (100,400 and 200µg.ml–1 protein and (1.44,2.88,and 2.16 mg.ml – 1) of 125I–anti CA125 Antibody.

2- Fifty microliter of the following halides (0.01M) (NaI, NaBr, NaCl, and NaF) was added to the mixture.

3- The volumes of the mixture were completed to 250µl with tris buffer (pH7.2, 7.8 and 7.8) for each group of homogenate respectively.

4- All the tubes were incubated at the following temperature and hours for the three groups (3hr.at5 oC, 7 hr. at 25 oC and 3 hr. at 5 oC) respectively.

5- A sample of each group of the three groups of tissue homogenate as a control was left without any addition of any halide and incubated at the optimum conditions for each group.

6- Steps 3, 4, 5 mentioned in experiment of (The effect of different protein concentration of homogenate on the binding) were repeated.

Calculations:

1 –The value of (B/T) % was calculated as mentioned in the experiment of (binding studies of Cancer Antigen CA125 in colorectal tumors homogenate with 125I – anti CA125 Antibody).

2 –The value of binding percent was plotted versus halides concentration.

Solutions:

1- Tris buffer was prepared as described in the experiment of (Binding studies of Cancer Antigen CA125 in colorectal tumors homogenate with 125I – anti CA125 Antibody) was adjusted to the corresponding pH for each group of tissue homogenate.

2- Halides solutions were prepared in concentration (0.01M) in tris buffer solution and the pH was adjusted to the corresponding pH for each group of tissue homogenate.

3- Four types of halides were prepared by dissolving 0.021gm of NaF, 0.0292gm of NaCl, 0.0515gm of NaBr, and 0.075 gm of NaI. Each type of halides was dissolved in tris buffer and the pH was adjusted to the corresponding pH of each group of tissue homogenate then the volume was completed to 50 ml with tris buffer.

2–10–6: The Effect of Divalent and Monovalent of Binding of CA125 with 125I–Anti CA125 Antibody:

1- Fifty microliter of (0.025M) of the following Monovalent and divalent cations (KCl, NH4Cl, CsCl, LiCl, CaCl2.2H2O, MgCl2.6H2O, MnCl2.4H2O, CuSO4.5H2O, ZnCl2, NiCl2.6H2O) were added to each group of tissue homogenate at the optimum conditions for each group.

2- The incubation was made up for each group at the optimum time and temperature.

3- A sample of each group of tissue homogenate at the optimum conditions was left aside without addition of any salt was used as a control.

4- Steps (3, 4, 5, and 6) in experiment of (The effect of different protein concentration of homogenate on the binding) were repeated.

Calculations:

1- The value (B/T)% were calculated as mentioned in the experiment of (Binding studies of Cancer Antigen CA125 in colorectal tumors homogenate with 125I – anti CA125 Antibody).The value of binding percent was plotted versus each Monovalent and divalent cations.

Solutions:

1- Tris buffer prepared as described in the experiment of (Binding studies of Cancer Antigen CA125 in colorectal tumors homogenate with 125I – anti CA125 Antibody) and adjusted to the corresponding pH for each group of tissue homogenate.

2- Monovalent and divalent were prepared by dissolving (0.0931gm of KCl, 0.0668gm of NH4Cl, 0.048gm of LiCl, 0.069gm of CsCl, 0.2541gm of MgCl2.6H2O, 0.1388gm of CaCl2.2H2O, 0.2474gm of MnCl2.4H2O, 0.3150gm of CuSO4.5H2O, 0.1703gm of ZnCl2 and 0.2588gm of NiCl2.6H2O) in tris buffer, the pH was adjusted to the corresponding pH for each group of tissue homogenate at the optimum pH for each group and the volume was completed to 50ml with tris buffer.

Results and Discussion:

Three groups of colorectal tumors were included in this study. These groups were classified according to their position (either in colon or rectum) and each type confirmed by histopathological examination (Stage B and C). The homogenates were centrifuged at 9000 r.p.m and 4oC to obtain the pellet and supernatant. The pellets represent the nuclear source, while the supernatants were used to obtain the cytosolic source (167). The Homogenization and centrifugation were carried out at 4C° in order to avoid protein denaturation (168).

The filtration of the tissue homogenate through several layers of nylon gauze was used to remove any suspended pieces of unhomogenized fragments and blood vessels, while the centrifugation of homogenate at 9000 r.p.m removed the unruptured cells and intact nuclei of the ruptured cells (169).

Determination of CA 125 Levels in Sera of Patients with Colorectal Tumors:

CA 125 levels in sera were measured with an Immuno Radiometric Assay (IRMA) in three groups of colorectal tumors matched with one group of control subject. Group I consisted of fifteen patients with benign colorectal tumors, group II included thirty nine patients with Colon Cancer Stage B and group III consisted of forty one patients of rectum cancer Stage C as summarized in table (2–3).

Table (2–4) shows that the CA125 levels in two malignant groups (CCB and RCC) were highly significant elevation ($P < 0.001$) and lowerly significant elevation ($P < 0.05$) for benign colorectal tumors (U.C) as compared with the control according to the student's T–test analysis (170).

The mean serum CA 125 level of the control was found to be

(21.3 U.ml±0.58) as shown in table (2 – 4) and the cut of values was found to be 35 U.ml–1 (171).

The elevations of CA125 in patients with colon and rectum cancer were in agreement with other studies found in this field (172,173).

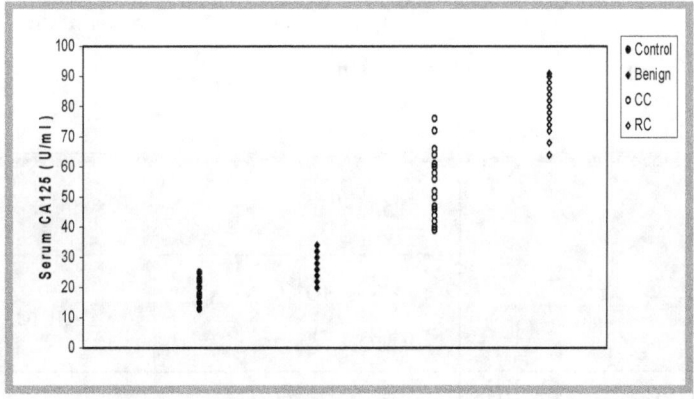

Figure (2 – 3): Distribution of CA125 level (U .ml – 1) in human sera by IRMA . (All other details are explained in the text).

Table (2–4): Sera CA125 levels (U.ml–1) in patients with benign and malignant colorectal tumors.

Group	Patients	No. of cases	Age range year	Sera CA125 U.ml–1	P values
I	Benign tumor U.C	15	16–38	25.86±1.38	P < 0.05
II	Colon Cancer Stage B	39	41–75	52.26±1.21	P < 0.001
III	Rectum Cancer Stage C	41	50–88	76.05±1.56	P < 0.001
IV	Control	30	30–65	21.3±0.58	

Binding Studies on CA 125 in Colorectal Tissue with 125I–Antibody

Preliminary Test of the Binding of CA 125 with 125I–Anti CA 125

Cytosolic and nuclear CA 125 were investigated in three groups of colorectal tumors homogenate (Ulcerative colitis (U.C), Colon Cancer Stage B(CCB) and Rectal Cancer Stage C (RCC)). In each group, CA 125 was detected by the incubation of 125I–anti CA125 Antibody with both cytosolic and nuclear fractions for 4 hr. at 25C° and the reactions were completed with tris buffer. The separation of the bound Antibody from the unbound was carried out at 4000 r.p.m for one hour. to precipitate the (125I–Antibody / CA 125) complex formed.

Table (2–5): Preliminary conditions of CA 125 in cytosol and nuclear fractions in three different colorectal homogenate.

Group	B/T %	
	Cytosolic fraction	Nuclear fraction
Ulcerative Colitis (U.C)	2.7	0.9
Colon Cancer Stage B	3.1	1.1
Rectum Cancer Stage C	4.5	1.4

Table (2–5) shows the amount of binding B/T % values in both cytosolic and nuclear fractions. The data revealed that CA125 was higher in cytosolic fractions than in nuclear and in general CA125 concentration in malignant tumor homogenate more than that in benign tumors tissue (i.e. U.C.). This observation is in good agreement with the results of several authors (174–176).

Optimum Conditions for the Binding of Cancer Antigen (CA 125) in Colorectal Tissue Homogenate with 125I–Anti CA 125:

Optimum Protein Concentration:

To estimate the suitable concentration of homogenates, 50 µL of 125I–anti CA125 Antibody were incubated with increasing concentration of cytosolic homogenate, according to the details in experiment of (The effect of different protein concentration of homogenate on the binding)

Figure (2 – 4) represents the formation of (125I–anti CA 125 Antibody / CA 125) complex in three groups of colorectal tumors (U.C, CCB and RCC).

The results revealed that the binding of CA 125 to 125I–anti CA 125 Antibody increases with increasing CA 125 homogenate. Figure (2–4) shows that 100µg, 400µg and 200µg.ml-1 protein were the most appropriate concentrations to give the maximum values of binding in U.C, CCB and RCC respectively. The decrease in binding after reaching the maximum binding may be due to the solubilization of the complex formed by the excess of CA125 added (177), or may be due to the conformational changes in CA125 and 125I–anti CA125 Antibody rather than the formation of reversible inactive (125I–anti CA125 Antibody / CA125) complex (178). Another opinion reported that the complex precipitate out solution, due to the multivalent nature of both molecules (179). The radioactive Antibody has two binding sites, it can cross link antigenic sites of two different CA125 molecules and can produce maximum complex formation and therefore maximum precipitate will occur (179).

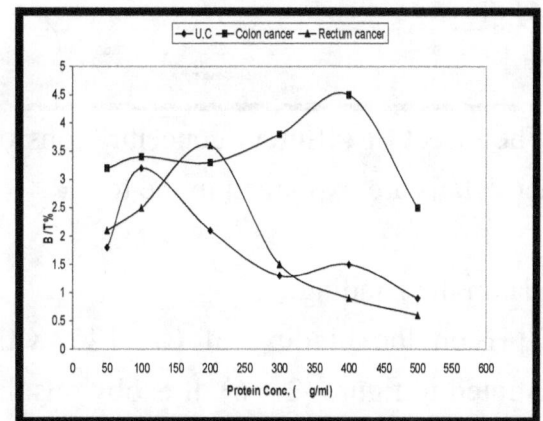

Figure (2–4): Influence of protein concentration on the binding with 125I–anti CA125 Antibody (All other details are explained in the text)

μ

The Effect of 125I–Anti CA125 Antibody Concentration on the Binding:

This experiment was carried out in the presence of fixed amount of protein concentration of the colorectal tumors homogenate and increasing concentration of 125I–anti CA125 Antibody. The results obtained are shown in figure (2–5). It is clear that the amount of (125I–anti CA125 Antibody / CA125) complex rises gradually and then the colorectal tumors protein was saturated with 125I–anti CA125 Antibody.

The maximum binding occurred when the concentrations of the Antibody were (1.44, 2.88 and 2.16 mg.ml–1) for the three groups of colorectal tumors (i.e. U.C, CCB and RCC) respectively. Then the binding percent decreased as the amount of 125I–anti CA125 Antibody increased.

The reason is due to all antigenic sites covered with Antibody and complex formation is inhibited (180). These results indicate that the binding is principally dependent on the amount of the Antibody in the reaction mixture (181), because one of the factors affecting the binding percent of Antibody – Antigen reaction is the concentration of the Antibody.

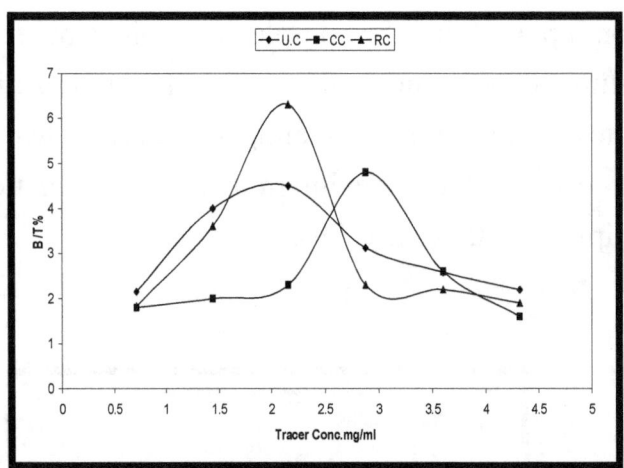

Figure (2–5): The effect of different concentrations of 125I– anti CA125 Antibody (All other details are explained in the text).

The Effect of pH on the Binding:

The effect of pH on the binding of CA 125 with 125I–anti CA125 Antibody was illustrated in figure (2 – 6). It is obvious that the binding occur when pH were (7.2, 7.8 and 7.8) respectively for the three groups of colorectal tumors (i.e. U.C, CCB and RCC) respectively.

Immunoprecipitation is usually performed at pH between 7.0 and 9.0; the immunoprecipitates are soluble below pH 4.5 and above pH 10.0. However these results indicate that the binding was pH dependent. The protein CA 125 binding site which is composed of ionizable groups that should be in the proper ionic form in order to maintain a proper conformation of the binding site to bind 125I–anti CA 125 Antibody (182). In addition, 125I–anti CA 125 Antibody itself may have ionizable groups and only at a certain pH the Antibody will have ionic form where it can bind to CA 125(183).

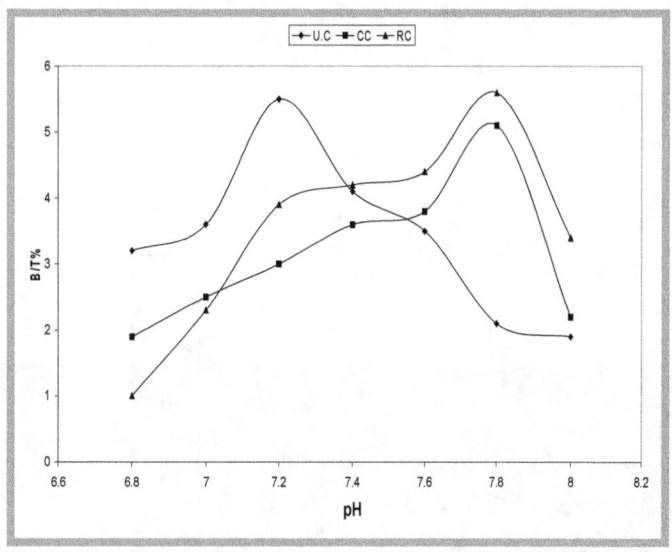

Figure (2–6): The effect of pH on the binding of 125I–anti CA125 Antibody with CA125 (All other details are explained in the text).

Time Course of the Binding of 125I–Anti CA 125 Antibody to CA 125 in Colorectal Tumors:

Figure (2–7) shows the results obtained from the time course pattern at different temperatures (5, 25, 37 and 45°C). The maximum binding occurred at 5°C after incubation for 4 hours in crude fractions of U.C and at 5°C after incubation for 3 hours, in rectum cancer Stage C, whereas the binding in crude fractions of Colon Cancer Stage B occurred at 25°C after incubation for 7 hours. These results indicate that 125I–anti CA125 Antibody binding to crude fraction of CA125 are temperature and time dependent process.

The decrease of the binding may be due to either the degradation of CA125 or irreversible dissociation of the (125I–anti CA125 Antibody / CA125) complex. At higher temperatures, denaturation and destruction tertiary structure may occur leading to loss of activity and conformational changes. At lower temperature, heat is not enough to overcome the energy barrier, even for catalyzed reaction (184). Heating more than 45C° disrupt the folded structure of the protein by increasing the vibrational and rotational motions of atoms was occurred(185).

The results obtained in this experiment were used in all subsequent experiments.

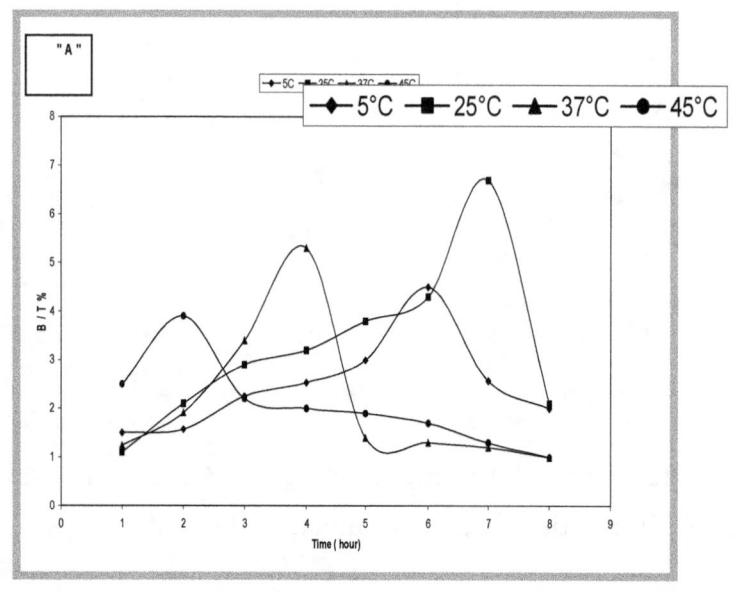

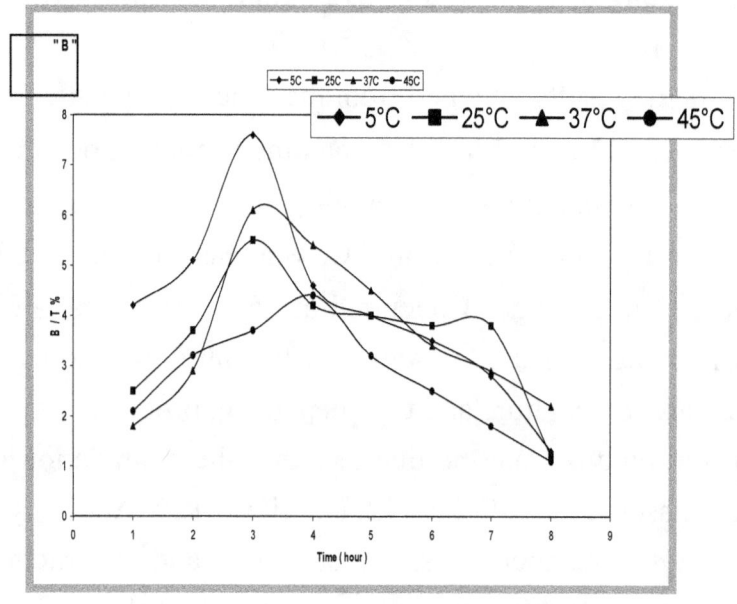

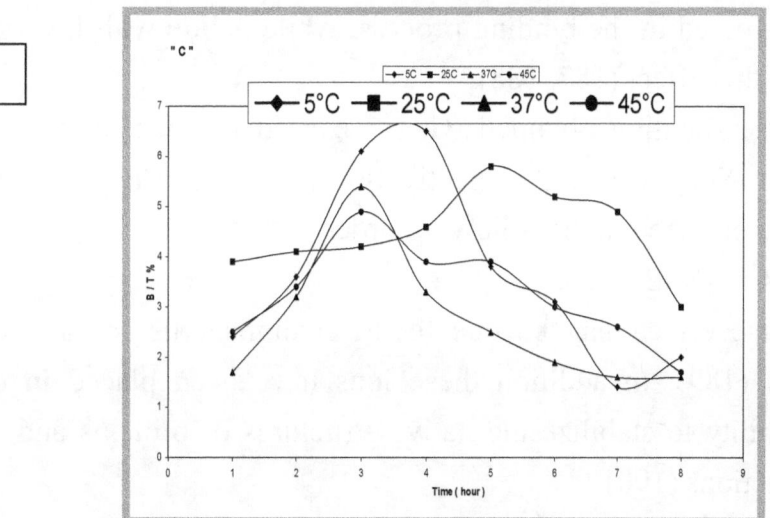

Figure (2–7) : Time course of the 125I–anti CA125 Antibody binding to CA125 in :

(A) Colon Cancer Stage "B"

(B) Rectum Cancer Stage "C"

(C) Ulcerative Colitis

(All other details are explained in the text).

The Effect of Different Halides on the Binding:

To study the effect of different halides on the binding of 125I–anti CA125 Antibody with CA125, (0.01 M) concentration of (NaI, NaBr, NaCl, NaF) were used. Figure (2–8) shows the effect of these halides. The results indicated that the sodium halides inhibit the Antibody–Antigen (Ab – Ag) binding according to the following order for the U.C (benign colorectal tumor): –

NaI < NaBr < NaCl < NaF

Due to the decreasing ionic radius and increasing radius of hydration. It seemed that fluoride ion causes lower binding, this could be due to higher electro negativity of fluoride ion that tend to interact with the positive residue in the binding site of the Antibody and/or the Antigen which lead to decrease the interaction between CA125 and 125I–anti CA 125 Antibody(186). The order corresponds to the increasing molar surface tension increment value and molar surface tension increment values (MSTI). Salt halide with high (MSTI) i.e., value will strengthen hydrophobic interaction which is essentially involved in the binding process, while halide with lower (MSTI) value reverse this effect (187, 188).

The reverse situation obtained when we used CA 125 from colon and rectum cancer (Stage B and C respectively). Inhibition of the binding by the sodium halide occurred in the following order

NaF < NaCl < NaBr < NaI

This reverse effect may be due to the malignant tissues and different target organs (189). In addition these ions have been placed in order of decreasing ability to stabilize the native structures of proteins and protein–protein interactions (190).

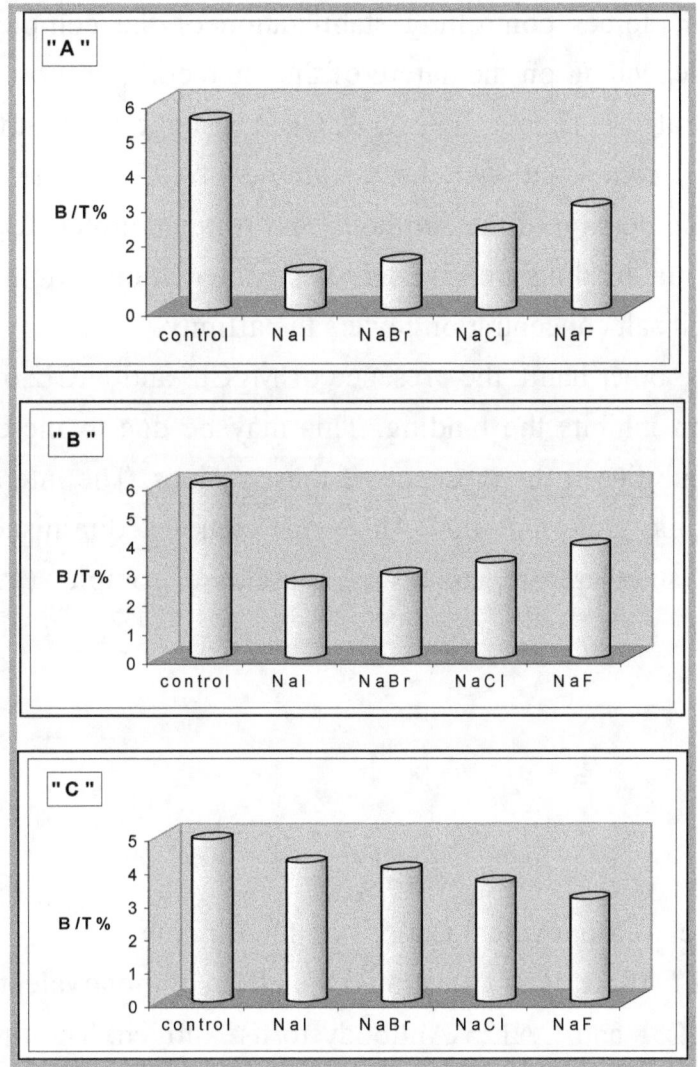

Figure (2–8): The effect of different halide on the 125I–anti CA125 Antibody binding to CA125 in:

(A) Colon Cancer Stage "B"

(B) Rectum Cancer Stage "C"

(C) Ulcerative Colitis

Control: Without halide addition.

(All other details are explained in the text).

The Effect of Divalent Cations on the Binding

The importance of ionic environment for the binding of 125I–anti CA 125 Antibody to CA 125 in colorectal tissue homogenate is shown in figure (2 – 9, A, B, C). The presence of divalent cations (i.e., CaCl2.2H2O, NiCl2.6H2O, CuSO4.5H2O, ZnCl2, MnCl2.4H2O and MgCl2.6H2O at 25mM concentration increase the binding. As shown in the figure ZnCl2 increases the binding more than other divalent cations for the three tissues homogenate. The reason may be due to the salt that may alter the nature of hydro phobic forces controlling stabilization of the complex formed and these vary depending on the nature of the interacting groups(191). From the results illustrated in figure (2–9, A, B, C), it is suggested that these salts may provide some conformational changes in the CA125 and the charged groups of the binding domain of the Antibody and Antigen molecule(192, 193), that hinder maximal binding are shielded. If the interaction is dominated by ionic strength, high salt concentration lowers the affinity.

On the other hand, the presence of $MgCl_2$ and $NiCl_2.6H_2O$ at 25mM concentration inhibits the binding. This may be due to increased (Ab–Ag) complex solubility in the presence of these cations. The interaction of these ions with ionic groups of the (Ab – Ag) complex diminishes the Ab, Ag interactions, and therefore, increasing solubility of complex (194).

The Effect of Monovalent Cations on the Binding:

Figure (2 – 10, A, B, C) illustrated the effect of monovalent cations on the binding of 125I–anti CA125 Antibody to its Antigen. The presence of four different monovalent (KCl, CSCl, NH_4Cl and LiCl) at the concentration 25mM caused to inhibit the binding of Antibody to its Antigen as shown in figure (2 – 10, A, B, C).

The explanation of this phenomenon may be due to the presupposition that the lesser degree of hydration permits greater interaction of the salt with an anionic group located in the Antibody combining site and then inhibits the complex formation (195). Another explanation is, the presence of these cations may be compete with proteins and change the conformation of the polar groups and then inhibit the complex formation (196).

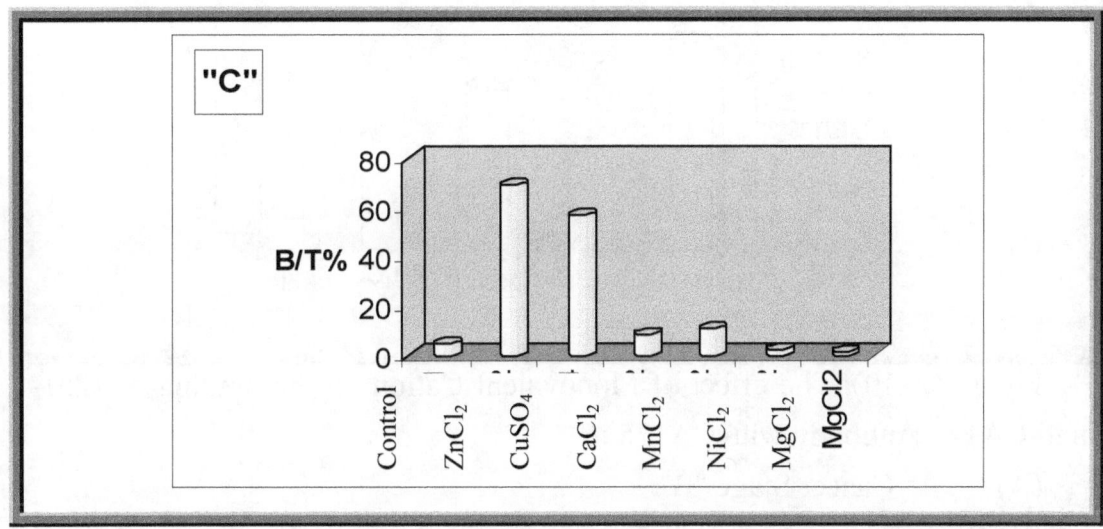

Figure (2–9): The effect of different divalent cation on the binding of 125I–anti CA125 Antibody withCA125 in:

(A) Colon Cancer Stage "B"

(B) Rectum Cancer Stage "C"

(C) Ulcerative Colitis

Control: Without divalent cation addition.

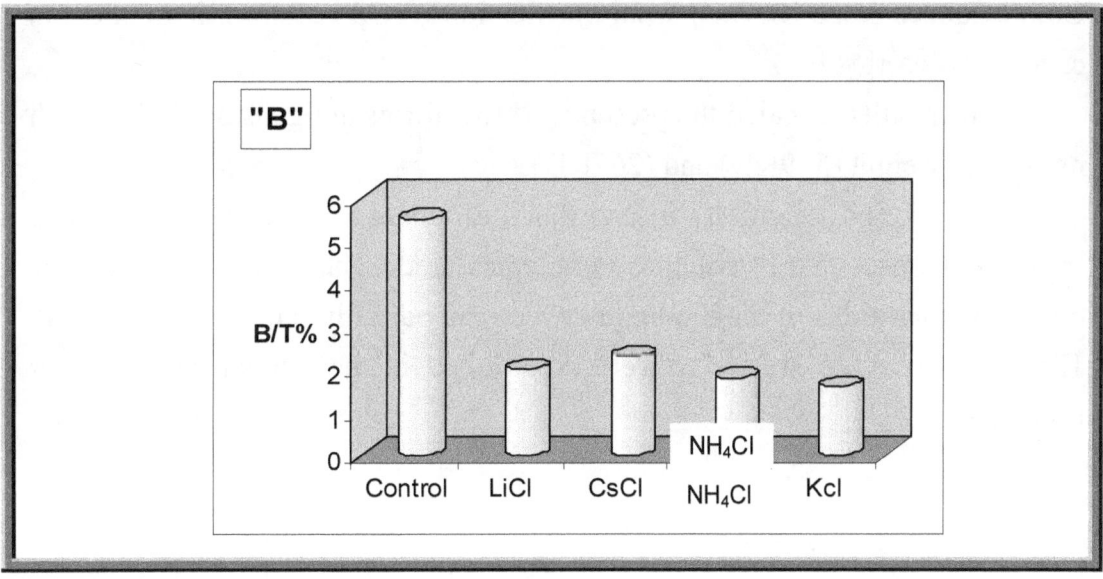

411

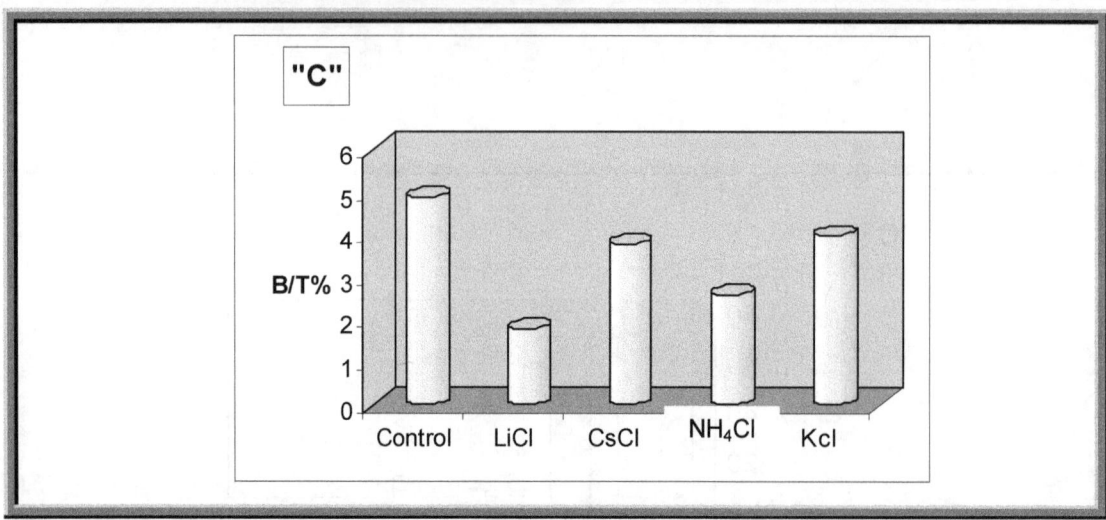

Figure (2–10): The effect of Monovalent Cation on the binding of 125I–anti CA125 Antibody with CA125 in

(A) Colon Cancer Stage "B"

(B) Rectum Cancer Stage "C"

(C) Ulcerative Colitis

Control: Without Monovalent cation addition.

(All other details are explaiopical studies on (h–CA125 antigens) and the complexes   (CA125/anti   CA125)   and   (125I   –

Chapter Three   Abstract:

Cancer Antigen (CA125) was partially purified from homogenate of Colon Cancer Stage B .The partial purification of CA125 from human colon cancer was carried out.

The results revealed the presence of two forms antigens of CA125 with molecular weight (579KD) and (267KD).

The elution volume (Vo) and the Kav values from elution of CA125 from Sepharose Cl–6B column were calculated. The experiments of the optimum conditions of the binding between the partially purified CA125 and 125I – anti CA125 Antibody were determined in the human colon cancer homogenate.

ChapterThree

Introduction

CA125 is a tumor Antigen that was defined by the monoclonal Antibody (MAb) OC125.

Only recently the primary structure of CA125 was elucidated, demonstrating that CA125 represent a gaint mucin–like glycoprotein (195). On this basis, CA125 has been termed Muc16 to reflect the nature of CA125 as a new member of the protein family of mucin (196). Full length CA125 contains more than 11,000 amino acids that form the protein aceous core structure and both N–and O glycosylated in its N–terminal extracellular domain(197,198), composed of stalk domain next to the trans membrane span, more than 60 repeat structures (each of which consist of 156 amino acids) and an N–terminal extension.CA125 C–terminal fragment of 1148 amino acids, representing less than 10% of the full length protein ,retains the ability to integrate into secretory membranes such as the endoplasmic reticulum (ER) and the Golgi, and is targeted to the plasma membrane by conventional secretary transport (199).

Using Sepharose 6B, CA125 was partially purified from patients with ovarian cancer (200), also affinity chromatography was used to purify CA125 in serum of ovarian, colon and digestive tract (201).

In this chapter CA125 was partially purified from patients with Colon Cancer Stage B. The factors that affect the binding of partially purified CA125 to its Antibody (125I–antiCA125 Antibody) were also studied.

Materials and Methods:

3–1: Materials:

Chemicals:

All chemicals and reagents mentioned in chapter two were used in the experiments of the chapter.

3–2: Instruments:

413

All instruments mentioned in chapter two were used in the experiments of this chapter.

3–3: Patients:

The same patients of Colon Cancer Stage B mentioned in chapter two were involved in the experiments of this chapter.

3–4: Partial Purification of CA125 by Sepharose-C1-6B Column:

Preparation of the Column:

The dimensions of the column were chosen according to the following equation (202):

$$\text{Diameter} = \sqrt[3]{m/10}$$

Where:

m: amount of protein in mg.

L= 30x diameter.

Where:

L: length of column.

Preparation of the Buffer:

Tris buffer (0.05M) was prepared by dissolving 3.0285 gm of tris (hydroxy methyl amino methane, 0.9306 gm of EDTA and 0.1 gm of sodium azide in 400 ml, the volume was completed to 500 ml with deionized distilled water, the pH was adjusted to pH 7.2.

Preparation of Gel:

The gel was prepared by allowing the preswollen gel to swell again in tris buffer pH7.2, then left to settle and the excess of buffer was decanted. The step was repeated several times. Suction was then used to degas the gel and slurry was left for 24 hrs. to equilibrate with buffer.

The swollen gel was suspended and carefully poured into a vertical glass column (0.9 x 27cm) down the wall using a glass rod. After the gel had settled the column was equilibrated with tris buffer for 72 hrs.

3–5: Determination of the Void Volume:

The void volume of the column was determined by using blue dextran 2000 at concentration of 2mg.ml–1 dissolving in tris buffer pH 7.2, the elution was carried out with the same buffer at a flow rate of 10ml, hr–1

Fractions of 1ml were collected and their absorbances were measured at 600nm. Figure (3–1) shows the elution profile of blue dextran 2000.The volume of the buffer required to elute the blue dextran, which represents the void volume, was (10 ml).

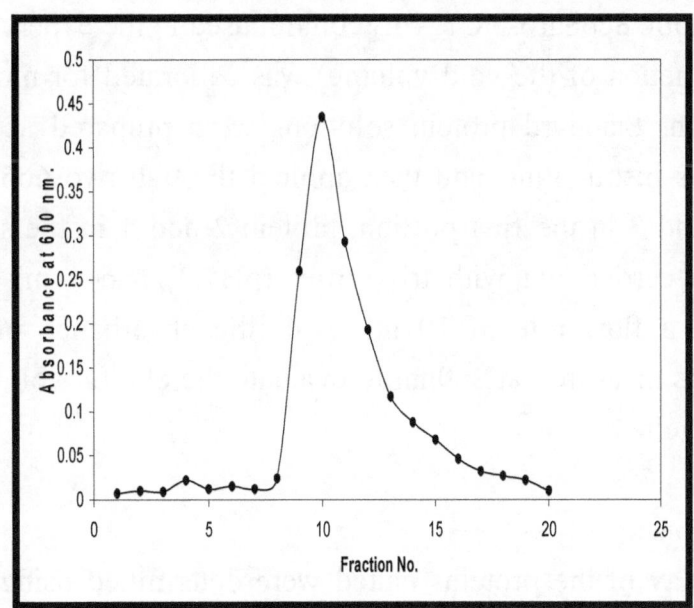

Figure (3–1): The elution profile of blue dextran 2000. (All other details are explained in the text).

3–6: Determination of the Molecular Weight by
    Gel Filtration Chromatography:

Pharmacia calibration kit was used for determination of the molecular weight of the isolated antigens by gel filtration. The kit comprises the highly purified proteins and their high molecular weight as detailed in table (3–1)

Table (3–1): Standard proteins and their molecular weights

Protein	Molecular Weight (KD)	Concentration mg.ml−1
Thyroglobulin	669	5.0
Ferritin	232	1.0
Catalase	440	5.0
Aldolase	158	5.0

Procedure:

The same Sepharose C1 – 6B column used in the experiment (Determination of the void volume) was calibrated for molecular weight determination. Standard protein solutions were prepared according to the manufactures instructions, and then applied through two 666μl of proteins, proteins 1 and 3 in the first portion, protein 2 and 4 in the second portion. Elution was carried out with tris buffer (pH7.2) and 1 ml fractions were collected at a flow rate of 10 ml.hrs−1, the absorbance of the fractions collected was measured at 280nm to evaluate the elution volume (Ve) of the standard protein.

Calculations:

The Kav of the proteins eluted were determined using the following equation (203):

$$Kav = \frac{Ve - Vo}{Vt - Vo}$$

Where:

Vo = Void volume

Ve = Elution volume

Vt = Total gel bed volume

The calibration curve of Kav values against log M .wt of the proteins was plotted.

3–7: Partial Purification Procedure:

Reagents:

Tris buffer (pH 7.2) contains 0.02% sodium azide was prepared as described previously in the experiment of (Preparation of the buffer).

Procedure:

The sample of tissue homogenate (666 μl) of Colon Cancer Stage B containing approximately (8 mg) proteins was applied to the surface of the gel. The elution was carried out using tris buffer (pH7.2) with a flow rate of 10 ml.hr–1., and fractions of one ml were collected, the elution was made at room temperature.

Calculations:

1 - In each fraction, the protein concentration was determined according to Lowry et.al(151) and the total binding was estimated at the optimum condition of Colon Cancer Stage B, as described in chapter two , the experiment of (Factors effecting 125I – anti CA125 Antibody binding to CA125 in colorectal tissue homogenate). The binding of each fraction was calculated and plotted against the elution volume. The specific binding activity percent was estimated from the following equation:

$$\textbf{Specific binding activity} = \frac{\textbf{Total binding B/T}}{\textbf{mg of protein}} \times \textbf{100}$$

2 - The isolation fold for CA125 was determined using the following equation:

$$\textbf{Isolation fold of CA125} = \frac{\textbf{Specific binding of purified CA125}}{\textbf{Specific binding of crude CA125}} \times \textbf{100}$$

3–8: The Choice of Optimum Conditions for the Binding of the Partial Purified CA125 to 125I–Anti CA125 Antibody:

The Choice of the Optimum Protein Concentration:

1- A volume of 40 μl of 125I–anti CA125 Antibody (2.88 mg.ml–1) was added to increasing amounts (5, 10, 15, 20, 25 and 30 μg.ml–1) of a polled fractions under the first peak of the partial purified Colon Cancer Stage B and (6, 12, 18, 24, 30 and 36 μg.ml–1) of a polled fractions under the second peak, the volume was completed to 250 μl with 0.05 M of tris buffer (pH 7.8).

2- All tubes were incubated for seven hours at 25°C.

3- Two additional tubes containing 40 µl (2.88 mg.ml–1) of 125I–anti CA125 Antibody only for total activity were set aside until counting.

4- Steps 4, 5 mentioned in chapter two the experiment of (The effect of different protein concentration of homogenate on the binding) were repeated.

Calculations:

The (B/T) % was calculated as described in chapter two, the experiment of (Binding studies of Cancer Antigen CA125 in colorectal tumors homogenate with 125I – anti CA125 Antibody), and was plotted against protein concentration.

Solutions:

Tris buffer (0.05 M) was prepared by dissolving 0.6057 gm of tris (hydroxy methyl amino methane in 50 ml of deionized distilled water and the pH was adjusted with HCl (1 ml) at (pH 7.8), the volume was completed to 100 ml with deionized distilled water.

The Effect of 125I–anti CA125 Antibody:

1- Increasing volume of 125 I–anti CA125 Antibody (10, 20, 30, 40, 50, and 60 µl) containing (0.720, 1.44, 2.16, 2.88, 3.60 and 4.32 mg.ml–1) was incubated with 25 and 18 µg.mL–1 for the first and second peaks respectively of partially purified CA125, the volume was completed to 250 µl with 0.05M tris buffer pH 7.8.

2- All tubes were incubated for seven hours at 25oC.

3- Steps 4, 5 mentioned in chapter two the experiment of (The effect of different protein concentration of homogenate on the binding) were repeated.

Calculations:

The (B/T)% was calculated according to chapter two the experiment of (Binding studies of Cancer Antigen CA125 in colorectal tumors homogenate with 125I – anti CA125 Antibody) and was plotted versus 125I–anti CA125 Antibody concentration.

The Choice of Optimum pH:

1- To choose the optimum pH for the partially purified CA125 from Colon Cancer Stage B (25µg.ml–1) and (18 µg.ml–1) of the first and second peak of partially purified CA125 were incubated with (30, 20 µl) (2.16, 1.44 mg.ml–1) respectively of125 I–anti CA125 Antibody. The volume of all tubes was completed to 250 µl with tris buffer (0.05M) of different pH (6.8–8.0).

2- All tubes were incubated for 7 hours at 25°C.

3- Steps 4, 5 mentioned in chapter two, the experiment of (Binding studies of Cancer Antigen CA125 in colorectal tumors homogenate with 125I – anti CA125 Antibody) were repeated.

Calculations:

The (B/T) % was calculated as described in chapter two the, experiment of (Binding studies of Cancer Antigen CA125 in colorectal tumors homogenate with 125I – anti CA125 Antibody) and was plotted against the corresponding pH.

Solutions:

Tris buffer (0.05M) was prepared as described in the experiment of (The choice of the optimum protein concentration) and the pH was adjusted from (6.8 – 8).

The Time Course of Partially Purified CA125:

1- To determine the time course of the partially purified CA125 from Colon Cancer Stage B, 25 µg.ml–1 protein of the first peak of partially purified CA125 was incubated with 30 µl of 125I–anti CA125 Antibody, while 18 µg.ml–1 protein of the second peak of the partially purified CA125 was incubated with 20 µl of 125I–anti CA125 Antibody, the volume was completed to 250 µl with tris buffer (0.05M, pH 7.4).

2- All tubes were incubated at 25°C at different time intervals (1, 2, 3, 4, 5, 6, 7, 8, 9, and 10) hours.

3- To determine the time course of the two peaks of partially purified CA125 at different temperature, steps 1, 2 in the same experiment were repeated at different temperature (5, 37and 45°C).

4- Steps 4, 5 mentioned in chapter two, the experiment of (The effect of different protein concentration of homogenate on the binding) were repeated.

Calculations:

1- The (B/T)% were calculated as described in chapter two , the experiment of (Binding studies of Cancer Antigen CA125 in colorectal tumors homogenate with 125I – anti CA125 Antibody)at different time and temperature.

2- The values (B/T) % was plotted against the time at different temperature.

3- The concentration of (125I–anti CA125/CA125) complex formed after time t is calculated from the following equation:

$$125\text{I-anti}\,CA125/CA125 = \frac{\text{count (c.p.m) of }^{125}\text{I-anti}\,CA125\text{ specifically bound after time (t)}}{\text{Total count (c.p.m) of }^{125}\text{I-anti}\,CA125\text{ used in the incubation}} \times \frac{\text{Concentration of }^{125}\text{I-anti}\,CA125}{\text{in the incubation}}$$

(in mg.ml^{-1} after time (t))   (mg.ml^{-1})

Solutions

Tris buffer (0.05M) was prepared as described in the experiment of (The choice of the optimum protein concentration) and the pH was adjusted to 7.4.

Results and Discussion:

Partial Purification of CA125:

Isolation of cytosol CA125 antigens were performed by gel exclusion chromatography technique. Colon Cancer Stage B homogenate was applied to Sepharose CL – 6B (0.9x27 cm). The void volume (Vo) of this column was (10 ml) as predicated from the elution profile of the blue dextran.

Figure (3 – 2) shows the elution profile of CA125 from malignant Colon Cancer Stage B. The resultant fractions of the homogenate were collected, polled and detected for the binding with 125I–anti CA125 Antibody. The binding of the polled fractions with 125I–anti CA125 Antibody revealed two antigens of CA125 (MI) and (M II).

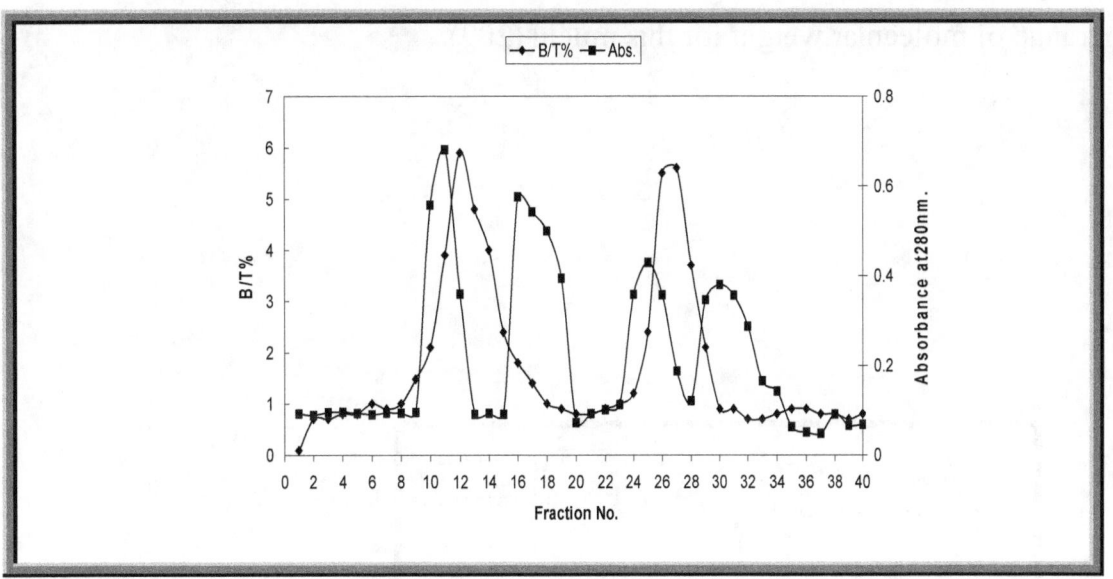

Figure (3–2): The elution profile of Human CA125 from malignant Colon Cancer Stage "B" (All other details are explained in the text).

Different standard proteins of known molecular weight were used to determine the molecular weight of the isolated antigens. The elution volumes (Ve) of the standard proteins are shown in figure (3 – 3). The Kav values for these standard proteins were calculated by using the formula represented in section (3 – 6) and then a calibration curve was plotted between Kav values of the standard proteins versus their logarithmic molecular weight as shown

421

in figure (3 – 4). The Kav of isolated CA125 antigens were measured and their molecular weights were determined.

The molecular weight of isolated antigens obtained from figure (3–4) was (579KD) and (267KD) for Antigens MI and MII respectively. The CA125 had been investigated and identified in different tissues and fluids by gel filtration technique and the molecular weight of the identified Antigen ranged between (50 – 200 KD)(204,206). Niloff et. al., and Timothyl et. al. have found that the amniotic fluid Antigen is composed of two subunits of approximately 240,000 and 180,000 Daltons as detected by 125 iodine labeled OC125 monoclonal Antibody.

The isolation fold of the two isolated antigens forms are illustrated in table (3 – 2) .The isolation fold of Antigen (MI) is 19.34, while for the second Antigen (M II) is 16.91. The glycosylation of the protein back bone may differ in carcinoma cells from normal epithelial cell causing a wide range of molecular weight for this mucin (209).

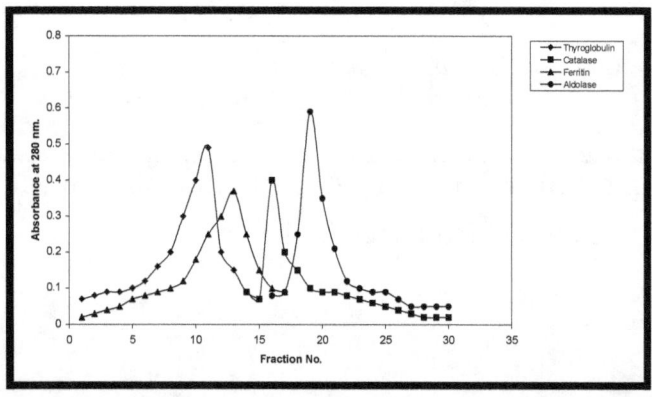

Figure (3–3) : Elution Profile of known molecular weight proteins (All other details are explained in the text) .

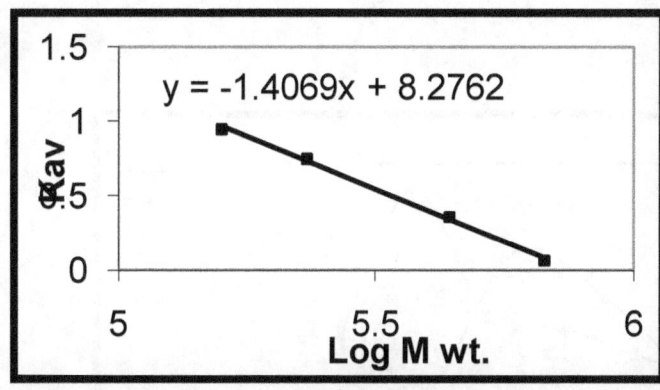

$$y = -1.4069x + 8.2762$$

Figure (3–4): Calibration Curve for determination of M.wt by gel filtration chromatography. (All other details are explained in the text).

Table (3–2): Partial Purification of CA125 by gel filtration technique

CA125 Source	Total protein mg.ml–1	Specifically Bound 125 I–anti CA125	Specifically Binding 125I–anti CA125/mg protein	Purification fold
Crude malignant homogenate	0.4	6.7	16.75	1.00
MI isolated fraction	0.025	8.1	324	19.34
MII isolated fraction	0.018	5.1	283.3	16.91

The Choice of the Optimum Conditions for the Binding of Partially Purified CA125 with 125I–anti CA125 Antibody:

The Choice of the Optimum Protein Concentration:

Figure (3–5) shows the optimum protein concentration for the two isolated forms of the malignant colon homogenate. This experiment was carried out by adding increasing amounts of the isolated forms to fixed amounts of 125I anti CA125–Antibody to produce (125I–anti CA125 Antibody/CA125) complex. The maximum binding occurred at 25 µg.mL–1 for (MI) isolated form, while 18µg.mL–1 was the optimum protein concentration for the binding of (M II) isolated form. Further addition of CA125 give rise to solubilization of complex formed (210).

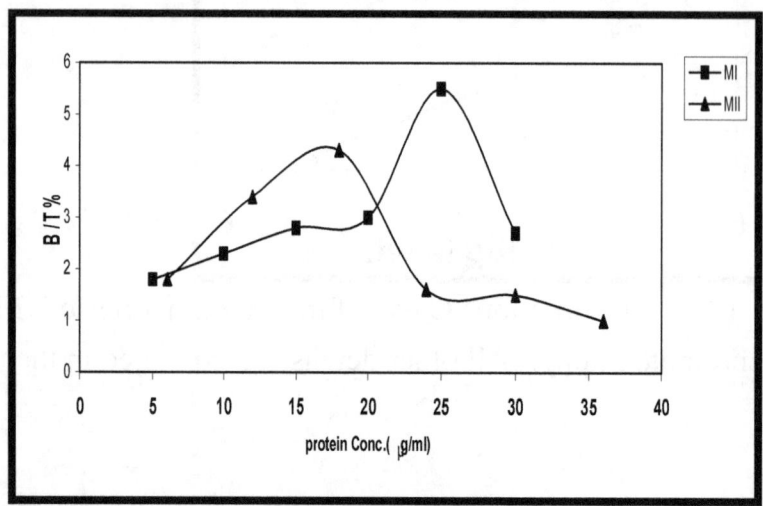

Figure (3–5): Influ   Protein Conc. μg/ml   ation on the binding of 125I–
anti CA125 Antibody with partially purified CA125 from Colon Cancer
Stage "B". (All other details are explained in the text).

The Effect of 125I–anti CA125 Antibody:

Figure (3 – 6) shows the effect of 125I – anti CA125 Antibody
concentration on the binding with isolated forms of the malignant colon
homogenate.

The maximum binding obtained at 2.16 mg.ml–1 for (MI) and 1.44
mg.ml–1 for (MII). It was found that the amount of 125I – anti CA125
Antibody required to bind with their isolated Antigen forms is less than in
malignant crude homogenate. This may be due to the increment of the epitop
(the part of an Antigen molecular that binds to any single Antigen combining
site)(211).

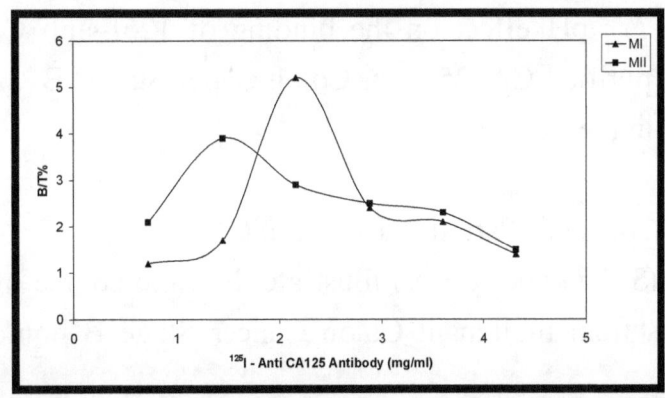

Figure (3–6): Effect of 125I–anti CA125 Antibody concentration on the binding with partially purified CA125 from Colon Cancer Stage "B". (All other details are explained in the text).

The Choice of the Optimum pH:

In order to choose the optimum pH 25 µg.mL–1 and 18 µg.mL–1 for (MI,MII) respectively of the two isolated forms of the malignant Colon Cancer Stage B homogenate were incubated with 2.16,1.44 mg.ml–1 respectively of 125I–anti CA125 Antibody. Figure (3 – 7) shows the optimum pH of the two isolated antigens forms. The results revealed that the optimum pH for MI and MII isolated antigens for the binding with its Antibody was 7.4.

The similarity in pH (7.4) suggests that the CA125 isolated forms possess the same epitopes in both cases. That means the induction of protonation – deprotonation process occurs with the same changed polar groups on the amino acid residues present in the binding domain (212).

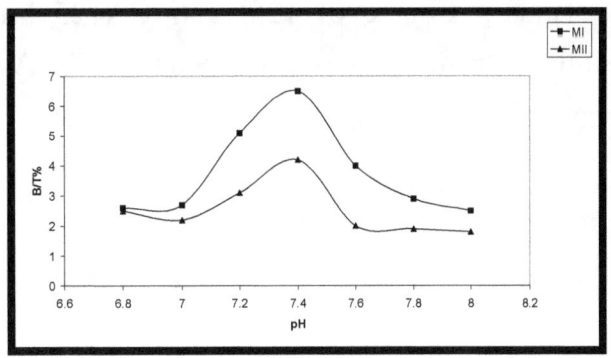

Figure (3–7) : pH effect on the binding of 125I–anti CA125 Antibody with partially purified CA125 from Colon Caner Stage "B".(All other details are explained in the text).

The Time Course of Partial Purification CA125:

Figure (3 – 8) and (3 – 9) illustrate the time course of the binding of isolated forms from malignant Colon Cancer Stage B homogenate to their Antibody.

The MI form Antigen binds to its Antibody in highest state after 4 hours at 37 °C, while MII form binds after 3 hours at 45°C.

In comparison with crude homogenate the optimum binding occurred at 25°C. After 7 hours, so the binding of 125I – anti CA125 Antibody to its Antigen is a time and temperature dependent process. (213)

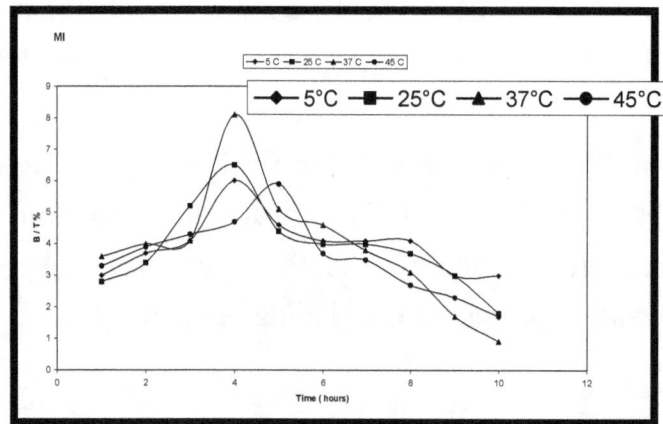

Figure(3–8) :Time – Course of 125I–anti CA125 binding to partially purified (MI) Antigen from Colon Cancer Stage "B". (All other details are explained in the text).

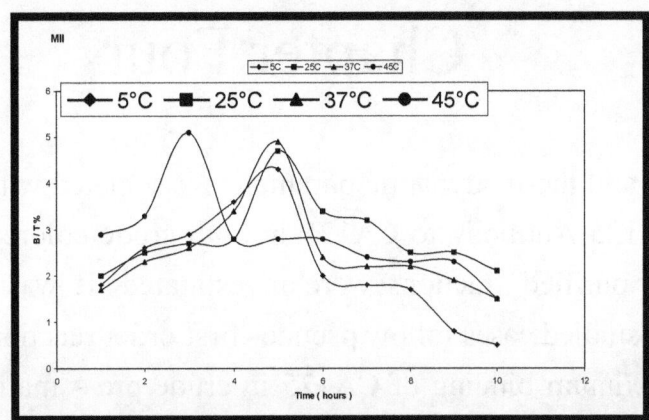

Figure (3–9) : Time – Course of 125I–anti CA125 binding to partially Purified (MII) Antigen from Colon Cancer Stage

427

Chapter Four

Abstract:

Kinetic and thermodynamic parameters associated with the binding of 125I- anti CA125 Antibody to CA125 in both crude colorectal homogenate and partially- purified fractions were investigated .It was shown that the reaction in all studied cases follow pseudo- first order reaction kinetics.

The maximum binding of CA125 in crude pre – malignant colorectal tumor homogenate , Ulcerative Colitis (U.C) occurred at 5°C , the association rate constant K+1 decreased from 4.59 mg -1 .ml.min -1   at 5oC to 3.23 mg –1 .ml.min –1 at 45oC . The values of affinity constant Ka also decreased from 0.828 x 10 3 mg –1.ml at 5°C to 0.558 x 10 3 mg –1 .ml at 45°C, while CA125 in crude Colon Cancer Stage B, the maximum binding occurred at 25°C3535, the rate of association constant K+1 decreased from 1.69 mg–1 .ml.min–1   at 25°C to 1.11 mg –1 .ml.min –1   at 45°C and the Ka value decreased from 0.505 x 10 3 mg–1.ml at 25°C to 0.353 x 10 3 mg-1 .ml at 45°C . On the other hand, the kinetic parameters of rectal cancer stage C, the maximum binding occurred at 5°C and the affinity constant Ka decreased from 1.095 x 10 3 mg –1 .ml at 5°C to 0.585 x 10 3 mg –1 .ml at 45°C, also K+1 value decreased from 7.69 mg–1 .ml.min–1 at 5°C to 3.72 mg–1 .ml. min –1 at 45°C.

The maximum binding of partially-purified colon cancer Antigens (MI and MII), occurred at 37°C and 45°C for MI and MII respectively . The Ka and K+1 values for (MII) Antigen increased with increasing temperature , while these values for MI reached the optimum at 37°C and decreased at 45°C .

The Van't Hoff plot demonstrated linear relationship between ln Ka and 1/T , using crude colorectal homogenate and MI ,MII as CA125 source . Plotting between log K+1 and 1/T gave linear relationship called Arrhenius relationship. The thermodynamic parameters $\Delta H°$ $\Delta G°$ and $\Delta S°$ for the formation of (125I- anti CA125 Antibody / CA125) complex at the standard state Ea, $\Delta H*$, $\Delta G*$ and $\Delta S*$ representing the transition state were determined.

Introduction:

Macromolecular interactions involve cooperative, independent and contiguous binding regions. The complexity caused by this is increased by the dynamic structural changes that the interaction and the equilibrium condition are influenced by the algebraic sum of the energies involved in reversible interacting energy components, namely electrostatic and hydrophobis , is best understood by a study of the thermodynamic parameters of the interaction .The method most widely used for such investigations is isothermal titration calorimetry (214 – 21 6) , which directly determines the heat changes during the binding process derives the thermodynamic parameters, enthalpy (ΔH), free energy (ΔG) and entropy (ΔS) . In the last two decades the method has been used to unravel the intricacies of the interaction between several ligands – ligate pairs, like protease – protease inhibitor (217), receptor – ligand (218), and Antigen – Antibody (215).

Kinetic parameters of the interaction of iodinated human Chorionic gonadotropin (125IhCG) with one of its monoclonal antibodies are sought and are determined after an analysis of the dissociation profile of IhCG – MAb (monoclonal Antibody) complexes in the presence of excess unlabelled hCG at various temperatures (219).

The idea of this chapter is to describe the basic mathematical analysis that could be used to explain the mechanism of binding of CA125 to its Antibody to form (125I – anti CA125 Antibody / CA125) complex in human colorectal tissues, using benign and malignant colorectal tissue homogenate and also partially purified colon tumors fractions, as CA125 source.

Materials and Methods:

4-1 Chemicals:

All chemicals and reagents mentioned in chapter two were used in the experiments of this chapter.

4-2 Instruments:

All instruments that are described in chapter two were used in experiments of this chapter.

4-3 Kinetic Studies:

Scatchard Analysis :

Determination of Affinity Constant Ka and the Maximal Binding Capacity (Bmax) of:

(A) CA125 in Colorectal Tissue Homogenate associated with 125I- anti CA125 Antibody:

1- One hundred μL of colorectal homogenate (U.C, Colon Cancer Stage B and Rectum cancer Stage C) containing (100, 400, 200 μg .ml −1) protein respectively were pipetted in each type of homogenate.

2- Increased volumes of 125I – anti CA125 Antibody for each group of colorectal homogenate i.e. , (4, 8, 12, 16 , and 20) μL , in the case of benign colorectal tumors (U.C) , (8 , 16 , 24 , 32 , and 40) μL for Colon Cancer Stage B , while (6 ,12 ,18 , 24 , and 30) μL for rectal cancer Stage C were added to each assay tubes for each case .

3- The volume of all tubes was completed to the final volume of 250 μl with tris – buffer (pH 7.2, 7.8, and 7.8) respectively to the three groups of tissue homogenate.

4- The time of the incubation required to reach the equilibrium state are reported in table (4 – 1)

5- After incubations of each group at each time and temperature required, all tubes were centrifuged at 4000 r. p. m. for one hour. at 4°C by using cooling centrifuge .

6- The supernatant was discarded and the complex formed was counted in gamma counter for one minute.

Table (4- 1): The time of incubation for benign and malignant colorectal tumor homogenate at different temperatures.

Temp .°C	Time (hour)		
	U . C	Colon Cancer Stage "B"	Rectum Cancer Stage "C"
5	3	6	3
25	5	7	3
37	3	4	3
45	3	3	4

Calculation :

1- The B/T ratio was computed for each tube , where :

B : is the bound radioactivity (mean counts c.p.m) , which represents the 125I – anti CA125 / CA125) complex .

F : is the free radioactivity (mean counts c.p.m), which represents (unbound or unreacted, 125I – anti CA125) .

T : is the total activity (mean counts)

F= T (total counts) – B (bound radioactivity) .

2- The concentration of (125I – anti CA125 / CA125) complex in mg.ml – 1 that formed after time (t) was calculated from the following equation :

$$B(mg\,ml^{-1}) = \frac{B(c.p.m)}{T(c.p.m)} \times concentration\ of\ ^{125}I\text{-}antibody\ in\ the\ incubation\ medium\ mg.ml^{-1}$$

The affinity constant and maximal binding capacity were determined according to Scatchard equation (220 , 221) :

$$\frac{B}{F} = \frac{1}{K_d}(B_{max} - B)$$

$$Ka = \frac{1}{K_d} = \frac{K_{+1}}{K_{-1}}$$

Where:

Ka = affinity Constant.

Kd = dissociation Constant.

B max = maximal binding capacity

The value of the affinity constant of the binding Ka at each temperature can be calculated from the slop of the straight line, While the value of the total concentration of CA125 (Bmax) in colorectal tissue for each group was calculated from the intercept on X – axis.

(B) Partially Purified CA125 in Colorectal Homogenate Binding with 125I – anti CA125 Antibody:

1- Increasing volume of 125I – anti CA125 Antibody (10, 15, 20, 25 and 30) µL was incubated with 25 µg. ml –1 of the first form of partially purified CA125 from Colon Cancer Stage B (MI) , while 18 µg . ml –1 of the second form of partially purified CA125 (MII) was incubated with increasing volume (4, 8, 12, 16 and 20) µL of 125I- anti CA125 Antibody.

2- All tubes were completed to 250µL with tris buffer (pH 7.4).

3- The time of incubation required to reach the equilibrium state are reported in table (4 – 2).

4- Steps 5, 6 in the experiment of (Kinetic studies of CA125 in colorectal tissue homogenate associated with 125I - anti CA125 Antibody).

Table (4- 2): The time of incubation for the partially purified CA125 from Colon Cancer Stage B

Temp .°C	Time (hour)	
	MI I	MI I
5	5	4
25	5	4
37	6	4
45	3	5

Calculation:

The steps of calculations outlined in experiment of (Kinetic studies of CA125 in colorectal tissue homogenate associated with 125I - anti CA125 Antibody), was followed exactly to obtain the values of Ka and Bmax at each temperature.

4-4 The Thermodynamic Studies:

The thermodynamic of 125I- anti CA125 Antibody Binding to its Antigen in Colorectal Homogenate and Partially Purified CA125 in Malignant Colorectal Tumors:

The same steps mentioned in chapter two , the experiment of (Time course of CA125 binding in colorectal tissue homogenate) and chapter three , the experiment of (The time course of partially purified CA125) for the colorectal homogenate and partially purified CA125 respectively were performed .

Calculation:

1- The thermodynamic parameters of the standard state obtained from Van,t Hoff , the values of the natural logarithm of equilibrium constant (affinity constant Ka) obtained at different temperature were plotted against the reciprocal values of the absolute temperature in Kelvin (1/T), according to the following equation :

$$Ln\ K_a = \frac{\Delta S^\circ}{R} - \frac{\Delta H^\circ}{RT}$$

Where:

ΔH° = the enthalpy change of the standard state .

ΔS° = the entropy change of the standard state .

R = the gas constant (8.31414 J. K – 1.mol – 1).

ΔH° value obtained from the slop , the linear relationship of the plot .

The change in Gibbs free energy of the standard state ΔG° was obtained from the following equation:

$$\Delta G^\circ = - R\ T\ ln\ Ka$$

Where Ka is the affinity constant, while the standard state entropy change was obtained from (222):

$$\Delta S° = \frac{\Delta H° - \Delta G°}{T}$$

2- The thermodynamic parameter of the transition state were obtained from Arrhenius plot of ln K+1 values against 1/T values that gives a linear relationship according to the following equation:

$$Ln\ K_{+1} = Ln\ A - \left[\frac{Ea}{RT}\right]$$

Where A = Arrhenius constant, some times called frequency factor or
per exponential factor.

The value of apparent energy of activation (Ea) of the binding reaction can be determined from the slop of the straight line . The enthalpy of transition state ΔH* was obtained from:

$$\Delta H^* = Ea\ -\ RT$$

Transition state free energy change ΔG* is calculated from the following equation:

$$\Delta G^* = -RT\ ln\ K_{+1} + RT\ ln\ \frac{KT}{h}$$

Where K and h were Boltzman and Plank, s constant which equal (1.38 x 10 – 23 J. K –1), (6.62 x 10 –34 J. sec –1) respectively.

The change in entropy of the transition state ΔS* is calculated from the following equation:

$$\Delta S^* = \frac{\Delta H^* - \Delta G^*}{T}$$

Results and Discussion:

Determination of Affinity Constant (Ka) and the Maximal Binding Capacity (Bmax) of CA125 in colorectal Tissue Homogenate Associated with 125I- anti CA125 Antibody

The concentration of CA125 in cytosolic fractions in the three groups of colorectal tissue homogenate (benign and malignant),Bmax and the affinity constant Ka of the binding to 125I-anti CA125 Antibody has been measured. The experiment was carried out at the optimum conditions that were obtained in previous experiments. Scatchard plot analysis gave straight line as shown in figure (4 – 1, A, B, C) , and the parameters obtained from Scatchard plot are shown in table (4 – 3).

Table (4 – 3) : The Kinetic parameters of CA125 binding to its 125I- anti CA125 Antibody in colorectal tissue homogenate

Temp °C	Ka x 103 mg . ml $^{-1}$			Kd x 10 – 3 mg . ml – 1			Bmax x 10 – 3 mg . ml – 3		
	U.C	Colon Cancer Stage B	Rectum Cancer Stage C	U.C	Colon Cancer Stage B	Rectum Cancer Stage C	U.C	Colon Cancer Stage B	Rectum Cancer Stage C
5	0.828	0.391	1.095	1.21	2.56	0.91	12.32	14.61	9.49
25	0.748	0.505	0.879	1.34	1.98	1.14	11.65	16.83	8.98
37	0.635	0.447	0.991	1.57	2.24	1.01	11.03	15.90	9.27
45	0.558	0.353	0.585	1.79	2.83	1.71	10.34	14.07	8.45

The values Ka and maximal binding capacity (Bmax) were calculated from Scatchard plot at four different temperatures.

It is clear from table (4 – 3) that the affinity constant (Ka) depends on the type of the tumor (i . e , benign and malignant) , stage of the malignancy (B or C) and on the temperature . The highest value of Ka occurred at 5°C in the case of U .C and rectum cancer stage C , while in the case of colon stage B , the optimum value of Ka was at 25°C , on the other hand the lowest values of Ka in the three groups of colorectal tissue homogenate were at 45°C . The kinetic and affinity constant were different due to the differences in one or more amino acid present in epitope domain(223).

The values of Kd were increased with increasing temperature as shown in table (4 – 3). In the case of U .C Kd increased with increasing temperature ordered 45°C > 37°C > 25°C > 5°C. On the other hand, determination of maximal binding capacity (Bmax) of CA125 to each type of tissue homogenate revealed similar result for Ka value; it is temperature dependent. In case of U. C, Bmax decreased with increasing temperature.

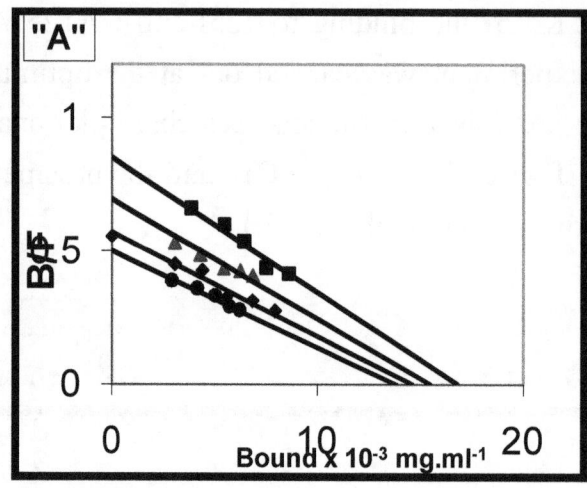

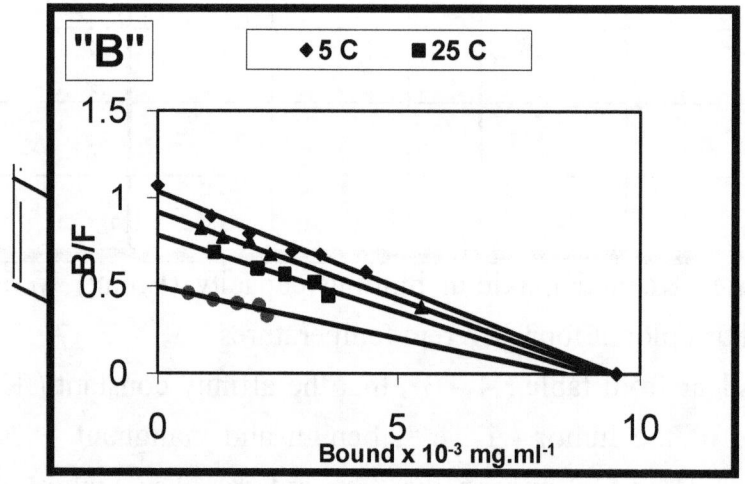

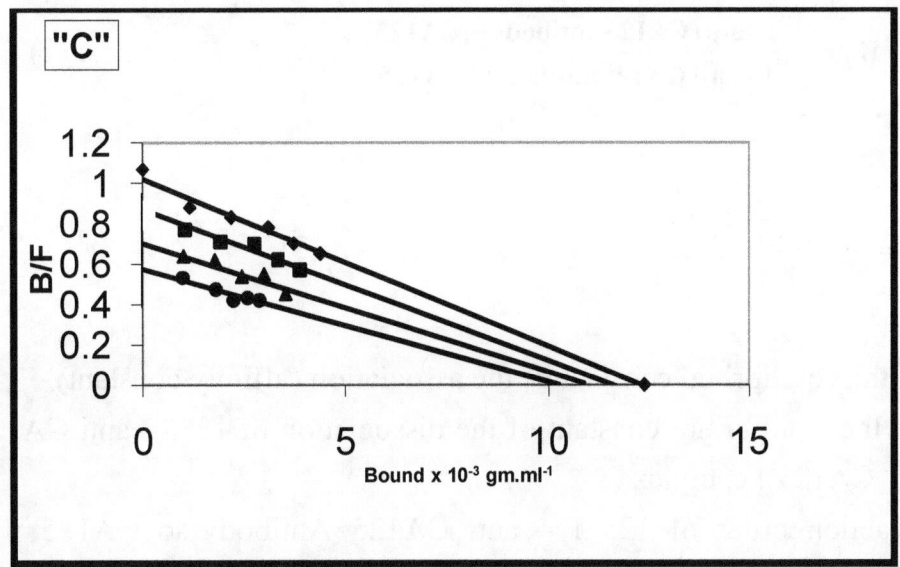

Figure (4-1): Scatchard plot of 125I – anti CA125 binding to CA125 in

(A) Colon Cancer Stage "B"

(B) Rectum Cancer Stage "C"

(C) Ulcerative Colitis

(All other details are explained in the text).

Determination of the Kinetic Parameters binding of (125I – anti CA125 Antibody / CA125) Complex Formation:

The simplest proposed model representing the binding of 125I – anti CA125 Antibody with CA125 could be expressed by the following equation

$$^{125}\text{I - Ab - Ag (CA125)} \quad \overset{k_{+1}}{\underset{k_{-1}}{}} \quad \left[^{125}\text{I} \rightleftharpoons \right]$$

Where:

K+1: is the rate of the association of 125I – anti CA125 Antibody with CA125.

K-1: is the rate of reverse reaction of dissociation of the complex formed under the same condition.

At equilibrium:

$$K_a = \frac{[^{125}\text{I - anti CA125 antibody / CA125}]}{[^{125}\text{I - anti CA125 antibody}] \, [\text{CA125}]} \quad \dots\dots\dots\dots\dots\dots \quad (1)$$

$$K_d = \frac{[^{125}I - anti\,CA125\,antibody]\,[CA125]}{[^{125}I - anti\,CA125\,antibody\,/\,CA125]} \quad\dotsb\quad (2)$$

Thus,

$$K_a = \frac{1}{K_d} = \frac{K_{+1}}{K_{-1}} \quad\dotsb\quad (3)$$

Where:

Ka: is the equilibrium constant of the association (affinity constant).

Kd : is the equilibrium constant of the dissociation of 125I – anti CA125 Antibody / CA125) complex .

The reaction order of 125 I – anti CA125 Antibody to CA125 was determined by using the following equation (224) :

$$\ln [Ab\,Ag]e \left[\frac{[Ab]t - [Ab\,Ag]t\,[Ab\,Ag]e\,/\,Ag]t}{[Ab]t\,[Ab\,Ag]e - [Ab\,Ag]e}\right] = K_{+1}\,t\left[\frac{[Ab] + [Ag]t\,[Ab\,Ag]e}{[AbAg]e}\right]\dotsb$$

(4)

Where:

K+1: is the kinetic association constant.

[AbAg] e: is the concentration of (125I – anti CA125 Antibody / CA125) complex formed at equilibrium.

[AbAg] t: is the concentration of (125I – anti CA125 Antibody / CA125) complex after time (t).

[Ab] t: is the total concentration of 125I – anti CA125 Antibody.

[Ag] t: is the total concentration of CA125.

Equation (4) represents the second order kinetics, but the percent of binding was in some cases, small and most labeled Antibody remains free and only small fraction binds even at equilibrium, i.e., [Ab]t >> [AbAg]e

Thus:

$$[Ab]\,t >> \frac{[Ab\,Ag]t\,[AbAg]e}{[Ag]t} \quad\dotsb\quad (5)$$

So that the following equation could be used in order to fit the pseudo-first order kinetics (225).

On the other hand figures (4 – 2, 4 – 3 and 4 – 4) show the plot of ln $\dfrac{[Ab\,Ag]e}{[Ab\,Ag]e - [Ab\,Ag]t}$ against time (t) gave a straight line with a slop equal to the observed value of the first rate constant (Kobs) in min-1. The rate of constant (K+1) in mg-1.ml.min was calculated at four different temperatures using the following equation(226).

$$\text{Kobs} = \text{K+1}\;\dfrac{[^{125}I\text{-}anti\,CA125]t\,[CA125]t}{[^{125}I\text{-}anti\,CA125\,/\,CA125]e}\quad\ldots\ldots\ldots\ldots\ldots\ldots(6)$$

Also, the value of K-1 at four temperatures were calculated using equation (3), whereas, the half life time of association (t 1/ 2)ass., which represented the time needed for the formation of half amount of the complex at equilibrium was determined from the concentration of the complex at equilibrium and the time course curve. The half-life time of dissociation (t 1/2) diss., was calculated from the following equation.

$$(\text{t 1/ 2 diss}) = \ln\dfrac{2}{K_{-1}} = \dfrac{0.693}{K_{-1}}$$

The values of Kobs., K+1, K-1, (t 1/2) ass., and t (1/2) diss., at different temperatures are summarized in table (4 – 4). The values in this table show the highest rate for the association reaction K+1, in benign colorectal tumors (U.C) and malignant colorectal tumors (CCB) and (RRC) occurred at 5°C, 25°C and 5°C respectively, while the lowest rate occurred at 45°C, so the reaction rate is a temperature dependent, while the rate constant for the reverse reaction K-1 which refers to the rate of dissociation of 125I– anti CA125 Antibody from its CA125 is temperature independent.

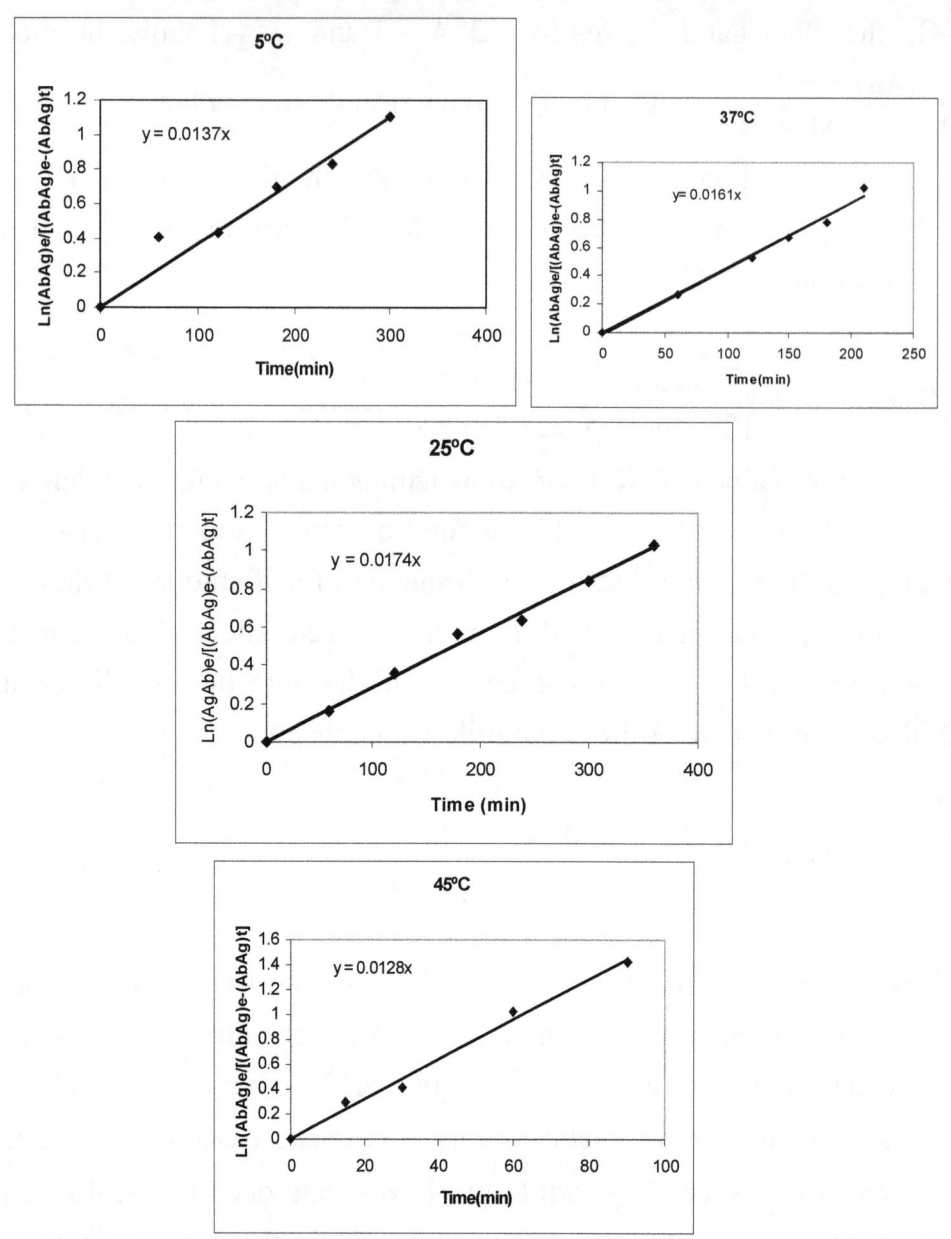

Figure (4 – 2) : Kinetics of 125I – anti CA125 Antibody binding to CA125 in Colon Cancer Stage "B". (All other details are explained in the text)

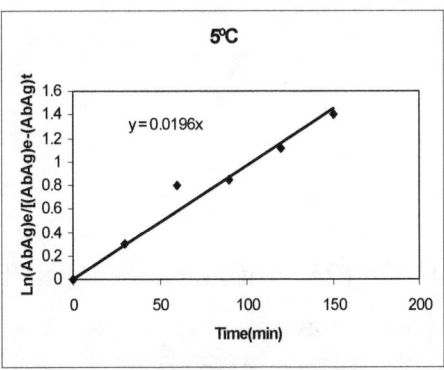

Figure (4 – 3) : Kinetics of 125I – anti CA125 Antibody binding to CA125 in Rectum Cancer Stage "C". (All other details are explained in the text)

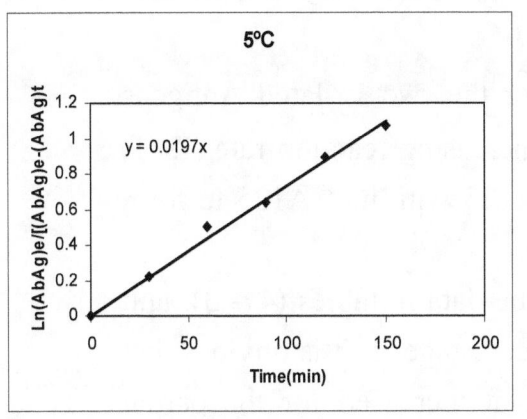

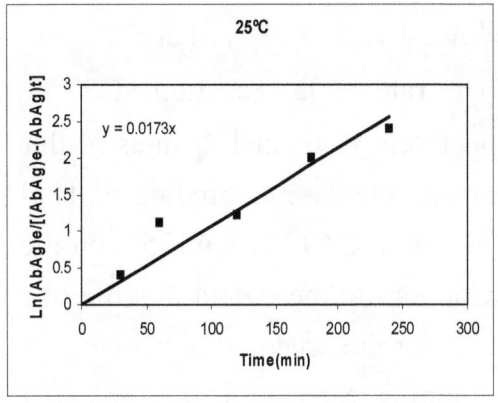

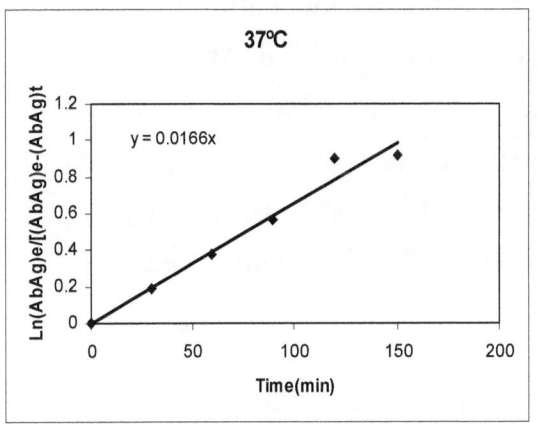

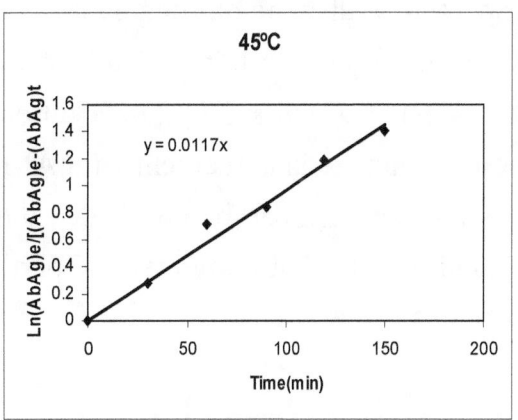

Figure (4 – 4) : Kinetics of 125I – anti CA125 Antibody binding to CA125 in benign colorectal tumor (Ulcerative Colitis). (All other details are explained in the text)

Kinetic of the Binding of 125I – anti CA125 Antibody to Partially – Purified CA125 from Colorectal Tumors Homogenate :

Table (4 – 5) illustrates the kinetic parameters of 125I – anti CA125 Antibody binding to partially purified malignant tumor homogenates (Colon Cancer Stage B). The results reveled that the maximal binding capacity (Bmax) and affinity constant Ka occurred at 37°C for the first form of partially purified Antigen (MI), while the second form of partially purified Antigen (MII) occurred at 45°C and decreased with decreasing temperatures the lowest value occurred at 5°C.

The rate of the reaction at 37°C and 45 for the two isolated Antigens respectively is about 1.4 times of that at 5°C. increasing reaction rate (K+1) means an increase of binding of 125I – anti CA125 with its CA125 to form (125I – anti CA125 / CA125) complex.

Comparing these data in table (4 – 5) with the data in tables (4 – 3) and (4 – 4) for the crude homogenate of Colon Cancer Stage B, it is obvious that the binding capacity Bmax and affinity constant increased for the partial purification CA125 Antigens than that of crude homogenate and the rate of the reaction increased about 2.5 and 2.2 times for two isolated Antigens respectively, also the binding capacity occurred at 25°C after incubation for 7 hours for the crude homogenate, while, for the partially purified Antigens (MI, MII) occurred at 37°C, 45°C after incubation for 4, 3 hours respectively, these results are in agreement with Al-Kazzaz observation(213).

Commonly, it can be concluded that the crude CA125 had lower affinity to bind with its Antibody than the partially – purified CA125 in both isolated Antigens.

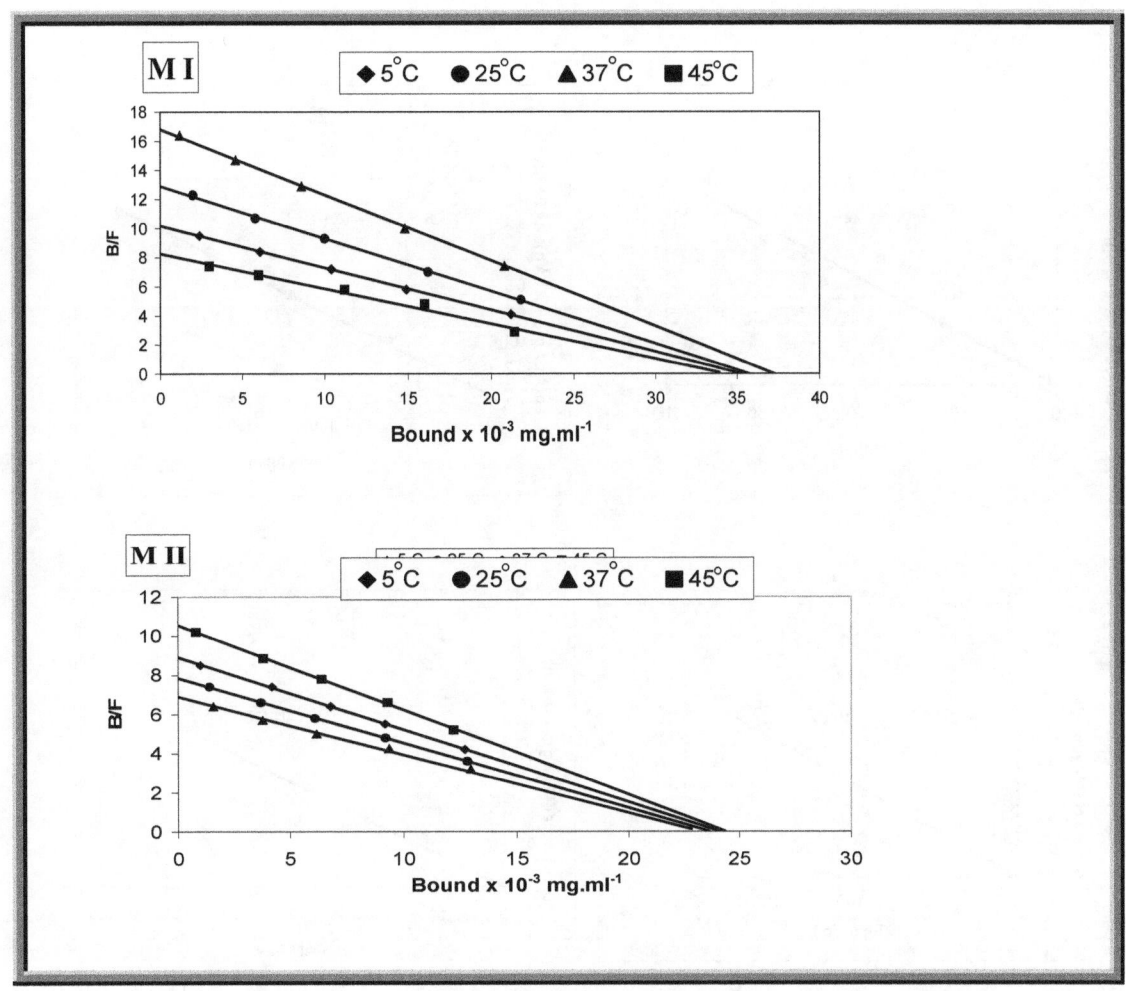

Figure (4 – 5) : Scatchard plot of 125I – anti CA125 binding to the partially purified CA125 Antigens in malignant colon tumors Stage "B" (All other details are explained in the text).

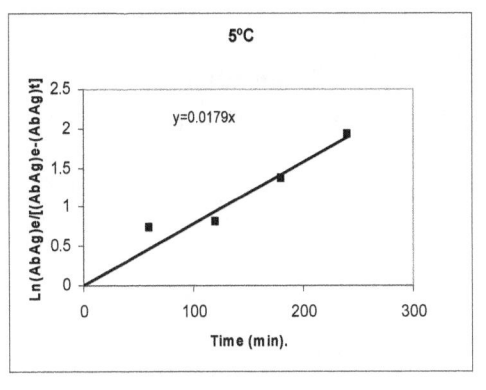

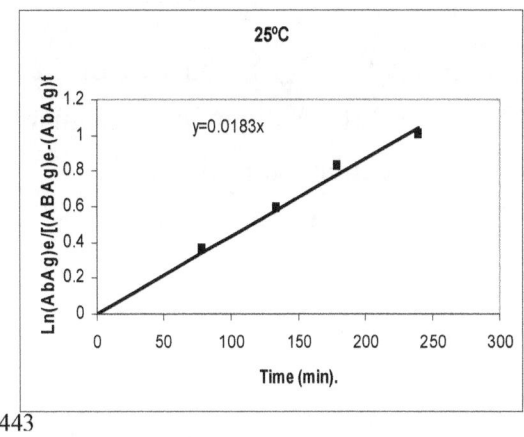

443

Figure (4 – 6) : Kinetics of 125I – anti CA125 Antibody binding to CA125 in MI Antigen of malignant colon tumors Stage "B". (All other details are explained in the text)

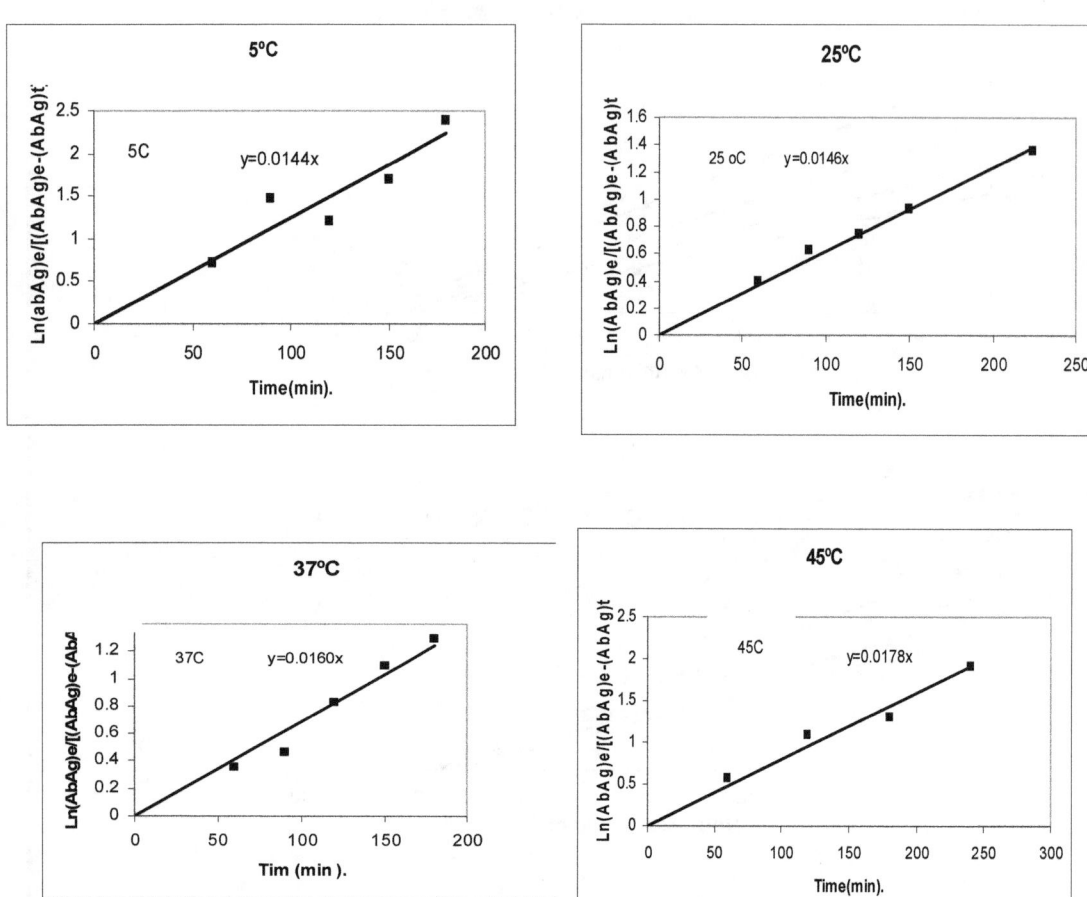

Figure (4 – 7) : Kinetics of 125I – anti CA125 Antibody binding to CA125 in MII Antigen of malignant colon tumors Stage "B". (All other details are explained in the text)

The Thermodynamics Studies of CA125 Binding in Colorectal Tissue Homogenate and Partially – Purified CA125 in Malignant Colon Cancer Stage B with 125I – anti CA125 Antibody

A: Thermodynamic Parameters of Standard State

The dependence of the equilibrium binding constant (affinity constant) for the binding of 125I – anti CA125 Antibody to the benign and malignant tissue homogenate (U.C, CCB and RCC) on the temperature can be observed from Van't Hoff plot, as shown in figure (4-8, A, B, C), while figure (4-9) shows the Van't Hoff plot for the partially purified Antigens from malignant Colon Cancer Stage B.

The results obtained from Van't Hoff plot indicates that $\Delta H°$ in general had small values, the negative value (for tissue homogenate (U.C, CCB and RCC ascertains that the reaction were nearly endothermic while, the positive sign (for partially purified Antigens of Colon Cancer Stage B) ascertains that the reaction were nearly exothermic.

The values of $\Delta H°$ may indicate a favorable interaction between 125I – Antibody and both CA125 in tissue homogenate and partially purified Antigens.

These include the non – covalent interaction which are fundamentally electrostatic in nature such as charge – charge, charge – dipole, dipole – dipole, and hydrogen bonds. The sum of these types of interactions can yield some stabilization to the folded structure of the complex (227).

Table (4 – 6) and (4 – 7) show the values of thermodynamic parameters of standard state of colorectal tissue homogenate and partially purified Antigens from malignant Colon Cancer Stage B at different temperatures. The negative value of $\Delta G°$ reflects the stability of the complex hence, the high affinity of the reactants.

So our system is characterized by the sole contribution of $\Delta S°$ to the stability of the complex formed, while $\Delta H°$ has little or no effect(228).

The high values of positive $\Delta S°$ suggest that the binding spontaneity was entropically driven. Entropy was the driven force for the occurrence of the binding; this indicates the hydrophobic interactions which played an important role in stabilization the complexes (229).

Table (4 – 6): Thermodynamic parameters at standard state of 125I – anti CA125 Antibody binding with CA125 in colorectal tissue homogenate.

Temp °C	$\Delta H°$ KJ. mol-1			$\Delta G°$ KJ. mol-1			$\Delta S°$ J. mol-1.K-1		
	U.C	Colon Cancer Stage B	Rectum cancer stage C	U.C	Colon Cancer Stage B	Rectum cancer stage C	U.C	Colon Cancer Stage B	Rectum cancer stage C
5	-7.17	-13.26	-11.51	-15.53	-13.8	-16.18	30.07	1.90	16.80
25	-7.17	-13.26	-11.51	-16.40	-15.42	-16.79	30.97	7.25	17.72
37	-7.17	-13.26	-11.51	-16.63	-15.73	-17.78	30.52	7.97	20.23
45	-7.17	-13.26	-11.51	-16.72	-15.51	-16.85	30.03	7.08	16.79

Table (4 – 7): Thermodynamic parameters at standard state of 125I – anti CA125 Antibody with CA125 in partially purified CA125 Antigens.

Temp °C	$\Delta H°$ KJ. mol-1		$\Delta G°$ KJ. mol-1		$\Delta S°$ J. mol-1.K-1	
	MI	MII	MI	MII	MI	MII
5	9.60	+10.12	-8.14	-18.49	100.76	102.91
25	+9.60	+10.12	-20.30	-20.09	100.34	101.38

| 37 | +9.60 | +10.12 | -21.69 | -21.18 | 100.94 | 100.97 |
| 45 | +9.60 | +10.12 | -20.59 | -22.14 | 94.93 | 101.45 |

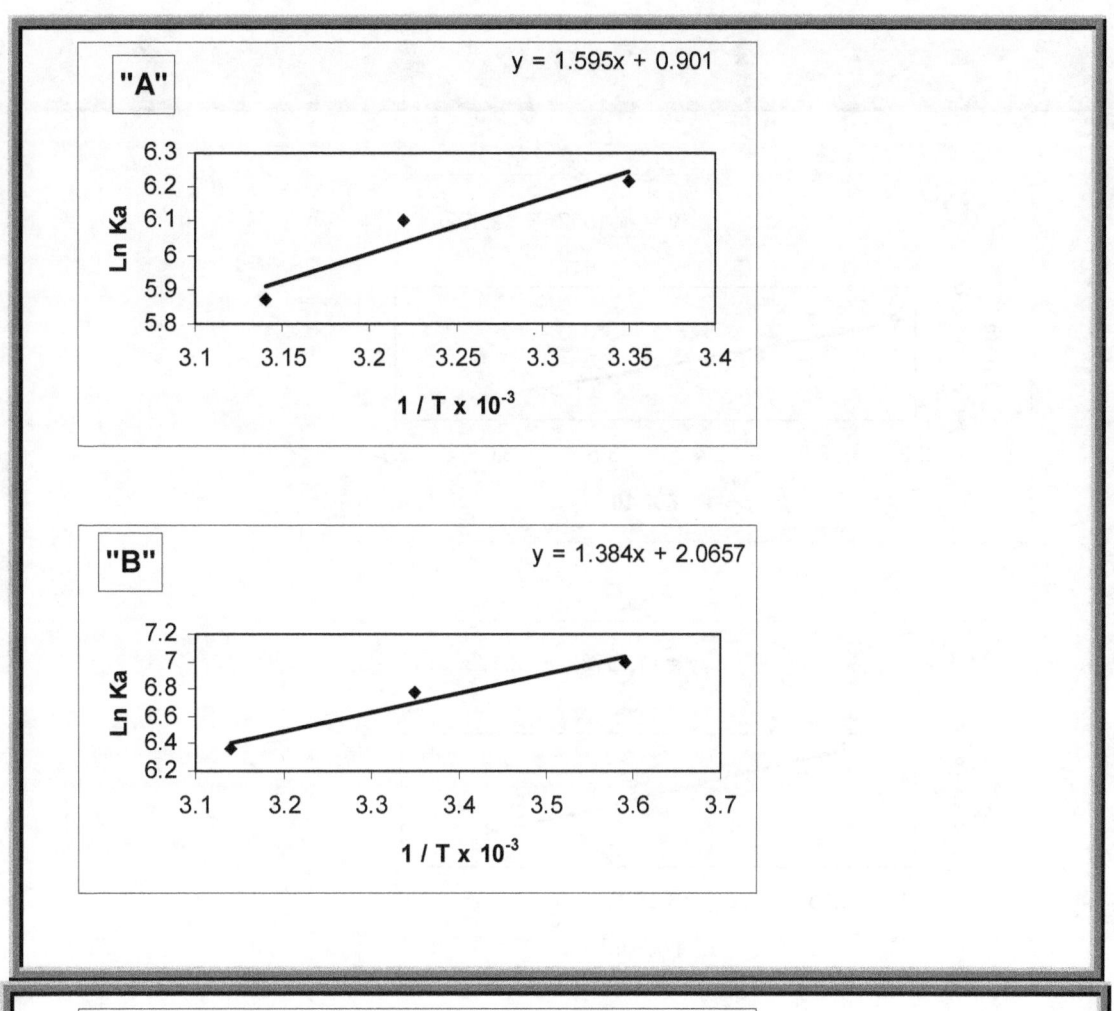

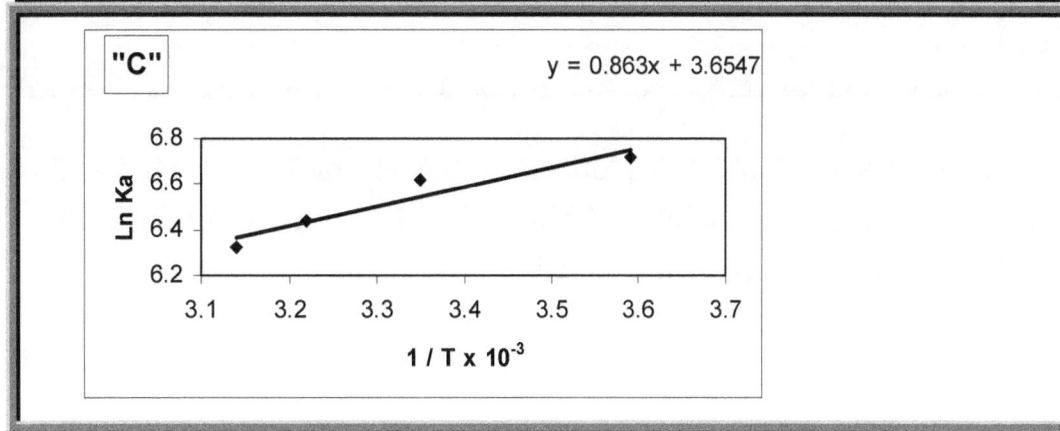

Figure (4 – 8) : Van't Hoff plot for the binding of 125I – anti CA125 binding to CA125 in

(A) Colon Cancer Stage "B"

(B) Rectum Cancer Stage "C"

(C) Ulcerative Colitis

(All other details are explained in the text).

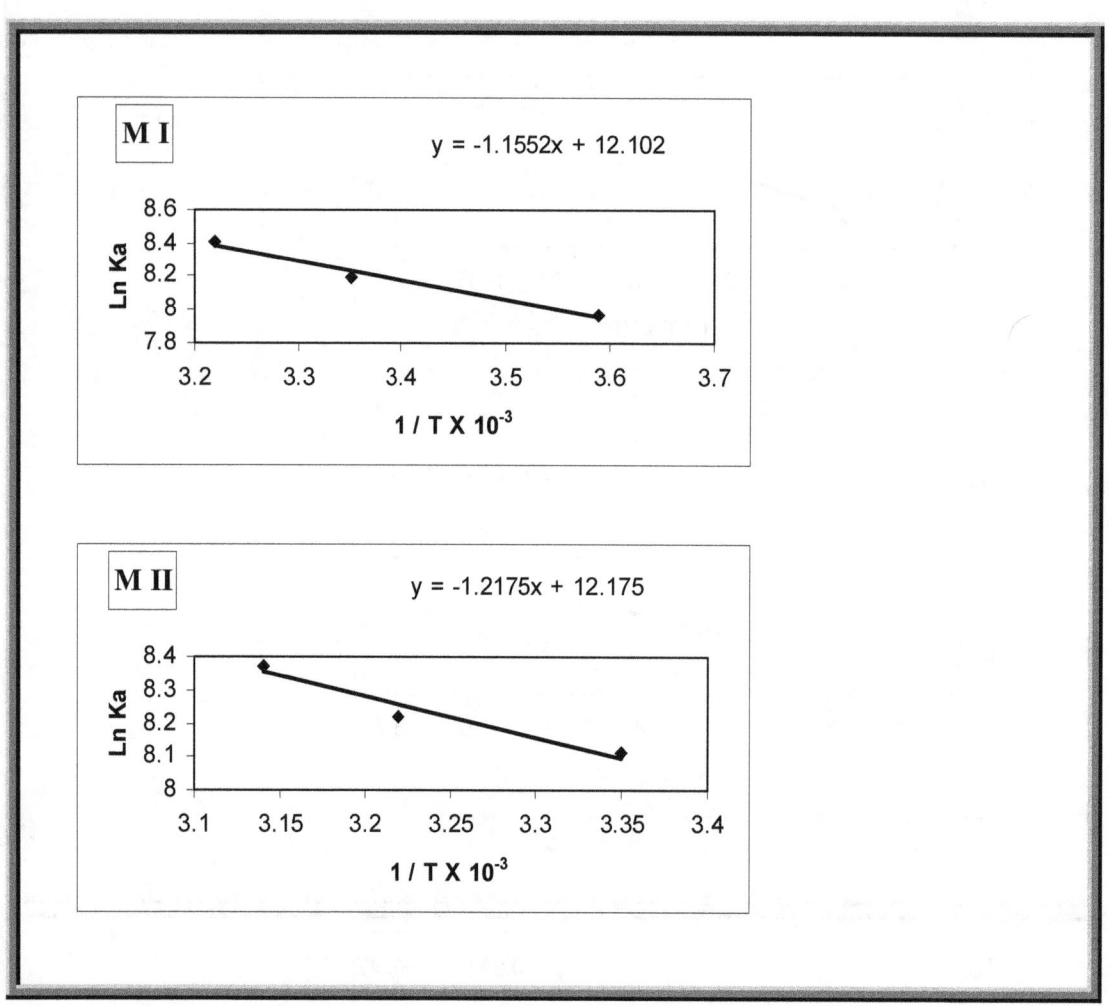

Figure (4 – 9) : Van't Hoff plot for the binding of 125I – anti CA125 binding to CA125 in partially purified (MI, MII Antigens) of malignant colon tumors Stage "B". (All other details are explained in the text)

B – Thermodynamic Parameters of Transition State

The transition state theory proposes that the association of two substances to form the final product proceeds through the formation of an activated complex (transition state). Consequently, the interaction of

125I – anti CA125 Antibody with colorectal tissue homogenate and partially purified Antigens can be represented as follows

$$^{125}\text{I - Ab} \quad + \text{Ag} \rightarrow [\,^{125}\text{I - Ab - Ag}\,]\,^* \rightarrow [\,^{125}\text{I - Ab - Ag}\,]$$

labeled CA 125 → an activated → Final product.
antibody   complex

The thermodynamic parameters of the transition state (ΔH^*, ΔG^*, and ΔS^*) could be determined from Arrhenius equation and the Kinetic constants.

Figures (4 – 10, A, B, C) and (4 – 11) show the Arrhenius plot of ln K+1 versus 1/T values. The slop of the straight line represents the activation energy (Ea).

Tables (4 – 8) and (4 – 9) show the values of thermodynamic parameters of transition state of colorectal tissue homogenate and partially purified Antigens from malignant Colon Cancer Stage B respectively at different temperature. The values of activation energy represents the required energy to overcome the energy barrier of the transition state for the formation of 125I – anti CA125 Antibody / CA125 complex. Also the value of activation energy is in accordance with the high positive values of ΔG^*, which indicates that the formation of the activated complex is a non – spontaneous process and requires a lot of energy (equal to Ea) to overcome the transition state energy barrier and giving the final product, whearse the high negative ΔS^* revealed that the activated complex had a more order structure than the reactants.

From the results obtained for the thermodynamic parameters in the transition state, it can be concluded that the positive values of ΔH^* and high positive values of ΔG^* are favorable to overcome the energy barrier of the transition state, the high negative values of ΔS^* mean more arranged structure for the activated complex. The positive values of ΔG^* is mainly attributed to the decrease in the entropy of the transition state ($\Delta S^* < 0$). In addition the positive value of ΔH^* shows that the heat content of the activated complex is more than that of isolated species(230,231).

The values of the thermodynamic parameters of the binding reaction, gave an over all idea about the nature of forces that regulate the formation of complex.

The formation of a complex occurs in two steps, the first is the stabilization of the complex by hydrophobic interaction and the second is the stabilization by short range interactions, such as electrostatic interaction, hydrogen bonding and Vander Waals interactions.

Hydrophobic interactions contribute to the complex stability via high positive entropy change ($AS^* > 0$), white electrostatic interactions, hydrogen bonding and Vander Waals interactions contribute to the stability of the complex via negative entropy change ($\Delta S^* < 0$)(232, 233).

The thermodynamic data indicate that the binding of 125I – anti CA125 Antibody to CA125 in colorectal tissue homogenate and partially purified Antigens are entropy driven agreement with the concept that hydrophobic interactions play an important role in (125I – anti CA125 Antibody / CA125) interactions.

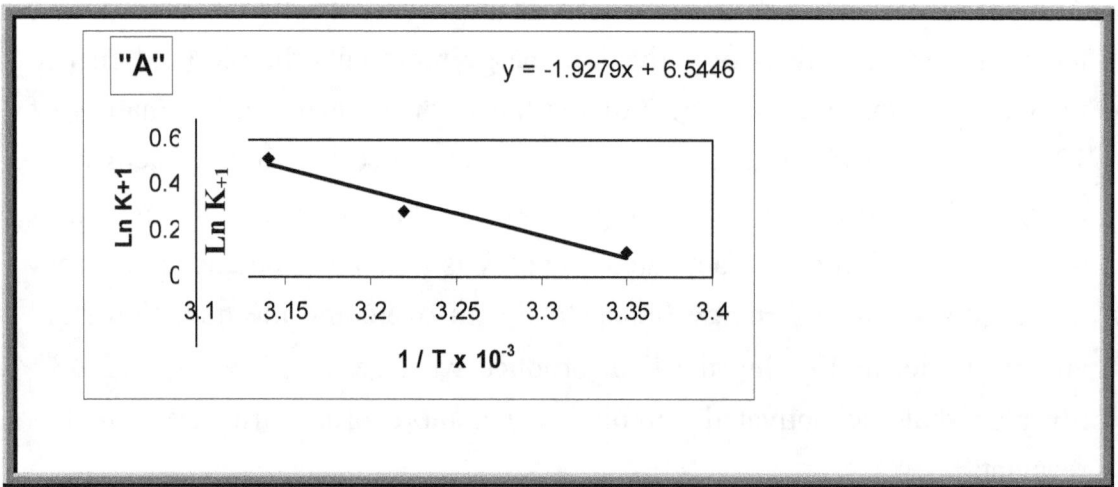

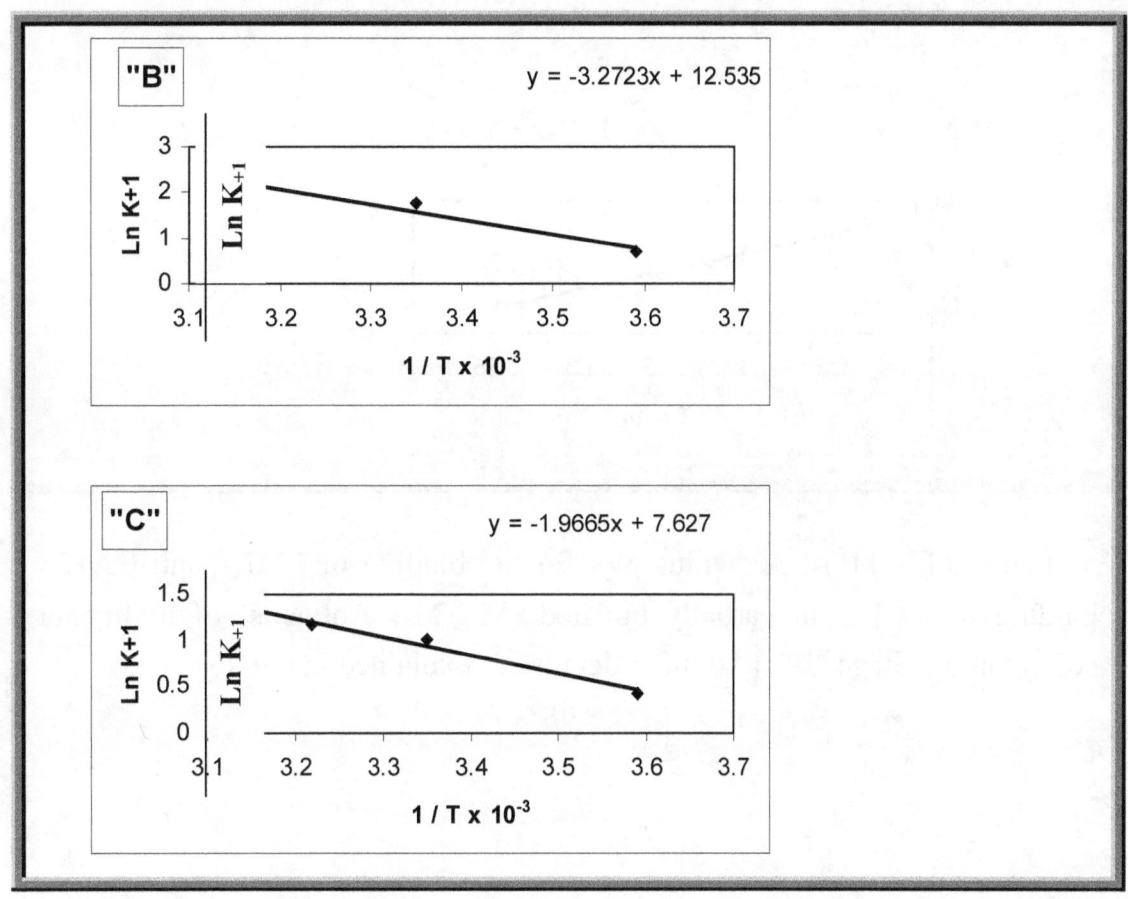

Figure (4 – 10) : Arrhenius plot for the binding of 125I – anti CA125 binding to CA125 in

(A) Colon Cancer Stage "B"

(B) Rectum Cancer Stage "C"

(C) Ulcerative Colitis

(All other details are explained in the text).

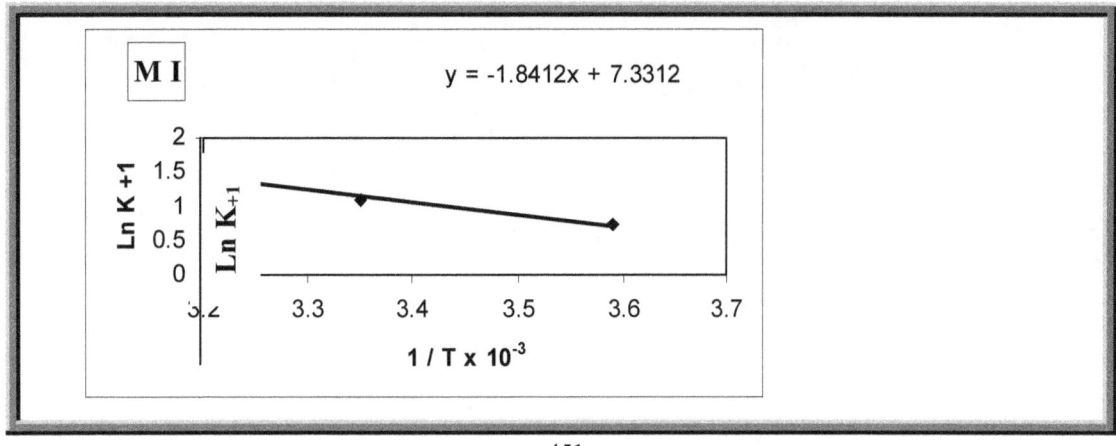

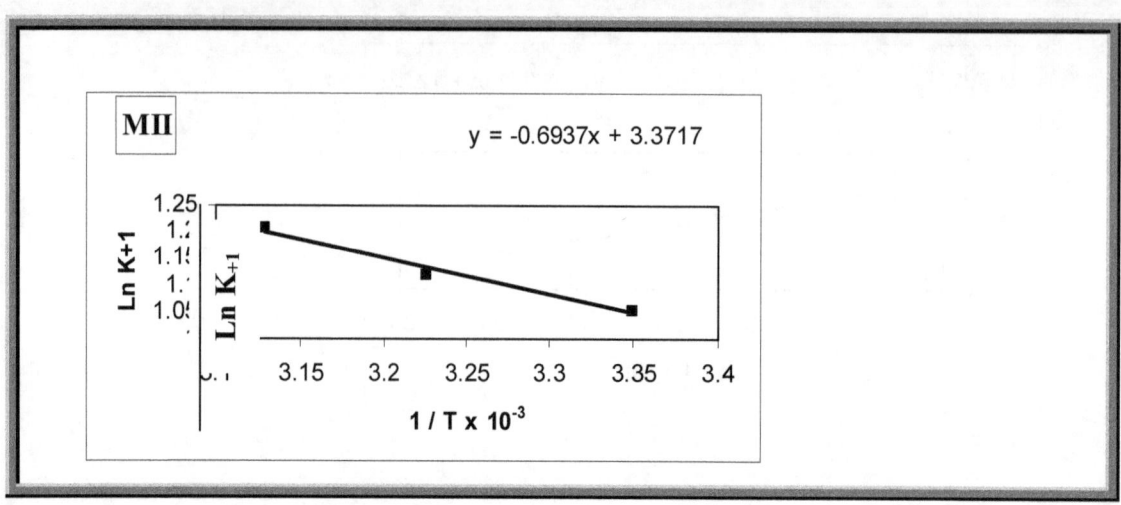

Figure (4 – 11) : Arrhenius plot for the binding of 125I – anti CA125 binding to CA125 in partially purified (MI, MII Antigens) of malignant colon tumors Stage "B". (All other details are explained in the text)

ChapterFive

Abstract

This chapter deals with the characterization of CA125 antigens, h-CA125 (CA125 / anti CA125) complex and (125I-anti CA125 Antibody/CA125) complex using partially purified CA125 from Colon Cancer Stage B and (standard solution) as h-CA125 and (CA125/anti CA125) complex.

Gel filtration technique was used to separate 125I-anti CA125 Antibody bound to crude colon cancer homogenate, partially purified antigens from Colon Cancer Stage B and standard solution of CA125 (as CA125 source) from unbound (free) 125I-anti Ca125 Antibody.

The characterization was carried out through spectroscopic studies using ultra violet absorption molecules. Factors affecting the absorption properties of the molecules under investigation of this chapter such as pH, solvent polarity (solvent perturbation, urea and KCL).

The thermal stability in the presence of different concentration of sodium chloride has been studied.

The spectrophotometric titration of (CA125/anti CA125) complex and (125I-anti CA125/CA125) complex show that about 53% and 67% of the histidine residues are located on the surface of the two complexes molecules, while 52% and 57% of tyrosine residues are located on the surface of the two complexes molecules.

:Introduction

Molecules absorb light, the efficiency of absorption depend on both the structure and environment of the molecules making absorption spectroscopy a useful tool for characterization of both small and large molecule.

The ultraviolet absorption spectra of protein solutions in the regions 250 to 310 nm are contributed from phenylalanyl, tyrosyl and tryptophanyl residues, but the shorter wavelengths; the contributions come from other groups such as histidyl residues and the peptide bond(234). Changes in the environment of these chromophores can lead to alteration in the absorption spectrum, and conformational changes of its chromophoric groups (235). A variety of environmental changes (e.g. pH, temperature) can affect the absorption spectrum, if the ground and excited states, the altered spectrum of the chromophore can be shifted to longer (red shift) or shorter (blue shift) wave lengths. The shift may or may not be accompanied by a change in intensity of spectrum (236,337).

The most common uses of spectroscopic technique in biochemistry employ the ultraviolet region spectrum (238). Although it might appear that changes in the U.V absorption of protein side chains could produce only a very limited amount information, the range of studies carried out using ultraviolet absorption prove to be very wide (239).

U.V spectral method remains one of the most important methods in immunology for the study of Antibody structure and specific ligand binding (240).

The solvent perturbation technique was introduced by Herskovits and Laskowski (241). In this procedure, chromophores, which are in contact with the solvent, are deliberately perturbed by the addition of another solvent.

In the absence of conformational changes of the protein, only those groups extending into the solvent alteration, and the perturbation becomes a measure of the number of chromophores "exposed" to the solvent (239). In other word, the fraction of the difference spectrum is a relative measure of the fraction of chromophoric groups (exposed) to the solvent.

The simplest of the difference is the effect of the size or bulk of the perturbing solvent and the second source of the difference arises from the range effect (242).

The interpertation of spectral change due to solvent perturbation is less ambiguous than that due to change in pH (acid difference spectra (243,244), denaturation to depend on changes in such factors as the polarity (dielectric constant), the polarizability (refractive index) (245,446), and the charge state of the immediate environment of chromophoric, residues and on changes in strong interactions such as hydrogen bonding (247).

The goal of this chapter is to use the technique of ultraviolet difference spectrophotometry, and study the factors affecting the absorbance at the region of U.V using partially purified CA125 from Colon Cancer Stage B as CA125 source.

:Materials and Methods
:Chemicals :1-5

All chemicals and reagents used in this chapter are mentioned in chapter two .

:Instruments :2-5

All instruments used in this chapter are mentioned in chapter two.

:Gel Filtration Technique for Separation of Free and Bound

1- Three hundred microliter of crude Colon Cancer Stage B (400 µg.ml-1) was incubated with 90µl of 125I-anti CA125 Antibody (2.16mg/ml), the volume was completed to 750µl with tris buffer (pH7.8), and the mixture was incubated for seven hours at 25 Co.

2- At the end of incubation 666µl of the mixture in step (1) was applied to the surface of Sepharose C1-6B column as described in chapter three, the experiment of (Partial purification of CA125 by Sepharose Cl - 6B) Elution was carried out using tris buffer (0.05M, pH7.2) to separate CA125 bound to 125I-anti CA125 Antibody from unbound, with a flow rate of 10ml.hr-1.

3- The ratio activity of each fraction was counted in gamma counter for 1min.

4- Seventy five microliter of standard Antigen (human, 500U.ml-1) provided with the kit from Immunotech Company) was incubated with 225µl of 125I-anti CA125 Antibody (2.25mg.ml-1), the volume was completed to 600µl with tris buffer (0.05M,pH7.8), the mixture was incubated for seven hours at 25Co. Steps 2,3 in this section were repeated.

5- One hundred and fifty microliter of the first peak from partially purified CA125 (25µg.ml-1) was incubated with 90µl of 125I-anti CA125 Antibody (2.16mg.ml-1), while sixty microliter of the second peak of partially purified CA125 (18µg.ml-1) was incubated with sixty microliter of 125I-anti CA125 Antibody (1.44 mg.ml-1), the volume of the two mixtures was completed to 600µl with tris buffer (0.05M, pH7.4). The first mixture was incubated for four hours at 37Co, while the second mixture was incubated for three hours at 45Co. Steps 2, 3 in this section were repeated.

6- Ninety microliter of 125I-anti CA125 Antibody was completed to 750µl with tris buffer (0.05, pH7.2), then this volume was injected to the column as mentioned in step 2 of this section, then steps 2,3 were repeated.

:Solution

Tris buffer (0.05, pH7.2) was prepared as mentioned in chapter three, the experiment of (Partial purification of CA125 by Sepharose Cl-6B)

:Calculations

1- Radioactivity (c.p.m) of each eluted fraction was plotted against the fraction number.

2- The experiment in step (2) gave profile of three peaks, the first and second peak represent the 125I-anti CA125 Antibody bound to CA125, while the third peak represents the unbound 125I-anti CA125 Antibody.

3- The experiment of step (4) gave profile of two peaks. The first peak represents the 125I-anti CA125 bound to CA125, while the second peak represent the unbound 125I-anti CA125 Antibody. This observation was repeated as in step (6).

4- The percent ratio activity of each peak was calculated by dividing the sum of ratio activity fractions under each peak by the sum of ratio activity of all peaks represented in the following formula:

$$\text{Percent Radioactivity of each peak} = \frac{\text{Radioactivity per peak (c.p.m)}}{\text{Sum of Radioactivity of all peaks (c.p.m)}} \times 100$$

5-4: The U.V Spectrum of (125I-anti CA125 Antibody / CA125) Complex:

The gel filtration experiments in section (5-3) gave multiple peaks, each peak was pooled and the absorption spectrum was scanned in U.V region using 0.5 cm cuvette against tris buffer (0.05M,pH7.2) in reference beam.

5-5: Factors Affecting the Absorption Properties of CA125 Antigens, h - CA125, (CA125 / Anti CA125) Complex and (125I-anti CA125 / CA125) Complex:

pH Effect on the Spectrum of:

A-CA125 Antigens:

Two hundred microliter of isolated Antigens, were completed to 1ml at different pH values (4, 7,9and 11). The samples were transferred to 0.5 cm cuvette in the sample beam and the buffer at the adjusted pH in reference beam, and then the absorption spectrum was scanned.

:125CA -h -B

A volume of 25µl of h – CA125 standard was completed to 1ml with required volume of different buffer at different pH values as mentioned in the experiment of (pH effect on the spectrum of CA125 Antigens) , then placed in 0.5cm cuvette in a sample beam and the buffer at the required pH in the reference beam, the absorption spectrum was scanned.

:Complex (125AntiCA/125CA) -C

1- Twenty-five microliter of h-CA125 standard provided by (CA125-IRMA Kit) was mixed with 75µl of 125I-antiCA125 Antibody. The volume of the mixture was completed to 250µl with tris buffer (0.05M, pH7.4).

2- The mixture was incubated at 25Co for four hours.

3- At the end of incubation, the mixture was centrifuged for 1hour at 4000r.p.m at 4Co.

4- The precipitate formed was dissolved to 1ml with different pH buffers values as mentioned in the experiment of (pH effect on the spectrum of

CA125 Antigens), then placed in a 0.5cm cuvette in a sample beam and the buffer at the required pH in the reference beam , then used the absorption spectrum was scanned.

:Complex (125CA/125antiCA-I125) -D

1- One hundred microliter of crude Colon Cancer Stage B (400µg.ml-1) was incubated with 40µl of 125I-antiCA125 Antibody (2.88mg.ml-1), the volume of the mixture was completed to 250µl with tris buffer (0.05M, pH7.8).

2- The mixture was incubated at 25Co for seven hours.

3- After incubation, the mixture was centrifuged for 1hour at 4000 r.p.m at 4oC.

4- The precipitate formed was dissolved to 1 ml with different pH buffer values as mentioned in the experiment of (pH effect on the spectrum of CA125 Antigens), then placed in a 0.5cm cuvette in a sample beam and the buffer at the required pH in the reference beam, the absorption spectrum was scanned.

:Solutions

1- Tris (acidic buffer (0.05M)), was prepared by dissolving 0.788gm of tris (hydroxy methyl amino methane hydrochloride), 0.186gm of EDTA and 0.2 gm of sodium azide in 50 ml of deionized distilled water, the volume of the mixture was completed to 100 ml with deionized distilled water. The pH was adjusted to 4 by adding few drops of NaOH.

2- Tris(basic buffer (0.05M)), was prepared by dissolving 0.6057gm of tris (hydroxy methyl amino methane) , 0.186 gm of sodium azide in 50 ml of deionized distilled water , the volume was completed to 100 ml of deionized water . The pH was adjusted to 7 and 9 by adding few drops of (0.1M) HCl, also few drops of NaOH was added to adjust the pH to 11.

The Effect of Solvent Polarity (Solvent Perturbation) on The U.V Spectrum of :

A – CA125 Antigens:

Two hundred microliter of isolated antigens (MI, MII) were completed to 1 ml with the following solvents dissolved in tris buffer

(pH 7.2, 0.05 M)

* 20 % DMSO.
* 20 % Ethanol.
* 20 % glycerol.
* 20 % Sucrose.
* 20 % Ethylene glycol.

The absorption spectrum of each sample was scanned against the corresponding solvent in reference beam using 0.5cm cuvette.

B-h– CA125:

Twenty five microliter of h–CA125 standard was completed to 1ml of the same solvent mentioned in the experiment of (The effect of Solvent polarity (Solvent Perturbation on the U .V spectrum of h–CA125). The absorption spectrum of each sample was scanned against the corresponding solvent in reference beam using 0.5cm cuvette.

C-(CA125/Anti CA125) complex:

The complex was prepared as mentioned in the experiment of (pH effect on the spectrum of (CA125/AntiCA125) complex), the complex was dissolved in the same solvents mentioned in the experiment of (The effect of Solvent polarity (Solvent Perturbation on the U .V spectrum of h – CA125). The absorption spectrum of each sample was scanned against the corresponding solvent in reference beam using 0.5cm cuvette.

:complex (125CA/125anti CA-I125)-D

The complex was prepared by the same steps mentioned in the experiment of (pH effect on the spectrum of (125I - anti CA125 Antibody/CA125) complex), the complex was dissolved in the same solvents mentioned in the experiment of (The effect of Solvent polarity (Solvent Perturbation on the U .V spectrum of Human CA125). The absorption spectrum of each sample was scanned against the corresponding solvent in reference beam using 0.5cm cuvette.

:Solutions

1 – 20 % sucrose was prepared by dissolving 5gm of sucrose in a final volume of 25ml of tris buffer (pH7.2, 0.05M).

2 – 20 % ethylene glycol was prepared by dissolving 5ml of ethylene glycol in a final volume of 25mlof tris buffer (pH7.2, 0.05M).

:Mixture on the Spectrum of (KCl ,Urea) ,KCl ,aEffect of Ure
:Antigens 125CA-A

Two hundred microliter of CA125 isolated antigens (MI, MII) were pipetted in a set of three tubes. The volumes were completed to 1ml with tris buffer at pH7.2 contained (0.03MKCl, 8M urea and mixture of 1:1 of both 0.03M KCl and 8M urea) respectively, then each of which was placed in 0.5 cm cuvette in the sample beam and the buffer at the same pH in the presence of the same salt in the reference beam, and the absorption spectrum of each sample was scanned.

:125CA-h -B

The same procedure mentioned in the experiment of (The effect of Urea, KCl, (Urea, KCl) mixture on the spectrum of CA125 Antigens) was repeated by using 25µl of standard human CA125.

C-(CA125/Anti CA125) Complex:

The complex was prepared as mentioned in the experiment of (pH effect on the spectrum of (CA125/AntiCA125) complex), the complex was dissolved in the same solutions mentioned in the experiment of (The effect of Urea, KCl, (Urea, KCl) mixture on the spectrum of CA125 Antigens) and the same procedure was repeated as mentioned in the experiment of (The effect of Urea, KCl, (Urea, KCl) mixture on the spectrum of CA125 Antigens).

D-(125I-Anti CA125/CA125) Complex:

The complex was prepared as mentioned in the experiment of (pH effect on the spectrum of (125I - anti CA125 Antibody/CA125) complex); the complex was dissolved in the same solutions mentioned in the experiment of

(The effect of Urea, KCl, (Urea, KCl) mixture on the spectrum of CA125 Antigens) and the same procedure was repeated as mentioned in the experiment of (The effect of Urea, KCl, (Urea, KCl) mixture on the spectrum of CA125 Antigens).

Solutions:

1- Eight molar of urea was prepared by dissolving 48.04gm of urea in a final volume of 100ml of tris buffer (pH7.2, 0.05M).

2- KCl (0.03M) was prepared by dissolving 0.5474gm of the salt in a final volume of 100ml of tris buffer (pH7.2, 0.05M).

5-6: The Effect of NaCl Concentration on the Thermal Stability of the Complex by U.V Spectral Studies:

1- The preparation of the two complexes were mentioned in the sections on the experiment of (pH effect on the spectrum of (CA125/AntiCA125) complex) and the experiment of (pH effect on the spectrum of (125I - anti CA125 Antibodyl/CA125) complex) respectively.

2- The two complexes were dissolved in a final volume of 1ml with 20% ethylene glycol and (0.01M NaCl dissolved in tris buffer (pH7.2, 0.05M).

3- Each mixture was placed in 0.5cm cuvette in the sample beam and the buffer in the reference beam.

4- The absorption was measured at the wavelengths of (292 and 295nm) at different temperatures (20, 30, 40, 50, 60, 70, 80, 90,100oC).

5- The experiment was repeated for each complex with another solution containing (20% ethylene glycol and 0.1M NaCl) dissolved in tris buffer (pH7.2, 0.05M).

6- The absorbance of each complex was plotted against the different temperature at two wavelengths (292, 295).

:Solutions

1- Twenty percent of ethylene glycol was prepared by dissolving 20ml of ethylene glycol in 80ml of tris buffer (pH7.2, 0.05M).

2- NaCl (0.01M) in 20% ethylene glycol was prepared by dissolving 0.05844gm of NaCl in 100ml of 20% ethylene glycol buffer.

3- NaCl (0.1M) in 20% ethylene glycol was prepared by dissolving 0.5844gm of NaCl in 100ml of 20% ethylene glycol buffer.

5-7: Spectrophotometric pH Titration of (CA125/Anti CA125) Complex, (125I-anti CA125 /CA125) Complex:

1- The preparations of the two complexes were mentioned in the experiment of (pH effect on the spectrum of (CA125/AntiCA125) complex) and the experiment of (pH effect on the spectrum (125I - anti CA125 Antibody/CA125)) complex respectively.

2- A series of the two complexes were dissolved in a final volume of 1ml with buffer at pH range from (7-12). The maximum absorbance of each sample was measured at 295 nm.

3- The absorbance of λ max at each pH values was plotted versus the corresponding pH.

4- Other series of complexes were dissolved in a final volume of 1ml with buffer at pH range (2-6). The maximum absorbance of each sample was measured at 211nm.

5- The absorbance of λ max at each pH values was plotted against the corresponding pH.

Results and Discussion:

Gel Filtration Technique for Separation of Free and Bound 125I-anti CA125 Antibody.

Figure (5-1) shows the results of gel filtration technique used to separate 125I-anti CA125 Antibody bounds to CA125 from crude Colon Cancer Stage (B), from this figure, it is obvious that there are two sharp peaks and another small peak which represent the isolated Antigen (MI) bound with 125I-anti CA125 Antibody, while the second peak represents the second Antigen (MII), while the small peak represents the unbound (free) 125I-antiCA125 Antibody.

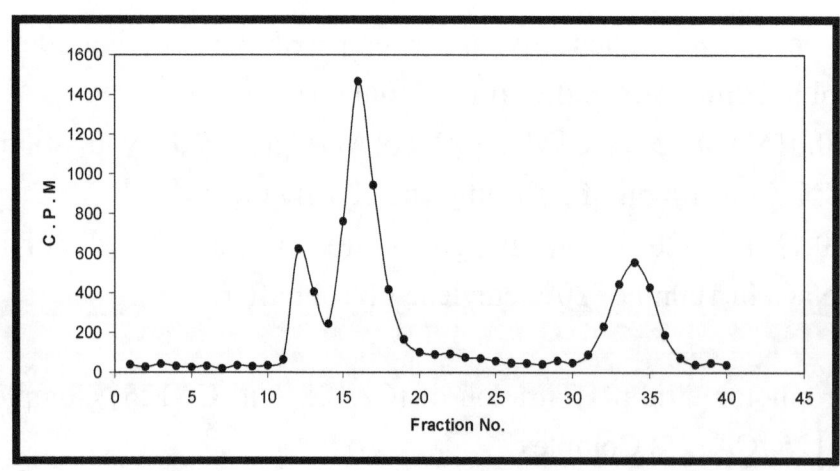

Figure (5-1): The Elution profile of (anti CA125 Antibody binding to CA125 in cytosolic fraction of malignant colon tumors using Sepharose Cl – 6B (All other details are explained in the text)

Figure (5-2) shows the complex formed from standard h-CA125, this figure gives two peaks, the first peak regards to the (Anti CA125/CA125) complex, while the second peak regards to the free 125I-anti CA125 Antibody. The comparison of these two figures is shown in figure (5-3); it is obvious that the complex of the crude Colon Cancer Stage B gives two peaks of two antigens complexes. This result is corresponding to that obtained in chapter three (Partial purification of CA125) that there are two antigens, while the complex of standard h–CA125 gives one peak, which means that there is only one Antigen, these difference may be due to the source of the isolated antigens (tissue or serum) and the case (normal or malignant)(248).

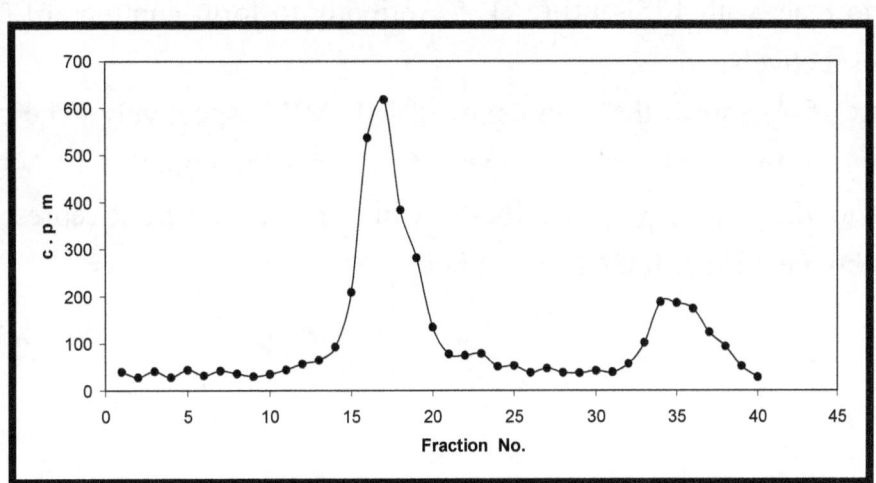

Figure (5-2) : The Elution profile of (CA125 / Anti CA125) Complex using Sepharose Cl – 6B (All other details are explained in the text)

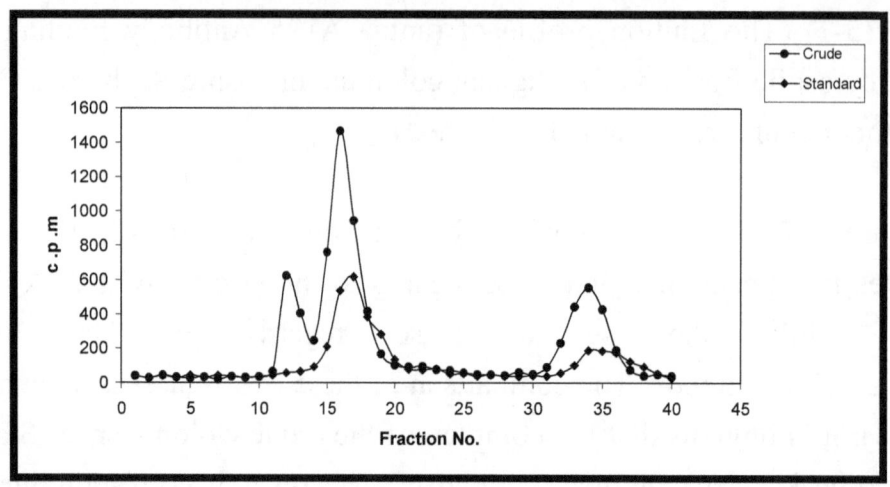

Figure (5-3) : The comparison of Elution profile of (CA125 / Anti CA125) complex and 125I – anti CA125 Antibody / CA125) complex using Sepharose Cl – 6B (All other details are explained in the text)

The isolated antigens from malignant Colon Cancer Stage "B" were submitted to react with 125I-anti CA125 Antibody to form complex of (MI and MII) respectively.

Figure (5-4) shows the complexes of MI, MII respectively. The two complexes gave two peaks, the first peak represents the complex of MI or MII bound to 125I-anti CA125 Antibody, while the second peak represents the free (unbound)125I-anti CA125 Antibody.

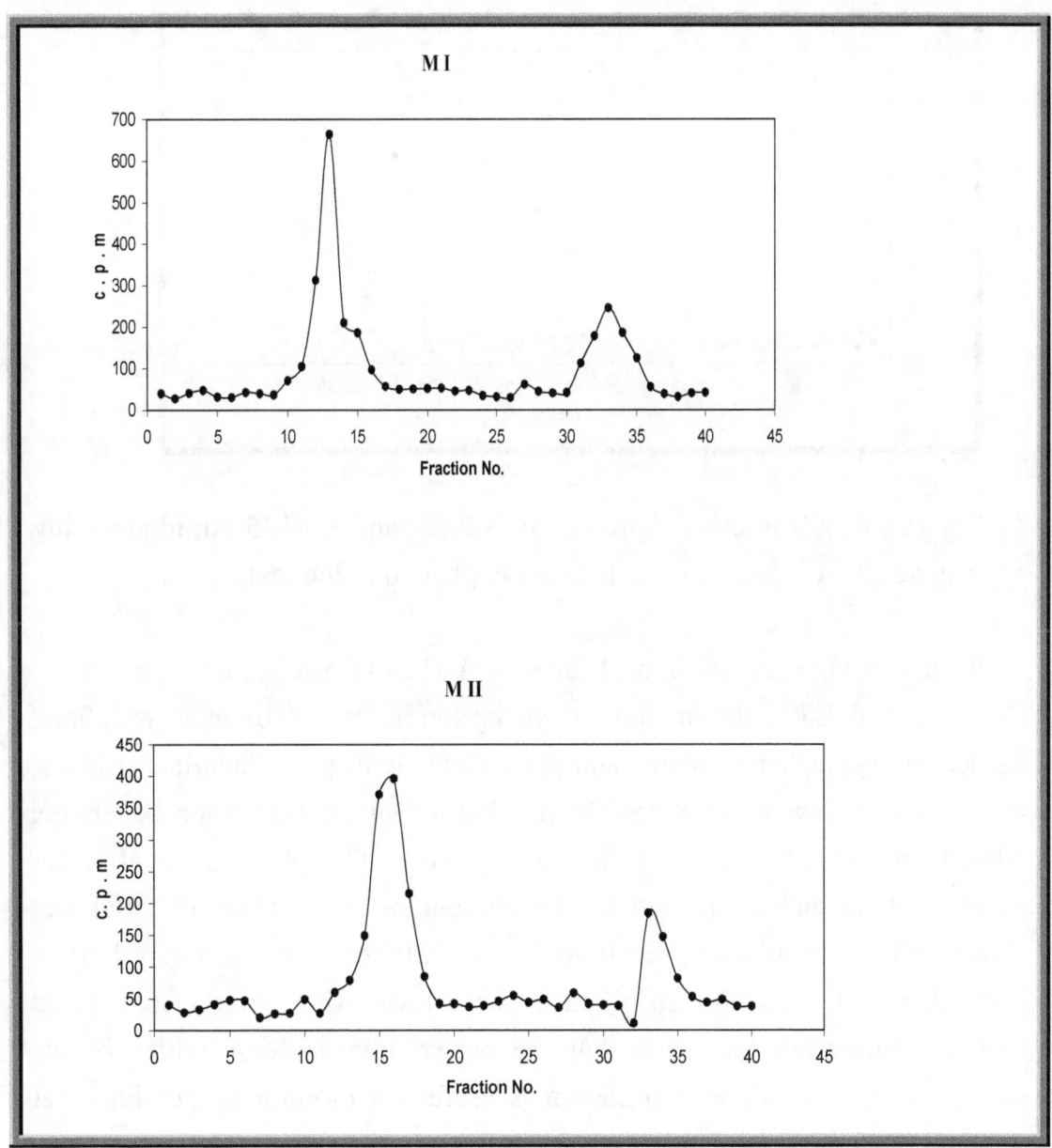

Figure (5-4): The elution profile of (125I – anti CA125 Antibody / MI CA125) complex and (125I – anti CA125 Antibody / MII CA125) complex using Sepharose Cl – 6B (All other details are explained in the text)

Figure (5-5) shows the gel filtration of 125I-anti CA125 Antibody, the result revealed only one peak in the same position of the peaks in figures (5-1, 5-2, 5-3 and 5-4), which represent the unbound 125I-antiCA125 Antibody.

465

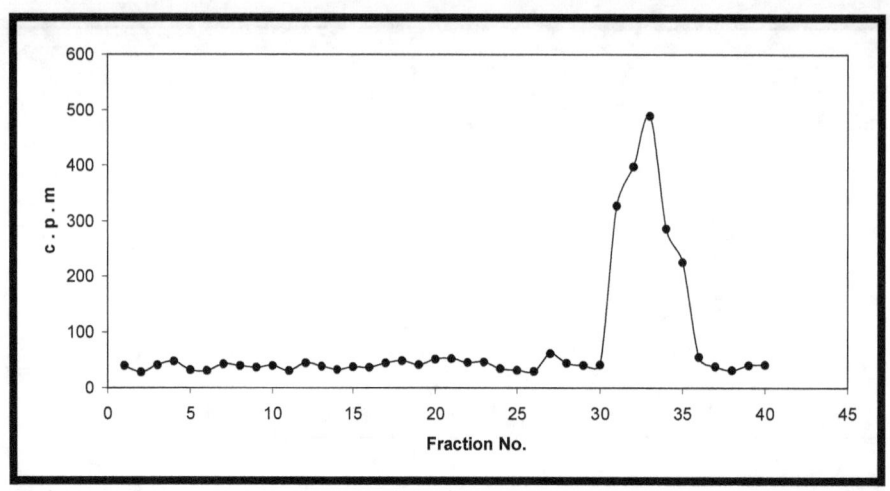

Figure (5-5): The elution profile of (125I – anti CA125 Antibody using Sepharose Cl – 6B (All other details are explained in the text)

:Complex (125CA/Antibody 125Anti CA-I125)V Spectra of .The U

Protein UV light maximum absorption is at approximately 280nm, caused by tryptophan, tyrosine and (to a less extent) phenylalanine residues, and at lower wavelength (215-230nm) due to polypeptide chain backbone. Absorbance at 280nm varies for each protein. The absorbance at lower wavelength is directly related to the amount of polypeptide material and usually considerably more sensitive than at 280nm. However many buffers and other molecules also absorbed at these lower wavelengths (phosphate and tris buffer are acceptable but the preservative sodium azide absorbs strongly). Absorbance at 215-230nm is useful for monitoring peptides that may not contain tryptophan or tyrosine (249).

The U.V spectra of partially purified antigens (MI, MII, h-CA125, (Anti CA125/CA125) complex, (125I – anti CA125 Antibody/MI (CA125)) and (125I-anti CA125 Antibody/MII (CA125)) complex were scanned from 200-350nm to determine the absorption spectra, and the alternation in the U.V spectra as a result of their interaction. Figure (5-6) and table (5-1) illustrate λ max values of the molecules under this study.

The U.V Spectrum of h-CA125:

Figure (5-6-(A)) illustrated the U.V spectrum of h-CA125 provided by CA125 IRMA Kit (Immunotech (France)) at neutral pH. As shown, the spectrum consisted of one broad peak at 280nm represents the side chain chromophore of tryptophyl residues (250).

The U.V Spectrum of (CA125/Anti CA125) Complex:

The U.V spectrum of (h-CA125/Anti CA125) complex has shown in figure (5-6-B). The spectrum consisted of two obvious peaks; the first sharp peak at 213nm represents the amide group in polypeptide bond with contribution of histidyl residues (251), while the second peak at (278nm) is assigned to the tyrosyl residue (250).

The U.V Spectrum of (125I-anti CA125 Antibody/CA125) Complex:

In the U.V spectrum of (crude homogenate/Anti CA125) complex, two peaks appeared at 220 and 257 respectively as shown in figure

(5-6-C). These two peaks represent the amide bond, which assigned to tyrosyl residue and phenylalanine residue, respectively.

MI /Antibody 125antiCA-I125) V Spectrum of MI Antigen and.The U :Complex ((125CA)

Figures (5-6-D and 5-6-E) show the U.V spectrum of MI Antigen and (125I-anti CA125 Antibody/MI (CA125)) complex. The spectrum of MI Antigen gives one peak at 221nm assigned to the tyrosyl residue (252), while the spectrum of MI Antigen complex gives one peak at 269nm assigned to the phenylalanine and tryptophan residues (253).

MII /Antibody 125anti CA-I125)V Spectrum of MII Antigen and .The U :Complex ((125CA)

The spectrum of MII Antigen and (125I-anti CA125/MII(CA125)) complex are shown in figure (5-6-F and 5-6-G). The spectrum of MII Antigen gives one peak at λ max 270nm assigned to the tyrosine residue (252), while the complex of MII Antigen gave two peaks, the first peak gave λ max at 230nm, while the second peak gave λ max at 278nm these two peaks assigned to the phenyl alanine and tyrosine residues respectively (254).

Table (5-1): The λ max of the U.V spectrum of CA125 antigens (MI,MII), h-CA125, CA125/anti CA125) complex and (125I-anti CA125Antibody/ CA125) complex at pH7.2

Sample	λ max(nm)
1-MI	221
2-MII	270
3-h-CA125	280
4-(CA125/anti CA125) complex	231, 278
5-(125I-antiCA125 Antibody/CA125) complex	220,257
6-(125I-anti CA125 Antibody/MI(CA125)) complex	269
7-(125I-anti CA125 Antibody/MII(CA125)) complex	230,278

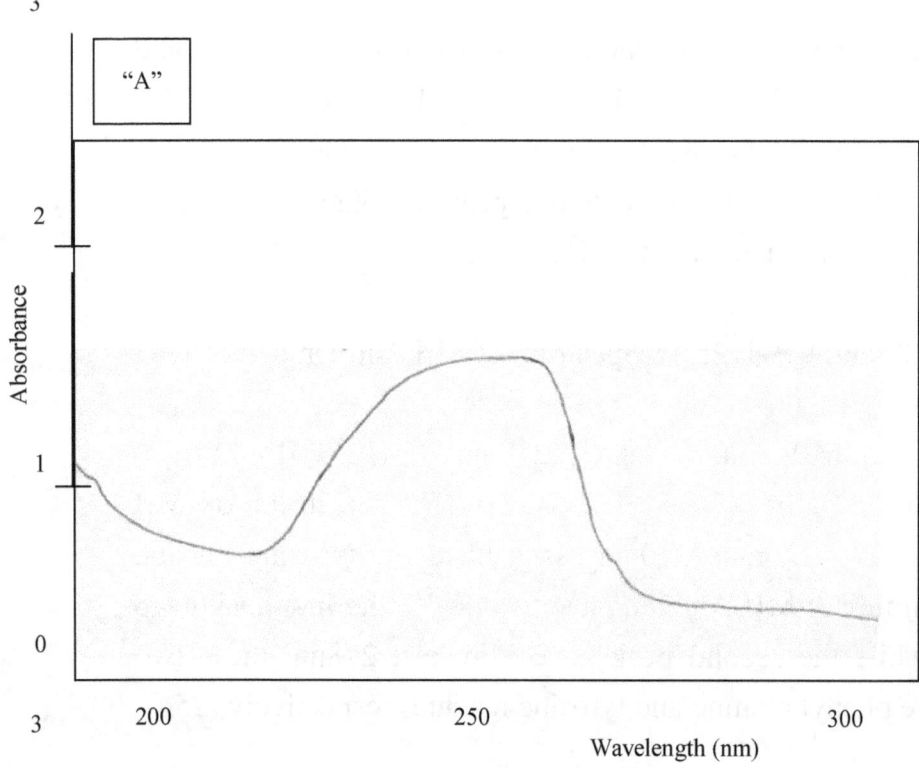

3

"A"

Figure (5 -6) The U. V. spectra of :

(A) h – CA125

(B) (CA125 / anti CA125) complex

(C) (125I – anti CA125 Antibody / CA125) complex

(D) MI Antigen

(E) (125I – anti CA125 Antibody / MI (CA125)) complex

(F) MII Antigen

(G) (125I – anti CA125 Antibody / MII (CA125)) complex

(All other details are explained in the text)

Factors Affecting the Absorption Properties of h - CA125, CA125 Antigens, (125I-anti CA125/CA125) Complex and (CA125/Anti CA125) Complex:

The absorption of a chromophore is primary determined by the chemical structure of the molecule. However, a large number of

environmental factors produce detectable changes in λ max(250,255 – 257).

The pH Effect

The pH of the solvent determines the Ionization state of the ionizable chromophore in the protein molecule. Table (5-2) shows the λ max values of CA125 antigens (MI, MII), Human-CA125, 125I-anti CA125 Antibody/ CA125) complex and (CA125/ Anti CA125) complex.

Table(5-2): The effect of different pH on λ max values on CA125 antigens, Human-CA125, (125I-anti CA125 Antibody/ CA125) complex and (CA125/Anti CA125) complex

	λ max(nm)					
H	I	MI	MII	h-CA125	CA125/anti (CA125) complex	(125I-anti CA125 Antibody/CA125) complex

469

			278	279	279
4	278	278	278	279	279
7	278	257	278	278,218	224
9	275, 229	270	278	279,229	220
11	276	270, 225	278	270,224	205

In this table λ max was measured at different range of pH (4, 7, 9, and 11). In the case of pH4.0, there were no changes in the λ max of the molecules under study; at this range λ max were 278 and 279 which were assigned to the tyrosine (258).

In the case of neutral pH(7.0) the MII and 125I-antiCA125 Antibody/ CA125) complex have a significant changes in λ max at 257 and 224 (blue shift) which were assigned to the phenylalanine and tyrosine respectively, this shift may be due to the conformational change in the protein (251). This behavior also shown for (125I-anti CA125 Antibody/ CA125) at pH 9 and pH 11 which was assigned to tyrosine and phenylalanine respectively.

The shifting in the protein spectrum which produced by pH can not by simply attributed to the inductive effect at vicinal charges, such spectral changes must therefore attributed to arrangement of secondary and tertiary structure, although, the possibility of field effects due to unusually close conjugation of charges of aromatic groups is not excluded (259).

The Effect of Solvent Polarity on CA125 Antigens, h-CA125, (125I-anti CA125 Antibody/ CA125) Complex and (CA125/Anti CA125) Complex U.V Spectrum (Solvent perturbation) Studies :

Table (5-3) shows the λ max values of CA125 isolated antigens, Human-CA125, (CA125/ AntiCA125) complex and (125I-anti CA125 Antibody/ CA125) complex by using 20% of different solvent at pH7.2. There was a shift towards longer wavelengths in the presence of dimethyl sulfoxide (DMSO) for all molecules. This behavior may be due to the inter molecular hydrogen bonding increase as the concentration of the solution increase and additional bands start to appear at longer or shorter wavelength(260). The blue shift indicates that the protein was defolded (rigid) and the exposed histidyl residues were buried interior the molecule in the presence of DMSO.

On the other hand the presence of 20% of ethanol, glycerol, ethylenglycol and sucrose, there were significant red shifts to (278, 268, and 258) which were assigned to tyrosine and phenylalanine respectively. This red shift is due to the $\pi \rightarrow \pi^*$ transition of aromatic ring of tyrosyl, while these solvent caused the absence of λ max for (125I - anti CA125 Antibody / CA125) complex, the proteins were denatured due to changes in the secondary and tertiary structures of protein. If there was no effect on the maximum absorbance, this indicated no interaction or any change that happens between the solvent and the molecules. When one band was absorbed, this may be attributed to the amino acids buried in the internal region of the protein and surrounded by non-polar amino acids (250).

The application of Spectrophotometric solvent perturbation on CA125 isolated antigens, h-CA125, Anti CA125/CA125) complex and (125I-anti CA125 Antibody/ CA125) complex molecules is to determined the local of tryptophyl, tyrosyl residues weather they are buried and inaccessible or exposed and accessible to the approach of solvent (242).

Laskowski (1966) (261) has listed the major assumptions of solvent perturbation experiments. These are (1) buried chromophore which are unperturbed, that is only the groups located on the surface or near the surface of the protein should experience the perturbing effects of the solvent; groups buried in the interior of the protein, not accessible to the solvent should not be affected and consequently could not contribute to the over all spectral shift observed (2) no conformational changes take upon additional of perturband, and (3) the solvation layer around the chromophore contains the same concentration of perturbant as the bulk of the solution(239). The most useful solvents for perturbation experiments when empled at convenient concentrations (often 20%), do not appear to produce conformational changes in protein studied under reasonable condition of pH, ionic strength and temperature. This concentration is large enough to cause measurable shifts in the spectra of chromophoric residues(262).

Table (5-3) : The effect of solvent polarity, solvent perturbation on CA125 antigens, h – CA125, (CA125 / anti CA125) complex and (125I – anti CA125 Antibody / CA125) complex on U.V spectrums.

Solvent	λ max nm				
	MI	MII	h – CA125	(CA125/anti CA125) complex	(125I – anti CA125 Antibody/CA125) complex
DMSO 20%	203 216 277	217 - 268	217 - 258	216 - 268	218 -
Ethanol 20%	277	278	-	-	-
Glycerol 20%	278	268	-	-	-
Ethylene glycol 20%	278	277	268	279	-
Sucrose 20%	277	268	258	268	-

Mixture on the Spectrum of (KCl ,Urea)The Effect of Urea and KCl anti –I 125)Complex and (125anti CA / 125CA) ,125CA-h ,Antigens 125CA :Complex (125CA /Antibody 125CA

The effect of 8M Urea, 0.03M KCl and mixture of 1:1 of 8M Urea and 0.03M KCl on the λ max of the CA125 antigens (MI, MII), Human– CA125, (CA125 / anti CA125) complex and (125I – anti CA125 Antibody / CA125) complex were examined. The values of λ max are illustrated in table (5-4).

The presence of 8M Urea caused a significant red shift from 224, 223, 226, and 225nm for MI, MII, h – CA125 and (CA125 / anti CA125) complex respectively which were assigned to the polypeptide bond to 270, 270, 275 and 270 respectively which were assigned to the tyrosyl residues, while the tyrosyl residues at (125I – anti CA125 Antibody / CA125) complex disappeared, new absorption peak appear at 280nm which could be assigned to the n - π* transition in the aromatic ring of the tryptophyl residues. These results indicate that the molecules solvated with Urea (dipole – dipole interaction) and produce a red shift and new chromophore come to the surface. The red shift is due to the intermolecular hydrogen bonding between the oxygen of the amide group and the solvent(247).

When 0.03M KCl was used, the polypeptide bond disappeared in MI Antigen and two λ max appeared at 208 and 270 which were assigned to phenyl alanine and tyrosine residues respectively, also phenyl alanine residues appeared in (125I – anti CA125 Antibody / CA125) complex, while these residues disappeared in MII Antigen and one λmax appeared at 213nm which was assigned to polypeptide bond.

There were a red shift in the cases of h – CA125 and (CA125 / anti CA125) complex from 213nm and 214nm respectively to 270nm which were assigned to polypeptide bond and tyrosyl residues respectively.

Such a blue or red shift can arise by introducing positive (K+) or negative (Cl-) charges near the chromophore (the amide group) which might interact directly with the π electron system of the amide group (247).

When 8M Urea was mixed with 0.03M KCl, the same shift in λmax was observed when 8M urea was used alone with each molecule under investigation, this means that the shift caused by the mixture may be due to the effect of urea, but not to KCl. The change in the absorption may be produced by change in the absorption and may be produced by changes in the n → π* absorption in the polypeptide bonds in the protein either because of change in their geometrical arrangement, or because of the environmental changes (239).

Table (5-4) : The effect of 8M Urea, 0.03M KCl and mixture of (1:1) Urea + KCl on the λ max of CA125 antigens, h – CA125, (CA125 / anti CA125) complex and (125I – anti CA125 Antibody / CA125) complex.

Solvent	λ max nm				
	M I	M II	h–CA125	(CA125/anti CA125) complex	(125I – anti CA125 Antibody/CA125) complex
8M Urea	-224 270	195 223 270	196 226 275	195 225 270	195 - 280
0.03 M KCl	208 270	213 274	214 277	212 270	205 276
Mixture of 1:1 Urea + KCl	194 222 276	194 221	195 225 278	194 222 279	194 221

anti /125CA)The Effect of NaCl Concentration on Thermal Stability of V .Complex by U (125CA/Antibody125anti CA -I125)Complex and (125CA :Spectral Studies

Figure (5-7) and (5-8) show the thermal stability of (CA125 / anti CA125) complex and (125I – anti CA125 Antibody / CA125) complex respectively using NaCl in the presence of 20% ethylene glycol, this concentration of ethylene glycol appear to have little effect on protein concentration and does not specifically interact with chromophore of protein(263).

Figure (5-7) shows that the internal tryptophan is completely exposed to the solvent at 60°C in 0.01N NaCl and 70°C in 0.1 N NaCl for (CA125 / anti CA125) complex. While, the internal tyrosine was exposed to the solvent at

70°C in 0.01 N NaCl and 80°C in 0.1 N NaCl for the same complex. The tryptophan residues are exposed to the solvent at 60°C in 0.01 N NaCl and 80°C in 0.1 N NaCl for (125I – anti CA125 Antibody / CA125) complex as shown in figure (5-8). On the other hand tyrosine residues are exposed to the solvent at 50°C in 0.01 N NaCl and 60°C in 0.1 N NaCl for (125I – anti CA125 Antibody / CA125) complex.

From these results it was concluded that these proteins are more stable at high NaCl concentration, this due to that each protein in solution containing salts will collect about it counter ion atmosphere entriched in oppositely charged small ion (Chloride ion, Sodium ion), and such a cloud of ions will tend to screen the protein. The larger the concentration of small ions present, the more effective this electrostatic screening will be, and decrement in the absorption intensity will be observed (238).

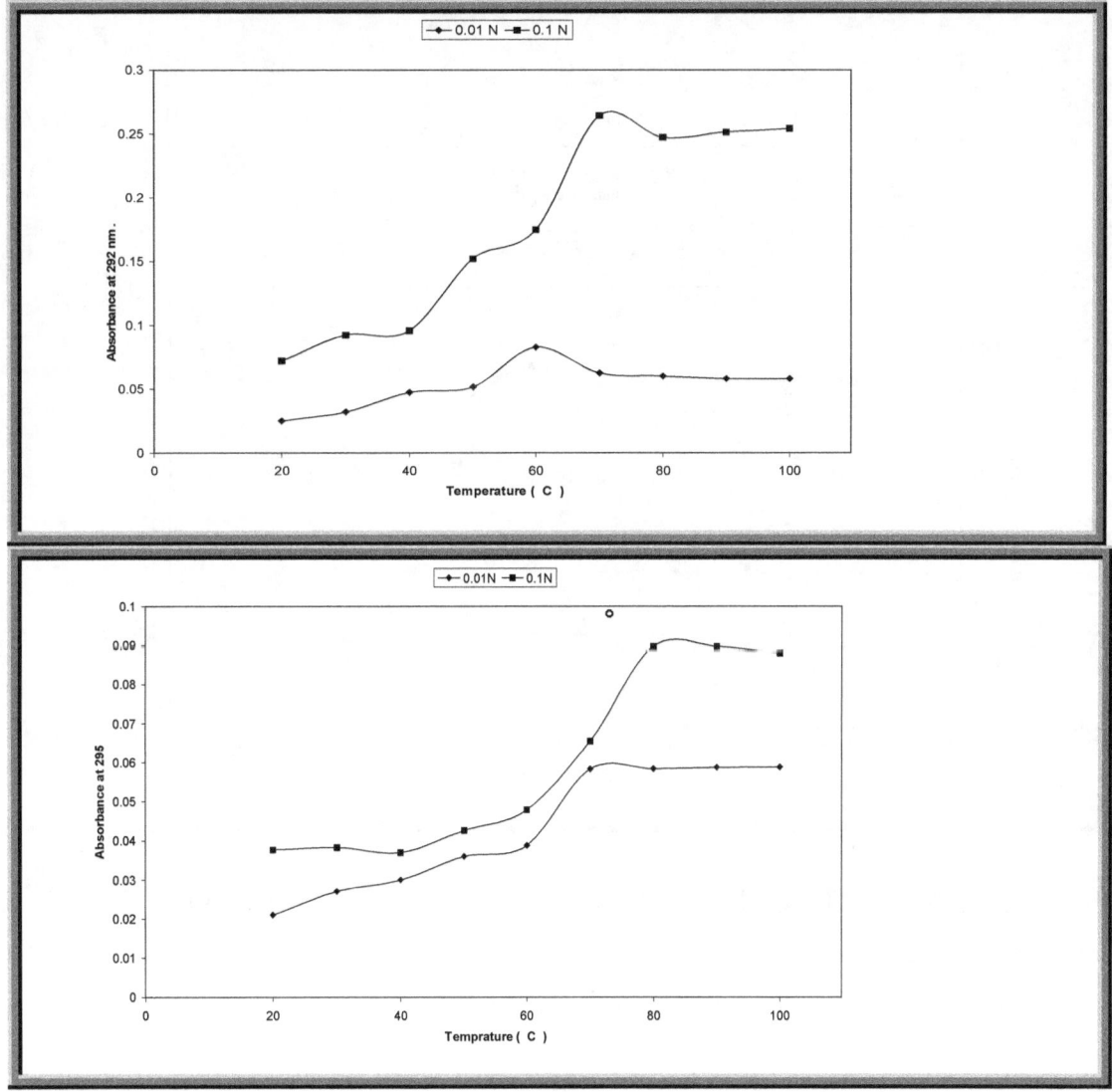

Figure (5–7): Thermal stability of (CA125 / anti CA125) complex at λ max 292 and 295 nm in the presence of 0.01 N NaCl and 0.1 N NaCl (All other details are explained in the text)

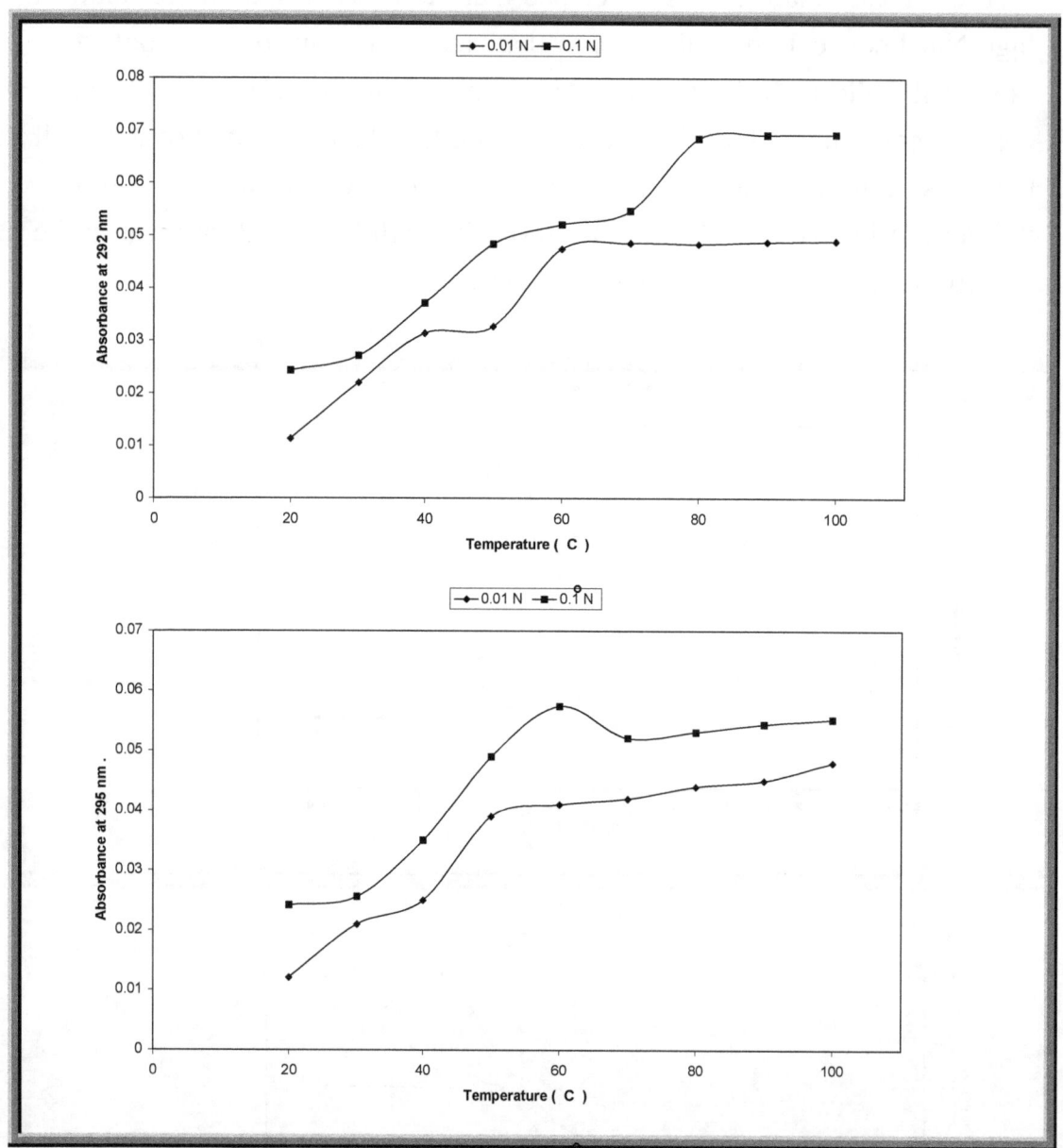

Figure (5–8): Thermal stability of (125I - anti CA125 Antibody / CA125) complex at λ max 292 and 295 nm in the presence of 0.01 N NaCl and 0.1 N NaCl (All other details are explained in the text)

Spectrophotometric Titration of (CA125 / anti CA125) Complex and (125I – anti CA125 Antibody / CA125) Complex:

Spectrophotometric pH titration is following the change in absorbance of the chromophore with increasing pH (250). Many studies of protein structure required the determination of pKa values for protein dissociation from ionizable amino acid side chains, because these values give an indication of the location of the amino acid in the protein. This can often be done spectrophotometrically because dissociation often changes the spectrum of one of the chromophors, the observation of tyrosine dissociation was performed by measuring the absorption at 295nm (λ max for the ionized form of tyrosine, and the observation of histidine dissociation was carried out by measuring the absorption at all 211nm.

Figure (5-9) show the pH titration curve of (CA125 / anti CA125) complex and (125I – anti CA125Antibody / CA125) complex. Figure (5-9 A) shows that the pKa values for histidine residues is (5.1) for (CA125 / anti CA125) complex and pKa (4.9) for (125I – anti CA125 Antibody / CA125) complex, while the pKa values for tyrosine are shown in figure (5-9 B). These values were 10.2 and 9.1 for both (CA125 / anti CA125) complex and (125I – anti CA125 Antibody / CA125) complex respectively.

From figure (5-9 A) it was found that about 53% of histidine residues are located on the surface of (CA125 / anti CA125) complex, while 47% of histidine residues are embedded in the interior region of the same molecule, also from the same figure, it was found that about 67% of histidine residues are located on the surface of (125I – anti CA125 Antibody / CA125) complex, while 33% of these residues were embedded in the interior region of the molecule.

From figure (5-9 B), it was found that about 52% of tyrosine residues are located on the surface of (CA125 / anti CA125) complex, while about 48% of tyrosine residues are buried in the interior of the folded structure. On the other hand the tyrosine residues of (125I – anti CA125 Antibody / CA125) complex were 57% located on the surface of the complex molecule and 43% are buried interior in the folded structure of the same complex molecule.

The histidine residues are largely present on the molecular surface of the two complexes molecules and the internal residues are in non-polar environment. On the other hand, the internal tyrosine in the two complexes molecules are on a polar environment (e.g., a tyrosine surrounded by carboxy groups) and the internal tyrosine are in non-polar environment (264).

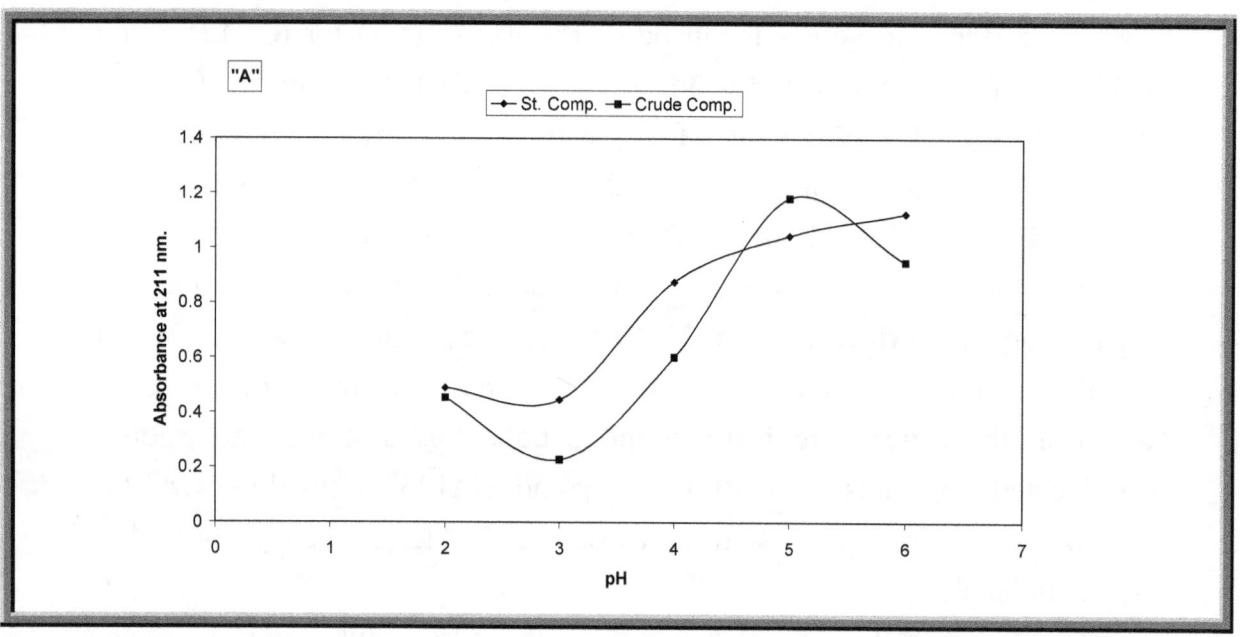

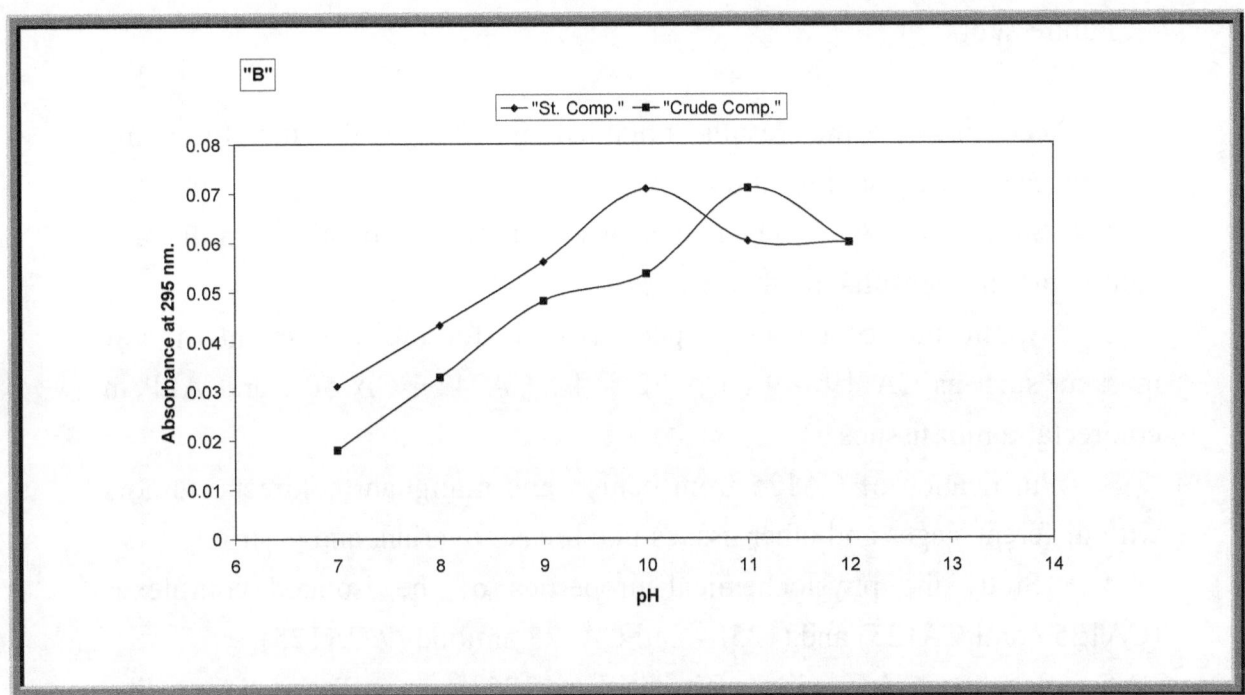

Figure (5-9) Spectrophotometric pH titration of (CA125 / anti CA125) complex (St. Complex) and (125I – anti CA215 Antibody / CA215) complex (Crude Complex)

(A) Histidine

(B) Tyrosin

Conclusion:

1– The level of CA125 increased in sera of patients with colorectal tumors.

2 – The procedure for the assessment of CA125 in benign and malignant colorectal tumors was developed.

3 –There is more than one immunoreactive isoform of CA125 in the colorectal tissue homogenate.

4 – The kinetic studies of 125I – anti CA125 antibody binding to both crude and partial purified colorectal tumors showed that the binding reaction is a temperature and time dependent, and the reaction is pseudo – first order at different temperatures.

5 – The Thermodynamic studies 125I – anti CA125 antibody binding to both crude and partial purified colorectal tumors were entropically driven.

6 – The spectroscopic study of h – CA125, CA125 antigens (isoforms) and their complexes have a characteristic spectrum. The spectrum is influenced by many fact

Future Work:

According to the results obtained in this work, the following researches are suggested for the future:

1 – Study the CA125 level in sera and tissue of ovarian tumors and comparing these results in other tissues.

2 – Application of the developed methods for the assessment of new markers such as CA 19 – 9 , CA 72 – 4 , CA242 , CA 50 , and AFP in colorectal tumor tissues.

3 – Purification of CA125 from benign and malignant colorectal tumors with different stages and other tissues like breast, ovarian, and gastric.

4 – Study the physiochemical properties of the isolated complexes (CA125 / anti CA125) and (125I – anti CA125 antibody / CA125).

5 – Spectroscopic studies of isolated CA125 from different tissues like breast, ovarian, and gastric.

ors such as pH, solvent polarity, urea and KCl.

Conclusion:

1– The level of CA125 increased in sera of patients with colorectal tumors.

2 – The procedure for the assessment of CA125 in benign and malignant colorectal tumors was developed.

3 –There is more than one immunoreactive isoform of CA125 in the colorectal tissue homogenate.

4 – The kinetic studies of 125I – anti CA125 antibody binding to both crude and partial purified colorectal tumors showed that the binding reaction is a temperature and time dependent, and the reaction is pseudo – first order at different temperatures.

5 – The Thermodynamic studies 125I – anti CA125 antibody binding to both crude and partial purified colorectal tumors were entropically driven.

6 – The spectroscopic study of h – CA125, CA125 antigens (isoforms) and their complexes have a characteristic spectrum. The spectrum is influenced by many factors such as pH, solvent polarity, urea and KCl.

Future Work:

According to the results obtained in this work, the following researches are suggested for the future:

1 – Study the CA125 level in sera and tissue of ovarian tumors and comparing these results in other tissues.

2 – Application of the developed methods for the assessment of new markers such as CA 19 – 9 , CA 72 – 4 , CA242 , CA 50 , and AFP in colorectal tumor tissues.

3 – Purification of CA125 from benign and malignant colorectal tumors with different stages and other tissues like breast, ovarian, and gastric.

4 – Study the physiochemical properties of the isolated complexes (CA125 / anti CA125) and (125I – anti CA125 antibody / CA125).

5 – Spectroscopic studies of isolated CA125 from different tissues like breast, ovarian, and gastric.

REFERENCES

1 – Burtis, C. A; Edward, R.; Ashwood, E. R.; (1999) "Tetiz Text Book of Clinical Chemistry". 3 rd. ed., Philadelphia, W. B. Saunders Co. Chap. 23. pp. 722 – 748.

2 – Kalstan, M. B. ; Onyekwere , O .; Sidransky , D .; Vogelstein , B .; Craig , R . W.; (1991). Cancer Res., 51: 6304.

3 – Daivid, W.; (2001) "Immunoassay Hand Book". 2 nd. ed. U. K. nature publishing Co. Chap. 63. pp. 635 – 662.

4 – http: // Nauvoo. byu. // Academy / micro biol. Tumor / table / htm / 10 / 1 / 1999.

5 – Koprwsk, H.; Herlyn, M.; Steplewise, Z.; Sears, H. F.; (1981). Science, 212: 53.

6 – Magnant, J. L.; Brockhus, M.; Smith, D. F.; Blaszrzyk, M.; et al., (1981). Science, 212: 55.

7 – Diezn. ; Cerdan, F. J.; Pollan, M.; Maestro, M. L.; Ortega, M. D.; et al., (1994). Anticancer Res. 14: 2819.

8 – Carpelan, H. M.; Haglund, C.; Kusela, P.; Jarvinen, H.; Roberts, P. J.; (1995). Br. J. Cancer, 71: 868.

9 – Doos, W. G.; Wolff, W. I.; Shinya, H.; et al. (1975). Cancer, 36: 1997.

10 – Loewenstein, M. S.; Zamchech, N.; (1978). Cancer, 42: 1412.

11 – Stevens, D. P.; Mackay, I. R.; (1973). Lancet, 2: 1238.

12 – Chu, T. M.; (1973). J .Natl. Cancer. Inst., 51: 1119.

13 – Vincent, R. G.; Chu, T. M.; (1973). Thorac Cardiovase Surg., 66: 320.

14 – Dittrich , C .; Jakes , Z .; Havelec .; et al ., (1985). Cancer, 8: 181.

15 – Ona, S. W.; Zamcheck, N.; Blair, P.; et al., (1973). Cancer, 31: 324.

16 – Van Nagell, J. R.; Donaldson, E. S.; Wood E. G. ; et al . , (1978). Cancer, 42: 1527.

17 – Goldenberg, D. M.; (1988). Arch. Pathol. Lab. Med., 112: 580.

18 – Wanebo, H. J.; Rao, B.; Pinsky, C. M.; et al., (1978). N. Engl. J. Med., 229: 448.

19 – Campo, E.; Munoz, J.; Miquel, R.; Palacin, A.; et al., (1994). Am. J. Pathol. , 145: 301.

20 – Jessup, J. M.; (1994). Am. J. Pathol. , 145: 253.

21 – Walach, N.; Guterman, A.; Zaidman, J. L.; et al., (1991). Tummori. , 77: 164.

22 – Verazin G.; Riley, W. M.; Gregory, J.; et al., (1991). Dis. Colon Rectum. , 33: 139.

23 – Barillari, P.; Rammacciato G.; De Angelis, R.; et al., (1989). Int. J. Colorectal. Bis. , 4: 230.

24 – Order, S. E.; Donahue, V. C. ; Knapp, R. C.; (1973). Cancer. , 32: 573.

25 – Order, S. E.; Kirkman, R.; Knapp, R. C.; (1974). Cancer. , 43:175.

26 – Knapp, R. C.; Berkowitz, R. C; (1977). Am. J. Obstetrics & Gynecology. , 12: 782.

27 – Bast, R. C.; Knapp, R. C.; Mitchell, A. K.; et al. , (1979). J. Immunol. , 123: 1945.

28 – Bast, R. C. Jr.; Berek, J. S.; Obrist, R.; et al., (1983) . Cancer Rese. , 43: 1395.

29 – Kohlar, G.; Milstein, C.; (1975). Nature. , 275: 495.

30 – Davis, H. M.; Zurawski, V. R. Jr.; Bast, R. C. Jr.; et al. , (1987) . Cancer Rese. , 46: 6143.

31 – "Tumor Marker " http // M. S. Ramaiah Orator / htm. / 6 / 12 / 2001.

32 – Saad, E.; Sohair, Sh.; (1998) "Tumor Markers ". 1 st. ed., U. K, Chapman & Hall. Chap. 2. pp. 51 – 86.

33 – Lanzone, A.; Marana, R.; Musctello, R.; et al., (1991). Gyncol. Oncol. , 36 (8): 603. (Midline, abstr.) .

34 – "CA125: History, Current Status, and Future Prospects " http: / www. asco Org. / prof. / pp / html / m – Tumor 10 htm.

35 – Ruddon, R. W.; Norton, S. E.; (1993). J. Tumor. Marker. Oncol. , 20: 251.

36 – Uirji, M. A.; Mercer D. W.; Heberman, R. B.; et al., (1989). Am. J. Gastroenterol. , 78: 13.

37 – Bast, R. C Jr.; Feency, M.; Lazarush .H.; et al., (1981). J. Clin. Invest. , 68: 1331.

38 – Jonathan. S. B.; Neville, F. H.; (2000). "Practical Gynecologic Oncology ". 3 rd. ed., Philadelphia, Lippincott Williams & Wilkins. Chap. 2. pp. 41.

39 – Caristed, I.; Lindgren, H.; Sheehan, H.; et al., (1983). Biochem. J., 211: 13.

40 – Cludio, SH.; Roland, A.; Newman, D.; et al., (1982). Am. J. Biol. Chem., 25: 10766.

41 – Suzanne, K.; Deborah, J.; Robert, C.; et al., (1985). Am. J. Obst. Gyn., 152: 911.

42 – Bast, R.; Klug, T. L.; John, E.; et al., (1983). N. Eng. J. Med., 309: 169.

43 – Masuho, Y.; Zalutsky, M.; Knapp, R. C.; et al., (1984). Cancer Rese. , 44: 2813.

44 – Nustad, K.; Bast, R. C.; Brien, T.; et al., (1996). Tumor Biol., 17: 176.

45 – Herbrt, A.; Fritsh, C.; Robert, A.; et al., (1998). Clin. Chem., 7: 1379.

46 – Margit, S.; Bernad, C.; Ingrid, S.; et al., (1999). Cancer letters. , 145: 133.

47 – Altug, M. U.; Akdas, A.; Ruacan, S.; et al., (2002). European J. of Cancer. , 38 (13): 1701.

48 – Jense, N. J.; Maclean, G.; Suresh, R.; et al., (1991). Cancer. , 6: 1.

49 – Haglund, C.; Kunsela, P.; Roberts, P.; et al., (1991). In. J. Cancer. , 47 (2): 170 (Medline, abst.).

50 – Nagel, H.; Bahlo, M.; Klapdor, R.; et al., (1999). Am. Heart. J., 137 (6): 1044.

51 – Canny, P. A.; Moor, M.; Wilkinson, P. M.; James, R. D.; (1984). Br. J. Cancer. , 52: 765.

52 – Crombach, G.; Scharl, M.; Vierbuchen, H.; Bolte, A.; (1989). Cancer. , 63: 1337.

53 – Rainer Klapdor. ; (1984). "Tumor Marker in Clinical Oncology" 1 st. ed., Hamburg – Germany, Sorin Biomedica S. P. A. Chap. 12. PP. 127.

54 – Marchal, F.; Berthiot, G.; Kritly, T.; Legrand, M. G.; et al., (1989). Anti cancer Res., 9 (3): 593.

55 – Kenemans, P.; Wobbes, T.; Thomas, C. M.; Bon, G. G.; et al., (1992). Tumor Biol., 13: 18.

56 – Taal, B. G.; Hageman, P. C.; Delemarre, J. F.; Bonfrer. ; Et al., (1992). Eur. J. Cancer. , 28: 394.

57 – Kozatsani, D.; Mylonakis, N,; Kosmidis, P.; et al., (1993). In. J. Biol. Markers. , 8 (2): 88.

58 – Markowitz, A. J.; Winawer, G. J.; (1997). J. Am. Cancer Soci. , 47 (2): 93.

59 – Lawrence, J. Bronelt. ; (1999) "Clinical Practice of Gastroentrology", vol. 1 2 nd. ed., Philadelphia: Cuuent Medicine Inc., Chap. 66, pp. 588 – 595 & Chap. 48, pp. 752 – 776.

60 – Bombi, J. A.; (1988). Cancer. , 61: 1472.

61 – Rickert, R. R.; Aucrbach, O.; Garfinkel, L.; et al., (1979). Cancer. , 43: 1847.

62 – O' Brien, M. G.; Winawer, S. J.; Zauber, A. G.; et al., (1990). , Gastroenterology. , 98: 371.

63 – Winawer, S. J.; Zauber, A. G.; O' Brien, M. G.; et al., Cancer. , 70: 1236.

64 – Match, W.; Demling. ; Hermanek, P.; (1986). Endoscopy. , 18: 17.

65 – Joseph, R.; Bertino. ; (1996) "Encyclopedia of Cancer". Vol. 1. 1 st. ed., California, Academic Press. pp. 441.

66 – Mayers, M. A.; (1998). " Neoplasms of the Digestive Tract : Imaging Staging & Management . " , Philadelphia : Lippincott – Raven Publishers , Chap . 19. pp. 203.

67 – Christopher, H.; Edwin, R. Ch.; John, A. H.; Nicholas, A. B. ; (1999) " Davidson's Principles and Practice of Medicine " 8 th . ed., U. K., Harcourt Brace & Company Limited. Chap 9. pp. 671.

68 – Bostick, R. M.; Slattery, M. L.; Potter, J. D; et al., (1993). Epidemilol. Rev., 15: 499.

69 – Chow, W.; Dwvesas. , (1993). Cancer. , 71: 3819.

70 – Schottenfeld D.; (1995). " Cancer of the Colon , Rectum and Anus " . , New York : Mc Grow – Hill . , pp . 11 – 24.

71 – Ministry of Health (1989). Results of Iraqi Cancer Registry. (1986 – 1988).

72 – Ministry of Health (1993). Results of Iraqi Cancer Registry. (1989 – 1992).

73 – Ministry of Health (1995). Results of Iraqi Cancer Registry. (1992 – 1994).

74 – Ministry of Health (2000). Results of Iraqi Cancer Registry. (1995 – 1999).

75 – Ministry of Health (2003). Results of Iraqi Cancer Registry. (1999 – 2002   ).

76 – Bos, J. L.; Fearon, E. R.; Hamilton, S. R.; (1987). Nature. , 327: 293.

77 – Muto, T.; Bussey, HJ. R.; Morson, B. C.; (1985). , Cancer. , 36: 2251.

78 - O'Brien, M. J.; O'kean, J. C.; Zauber, A.; Gottlieb, L. S. ; et al . , (1992). Cancer. , 70: 1317.

79 – Harnden, D. G.; (1984). Carcinogenesis. , 5: 1535.

80 – Hamilton, S. R.; (1993). Gastroenterology. , 105: 3.

81 – Beazer, B. Y.; Zilz, N.; Powell, S .M.; (1992). Nature. 359: 235.

82 – Schaid, D. J.; Thibodeaus, S. N.; Shattuch, B. R.; Burgart, L. J. ; et al . , (1998). , Cancer Res., 58, 23: 5473.

83 – Couture, J.; Swallow, C.; Redston, M.; Gallinger, S.; et al., (1997). Cancer. , 21 (5): 233.

84 – Kato, H.; Tamaik, K.; Morioka, M.; Najai, T.; et al., (1999) Cancer., 54 (3): 1544.

85 – Bishop, J. M.; (1987). Science. , 233: 305.

86 – Carins, J.; (1981). Nature. , 289: 353.

87 – Kelin, G.; (1981). Nature. , 294: 313.

88 – Loser, C.; Folsch, V. R.; Paprotny, C.; Creutzfeldt, W.; (1990). Cancer. , 65 (4): 958.

89 – Tsavaris, N.; Vonortak, K.; Tsontsos, H.; Kozatsani, H. D.; (1993). Int .J. Biol. Markers. , 8 (2): 88.

90 – Wanebo, H. J.; Unger, S. W.; (1983). Am. J. Surg., 145: 71.

91 – Sleisenger, M. H.; Toribara, N. W.; (1995). N. Engl. J .m Med., 332: 861.

92 – Willett, W. C.; Hunter, D. J.; Colditz, G. A.; Fuchs, C. S.; (1994). N. Engl. J. Med., 331: 1669.

93 – Adami, H. B.; Zack, N.; Helmick, C. E.; (1990). Lancet. , 336: 357.

94 – White, R.; Lalouel, J. M.; Gardner, E.; et al., (1990). N. Engl. J. Med., 332: 904.

95 – Baily, C. J.; Bodmer, W. F.; Bailey, C. J.; et al. , (1987) . Nature. , 327: 298.

96 – Boyd, P. A.; Peterson, G. M.; (1995). Cancer. , 17: 67.

97 – Schuman, L.; Williams, S. E.; Gilbertson, V. A., et al., (1980) Cancer. , 45: 2899.

98 – Zauber, A.; Winawer, S. J.; Diaz, B.; et al., (1988). Prog. Clin. Biol. Res., 279: 35.

99 – Anderson, J.; (2000). Geriatrics. , 55, (2): 67.

100 – Watson, F. R.; Kyle, K.; Turnbull, R. B.; et al., (1987). Ann. Surg., 166: 420.

101 – Winawer, G. J.; Markowitz, A. J.; (1997). J. Am. Cancer. Soc., 47, (2): 93.

102 – Warell, D. A.; Leadingham, J. G. G.; Weatherall, D. J.; (1988). "Oxford Text Book of Medicine". , Vol . 1, London: English Language Book Society Oxford University Press. pp. 12, 146, 157.

103 – Pelegrin, A.; Mach, J. P.; Bischof, D. A.; Gillet, M.; et al., (1996). Cancer Res., 141: 19.

104 – Smith, A.; Match, J. P.; Bischof, D. A.; Gillet, M.; et al., (1997). J. Nucl. Med., 38: 847.

105 – Folli, S.; Westerman, P.; Braichott, D.; Pelegerin, A.; et al., (1996). " Immuno photo detection of Cancer by Antibody – Inodcyanan Conjugates , Experimental and Preliminary Clinical Results in Analytical Use of Fluorescent Probes in Oncology " . , New York : Plenum Publishing Co., Series : 286 , pp . 189 – 204.

106 – Monnier, P.; Wagnieres, G. A.; Forrer, M.; Mach, J. P.; et al., (1998). Int. J. Cancer. , 67: 842.

107 – Mach, J. P.; Deperthes, D.; Finnern, R.; Couty Jouve, S. ; Houimel , M . ; (1999). , http: // www. isrec. ch / reports /mach. asp. , 09 / 24 / 1999, pp. 1 – 6.

108 – Temple, W. G.; Sugarbaker, A. W.; Thornthweite, G .T.; et al., (1980). J. Surg. Res., 28: 314.

109 – Fischbach, W.; Seyschab, H.; (1990). Cancer. , 65: 1820.

110 – Jaun Rosai. ; (1989) "A ckerman's Surgical Pathology" 7 th. ed., Vol. 1, New York. The C. V. Mosby Company, Chap. 3, pp. 35 – 44.

111 – Janssen, A.M ; Bosman, C. B.; amers, C. B.; Vankrieken, J. M.; Kruidenier , L, (1999). J. Cancer. Res. Clin. Oncol. , 125 (5): 327.

112 – Donald, A. P.; Steven, C.; Vijaya, B.; et al., (1994). J. Clin. Oncol. , 12 (3): 489.

113 – Goldenberg, D. M.; (1994). CA. Cancer. J Clin. , 44: 43.

114 – Goldenberg, D. M.; Larson, S. M.; Reisfeld, R. A.; Schlom, J.; (1995). Immunol. Today. , 16 (6): 261.

115 – Goldenberg, D. M.; Goldenberg, H.; Shrky, R. M.; et al., (1989). Semn. Nucl. Med., 19: 262.

116 – Flampen, P.; Dupont, P.; Bormans, Guy. ; Cutsem, E. V.; et al., (1999). J. Clin. Oncol. , 17 (3): 894.

117 – Meyers, M. A.; (1998). "Neoplasms of the Digestive Tract Staging & Management". , Philadelphia , Lippincott Raven Publishers . Chap. 21, pp. 237 – 266 & Chap. 43: pp. 523 – 546.

118 – Yactayos. ; Foultier, M. T.; Patrice, T.; et al., (1990). Dig. Dis. Sci., 35: 545.

119 – Arroyop, J.; Stern, J. D.; Unger, S. W.; et al., (1990). Am. Surgeon. , 56: 153.

120 – Wiand, H. S.; Martenson, J.; O 'Connell, M.; (1994). N. Eng. J. Med., 331: 502.

121 – Macmillan, W. E.; Wolberg, W. H.; Welling, P. G.; (1978) Cancer Res., 38: 3479.

122 – Ullman, B.; Lee, M.; Martin, D. W. Jr.; Santi, D. V.; (1978). Proc. Natl. Acad. Sci., 35: 123.

123 – Horton, J.; Olson, K. B.; Sullivan, J.; Reilly, C.; et al., (1970). Ann. Intern. Med., 73: 897.

124 – Siefert, P.; Baker, L. H.; Reed, M. L.; Vaitkevicius, V.; (1975). Cancer. , 35: 123.

125 – Ansfiel, D. F.; Klotz, J.; Nealon, T.; Ramirez, G.; et al., (1977). Cancer. , 39: 34.

126 – Erlichman, C.; Fine S.; Wong, A.; Elhakim, T.; (1988). J. Clin. Oncol. , 6: 469.

127 – Lokich J. J.; Anlgren, J. D.; Gullo, J. J.; Phillips, J. A.; Fryer, J. G.; (1989). J. Clin. Oncol. . 7: 425.

128 – Leichman, C. G.; Leichman, L.; Spears, C. P.; Rosen, P. J. ; et al ., (1990). Pharmacol. , 26: 57.

129 – Poplin, E. A.; Kraut, M.; Baker, L.; Brodfuehrer, J.; Vaitkevicius V.; (1991). Cancer. , 67: 367.

130 – Inglis, J. K.; (1989) "A Text Book of Human Biology". 3 rd. ed., New York: Pergamon Press, Chap. 7, pp. 114 – 115.

131 – Gylys, B. A.; Wedding, M. F.; (1988). "Medical Terminology a Systems Approach". 2 nd. Ed. Phiiladelphia: F. A. Davis Company. Chap. 6 pp. 92.

132 – Ferguson, J. E.; Hulse, P.; Jayson, G.; Lorigan, P. ; Scarffe, J. H . ; (1995). B. J. Cancer. , 72: 193.

133 – Presant, C. A.; Wolf, W.; Waluch, V.; Wiseman, C. L.; Weitz, I.; and Shani, J.; (2000). J. Am. Soc. Clin. Oncol. , 8: 107.

134 – O 'Dwyer, P. J.; Panal, A. R.; Weiner, L. M.; Comis, A. L. ; (1989) . Proc. Am. Soc. Clin. Oncol. , 8: 107.

135 – Holland, J. F.; Bast, R. C.; Morton, D. L.; (1997). "Cancer Medicine". , 4 th . Ed. London: Willians & Wilkins. Vol. 2, Section XXXI, Chap. 121. pp. 2029 – 2072.

136 – Moertl, C. G.; (1988). J. Clin. Oncol. , 6: 934.

137 – Bleiberg, H.; Rougier, P.; Wilker, H. J.; (1998). "Management of Colorectal Cancer". London: Martin Dunitz Ltd. Chap. 3. pp. 35 – 54.

138 – Carpelan, H. M.; Hagluned, C.; Kusela, P.; Jarvinen, H.; Roberts, P. J. ; (1995) . B. J. Cancer. , 71: 868.

139 – Sadler, R. S.; Freund, D. A.; Herbst, C. A. Jr. ; Sandler, D. P (1984). Cancer. , 53: 193.

140 – Giuseppe, C.; Evarsto, M.; Vittorio, G.; Francesco, G., et al., (1999). Cancer. , 85 (3): 535.

141 – Koprwsk, H.; Herlyn, M.; Sears, H. F.; Steplewise, Z.; (1981). Science. , 212: 53.

142 – Osborne, B. A.; Goldsby, R. A.; Kindt, T. J.; (2000). "KUBY Immunology". 4 th. ed., New York: W. H.; Freeman & Company. Chap. 22. pp. 539.

143 – Anonymous. ; (1995). J. Clin. Oncol. . 13: 921.

144 – Lin, B. Y.; Savona, S.; Mittelman, A.; Galney, E.; et al., (1989). J. Biol. Response. Mod. , 8: 468.

145 – Odchimar, R.; Holland, J. F.; Pacincci, P. A.; Glidewell. O.; (1989). J. Clin. Oncol. , 7: 869.

146 – Muul, L. M.; Lotz M. T.; Rosenberg, S. A.; Change, A E.; et al., (1987) .N. Engl. J. Med., 3416: 889.

147 – Holland,; Ryder, J. S.; Motwani, B.; Paciucci, P. A.; (1989). Proc. Am. Assoc. Cancer. , 30: 33.

148 – Huber, B. E.; Austin, E. A.; Richard, C. A.; (1994). Ann. NY. Acad. Sci., 716: 104.

149 – Levitsky, H.; Brose, K.; Jackson, V.; Jafee, E.; et al., (1993). Proc. Nat. Acad. Sci., 90: 3539.

150 – Willianj, J.; John, M. D.; John, R.; Neefe, M. D.; John, S.; et al., (1993) . Cancer. , 72 (11): 3191.

151 – Rowry, O. H.; Farr, L.; Randell, R.; Rosebrough N. J. ; (1951) . J. Biol. Chem., 193: 265.

152 – Klug, T. L.; Bast, R. C. Jr.; Niloff, J. M.; et al., (1984). Cancer. Res. , 44: 1048.

153 – Brioschi, P. A.; I rion, O.; Bischof, P.; et al., (1987). B. J. Obs. Gyn., 94: 196.

154 – Finkler, N. J.; Benacerraf, B.; Lavin, P. T.; et al., (1988). Obs. Gyn., 72: 659.

155 – Niloff J. M.; Klug, T. L.; Schaetzel E.; et al., (1984). Am. J. Obs. Gyn., 148: 1057.

156 – Malkasian, G. D. Jr. Podratzk, C.; Stanhop, C. R.; et al., (1986). Am. J. Obs. Gyn., 155: 515.

157 – Goldenberg, D. M.; Nevill, M.; Carter, A. C.; et al., (1998). Clin. Chem., 44 (6): 529.

158 – Yoichiro, M. D.; Keigo, M. D.; Yasutak, M. D.; et al., (1990). Cancer. , 65 (3): 506.

159 – Niloff, J. M.; Knapp, R. C.; Scheetzel E.; et al., (1984). Obs. Gyn., 164: 703.

160 – Pittaway, D. E.; (1986). Fertile. St., 46: 79.

161 – Pittaway, D. E.; Fayez, J. A.; (1987). Am. J. Obs. Gyn., 156: 75.

162 – Barbieri, R. L.; Niloff, J. M.; Bast R. C. Jr. ; et al ., (1986). Fertil. St., 45: 630.

163 – Bergmann, J. F.; Bidart, J. M.; George, M.; et al., (1987). Cancer. , 59: 213.

164 – Kennett, W.; Ryder. ; Tjien, O.; et al., (1988). Clin. Chem. 34 (12): 2513.

165 – Ziola B. R.; Matikaineu, M. T.; Salmi, A.; (1988). J. Immunol. , 17: 309.

166 – Boerman, O. C.; Thomas, M. G.; Segers, P. K.; et al., (1987). Clin. Chem., 33: 2191.

167 – Janson, J. C.; and Pyden, L. ; (1998) " Protein Purification (Principles , High – Resolution , Methods and Applications) " . , 2 nd . ed.; John Willey and Sons, Inc; New York. PP. 30, 79.

168 – Al – Khayt, T. H.; (1991). "Molecular Characterization of Prolactin Receptors in Human Prostate". Ph. D Thesis Supervised by Al – Mudhaffar S. A.; College of Science, Baghdad Univ.

169 – Chamberlain, J.; Jargarince, N.; Ofher, P.; (1966). Biochem. J., 99: 610.

170 – Farrant, T. J.; (1997). "Practical Statistics for the Analytical Scientist". L G C. pp. 16, 49.

171 – Rittenhouse, H. G.; Manderino, G. L.; and Hass, M.; (1985). J. M. Medicine. , 16: 556.

172 – Colakovic, S.; Lukic V.; Mitrovic, L.; et al., (2000). ; In. J. Biol. Markers. , 15: 147.

173 – Paul, K. B.; Mark, O. M. D.; Drake, R.; et al., (1990). J. Surgi. Oncol. , 44: 97.

174 – Fendrick, J. L.; Konishi, I.; Geary, S. M.; Parmley, T. H.; et al., (1997). Tumor Biol., 18: 278.

175 – Einhorn, N.; Ovall K.; Knapp, R. C.; Hall, P.; et al. , (1992) . Obs. Gyn., 80: 14.

176 – Know, S. K.; et al.; (1973). Int. J. Cancer. , 11: 681.

177 – Roitt, I.; Brostoff, J.; Male, D.; (1998). "Immunology".

178 – Changux, J. P.; (1966). Mol. Pharmacol. , 2: 369.

179 – Bryant, N. J.; (1986). "Laboratory Immunology and Serology" 2. nd. , Philadelphia, W. B. Saunders Co. Chap. 5. pp. 49 – 52.

180 – Helen, Ch.; Mansel, H.; Siraj, M.; Neil, S.; (1999). "Essential of Clinical Immunology". 4 th. ed., U .K., Blackwell Science Ltd., Chap. 19 pp. 314 – 321.

181 – Dadliker, W. B.; and Satussure, V. A.; (1970). Immu. Chem., 7: 799.

182 – Segal, I. H.; (1975). "Enzyme Kinetics: Behavior and Analysis of Rapid Equilibrium and Steady – State Enzyme System" John Wiley and Sons, New York. , p. 100.

183 – Dixon, M.; and Webb, E.; (1979) "Enzyms". 3 rd .ed., London, Long man Group Limiteded; pp. 273.

184 – Devilin, T. M.; (1986) "Text Book of Biochemistry with Clinical Correlation". 2 nd. ed., New York, Inc., John Wily and Sons. , pp 273.

185 – Price, N .C.; and Stevens, L. (1989); "Fundamentals of Enzymology". 2 nd. ed. New York, Oxford University Press. , pp. 125.

186 – Scheraga, H. A.; (1961). "Protein Structure". New York. , Academic Press. , pp. 365, 571.

187 – Melander, W.; Horvath, C.; (1977). Arch. Biochem. Biophys. , 183: 200.

188 – Williams, C. A.; and Chas, M. W.; (1971). "Methods in Immunology and Immunochemistry". 5 th. ed. New York, Academic Press. , Vol. III, Chap. 13.

189 – Shiu, R. P. C.; Friesen, H. G.; (1971). J. Biol. Chem., 294: 7902.

190 – Damodaran, S.; and Kinsella, J. E.; (1980). J. Biol. Chem., 255 (18): 8503.

191 – William, E. P.; (1998). "Fundamental Immunology". 4 th. ed., Philadelphia, Lippicott. Raven, Chap 4, pp. 75 – 110.

192 – Mellor. ; Maley. ; (1947). Nature. , 159: 370.

193 – Williams, R. J. P.; (1959). "The Enzymes" 2 nd. ed., New York, Academic Press, Vol. I, pp. 391.

194 – Al – Gurnawi, Z. A.; (1999). "Physical and Chemical Properties of Prostate Specific Antigen in Some Prostate Diseases". M .Sc. Thesis Supervised by Al – Mudhaffar S. A.; College of Science, Baghdad Univ.

195 – O 'Brien, T. J.; Beard, J. B.; Unerwood, L. J.; Dennis, R. A.; (2001). Tumor Biol., 22: 348.

196 – Yin, B. W.; and Lloyd, K. O.; (2001). J. Biol. Chem., 276: 27371.

197 – Zurawski, V.; Davis, H.; Finkler, N.; Harrison, C.; et al., (1988). Cancer Rev., 11 – 12, 102 – 118.

198 – Nagata, A.; Hirotan, N.; Sakai, T.; Komod T.; et al., (1991). Tumor Biol., 12: 279.

199 – Clandia, S.; Sabin, W.; Johannes, L.; Walter, N.; (2003). J. Cell. Science. , 116: 1305.

200 – Hidde, J.; Haisma, H.; (1987). In. J. Cancer. , 40: 758.

201 – Ursula, T.; and Pentti, L.; (1990). Chlin. Chem., 36 (7): 1992.

202 – Scopes, K. ; (1982) " Protein Purification , Principles and Practice " . , New York , Springer Verlage , pp . 162, 197.

203 – Price, N. C.; and Stevens, L.; (1986). "Fundamentals of Enzymology". 2. nd ed ., New York, Oxford University Press. , pp. 125.

204 – Stacker, S. A.; Tjanda, J. J.; Xing, P. X.; Walker, I. D. ; et al ., (1989). B. J. Cancer. , 59: 544.

205 – Hilkens, J.; Kroezn, V.; Bonfrer, J. M. G.; Hilgers, et al., (1985). Protides of Biological Fluids. , 2: 651.

206 – Abe, M.; Dufe, D.; (1987). J. Immunol. , 139: 257.

207 – Gary, A.; Bannon. ; et al., (1986). Am. J. Obst. Gyn., 155: 50.

208 – Niloff, J. M.; Knapp, R. C.; Schaetzal, E. M.; et al., (1984). Obst. Gyn., 64: 703.

209 – Bonfrer, J. M.; (1995). J. Clin. Chem., 20: 301.

210 – Al – Rubae 'I, S. H.; (2002). "Biochemical Characterization of CA 15 – 3 in Sera and Tissues of Breast Tumors". Ph. D Thesis Supervised by Al – Mudhaffar S. A.; College of Science, Al – Mustansiriyah Univ.

211 – Brostoff, J.; and Male, D.; (1994). "Clinical Immunology, an Illustrated Outline". Philadelphia. , Mosby. , Chap. 8, pp. 112.

212 – Shiu, R. P. C.; Friesen, H. G.; (1974). J. Biol. Chem., 249: 7902.

213 – Al – Kazzaz, F. F.; (2000). "Molecular Characterization of Carcinoembryonic Antigen (CEA) in Some Colorectal Tumors". Ph. DThesis Supervised by Al – Mudhaffar S. A.; College of Science, Al – Mustansiriyah Univ.

214 – Wiseman, T.; Williston, S.; Brandts, J. F.; Lung – Nan, L.; (1889). Anal. Biochem. , 179: 131.

215 – Wibdenmeyer, J. A.; Schuck, P.; and SmithGill, S. J.; (1999). J. Biol. Chem., 274: 26838.

216 – Sundberg, E. J.; et al, (2000) .Biochem. , 39: 15375.

217 – Gomez, J and Freire. ; (1995). J. Mol. Biol. 252: 337.

218 – Myszaka, D. G.; et al., (2000). Proc. Natl. Acad. Sci. USA. , 97: 9026.

219 – Tamilselvi, P.; Banerjee, A.; and Murthy, G. S.; (2002). Current Sci., 8 (12):1442.

220 – Scatchard, G.; (1949). Ann. N. Y. Acad. Sci., 51: 660.

221 – Chambelaing, J.; Jargarinece, N.; Ofner, P.; (1966). Biochem. J., 99: 10.

222 – Adams, A.; Karrott, D.; (1985). Biochem. Biophys. Res. Commun. , 128 (2).

223 – Jose, M.; Tomothy. A. S.; Joann, A. K. B.; et al., (1998). , J. Virol., 72 (7): 6244.

224 – Weiland, G. A.; Molinof, P. B.; (1981). Life Sci., 29: 313.

225 – Seely, G. A.; Wang, W. Y.; Sathanick, H. A.; (1980). Biochem. Biophy. Acta. , 632: 535.

226 – Segel, I. H.; (1979). "Biochemical Calculation". 3 rd. ed. John Willey & Sons, Inc. pp. 311.

227 – Waelbroeck, M.; Van – Obbergham, E.; De – Meytes, P.; (1979). J. Biol. Chem., 254: 7736.

228 – Nemthy, G.; and Scheraga, H. A.; (1962). J. Phys. Chem., 66: 1773.

229 – Haro, L. S.; and Talamaaantes, F. J.; (1985). Mol. Cell. Endocrinol. , 43: 199.

230 – Brown, E. M.; Hauser, D.; Troxler, F.; et al., (1976). J. Biol. Chem., 251: 1232.

231 – Villacampa, M. J.; Moro, R.; Uriel, J.; et al., (1984). Cancer Res., 44: 5314.

232 – Stull, J. T.; and Blumenthal, D. K.; (1982). Biochem. , 21: 2386.

233 – Storm, D. I.; Wierman, E. M.; Laport, D. C.; et al., (1980). Biochem. , 19: 3814.

234 – Sesaki, H.; Wong, E.; Siu, C.; (1997) J. Cell. Biol., 138: 939.

235 – Green, E.; Raman, E.; Riley, N.; Spiro, D.; et al., (1997). Biochem .Biophys. Res., 239: 612.

236 – Nolta, K.; and Steck, T.; (1994). J. Biol. Chem., 269: 2225.

237 – Zimmerman, A. L.; Karpen, J. W.; Baylor, D. A.; (1988). Biophys. J., 54: 351.

238 – Mathews, Ch K.; Holde, K. E.; (1990). "Biochemistry". Callifornia: The Benjamin / Cummings Publishing Co.

239 – Leach, S. J.; (1969). "Physical Principles and Techniques of Protein Chemistry". Part A. 5 th. ed., London: Academic Press Chap 3, pp. 102 – 170.

240 – Chanse, M. W.; Williams, C. A.; (1968). "Methods in Immunology and Immuno Chemistry" New York: Academic Press. Vol. II. , Chap. 10. , pp 163.

241 – Laskowski, M. J.; Herskovits, (1960). J. Biol. Chem., 235: 57.

242 – Herskovits, T .T.; Laskowski, M. J.; (1962). J. Biol. Chem., 237 (8): 2481.

243 – Foster, J. F.; Williams, E. J.; (1959). J. Am. Chem. Soci. , 81: 865.

244 – Laskowski, M. J.; Widom, J. M.; Scheraga, H. A.; et al., (1956). Bio chem. et Biophys. Acta. , 19: 581.

245 – Bayliss, N. S.; Mc Rae, E. G.; (1954). J. Phys. Chem., 235: 2827.

246 – Inuzuka, K.; Ito, M.; Imanishi, S.; et al., (1960). J. Am. Chem. Soc., 82:1317.

247 – Scheraga, H .A.; Leach, S. J.; (1960). J .Biol. Chem., 235: 2827.

248 – Armustrong, S. A.; Staunton, J. E.; Silverman, L. B.; et al., (2002). Nat. Genet. , 30: 41.

249 – Johuston, A.; Thorpe, R.; (1996). "Immuno Chemistry in Practice". 3 rd. ed. Blackwell Science Ltd., pp. 1 – 4, 292 – 311.

250 – Freifrlder, D. (1982). "Physical Biochemistry, Physical Application to Biochemistry Molecular Biology". 2 nd. ed., San Fracisco: W. H. Freeman & Company. Chap. 14. , pp. 494 – 591.

251 – Lubin, D.; Jensen, E. H.; (1995). Nature. , 377: 710.

252 – Bothwell, M. L.; Sherbot, D. M. J.; Pollock, C. M.; et al., (1994). Science. , 265: 97.

253 – David, L. N.; Michael, M. C.; (2000). "Lininger Principles of Bio Chemistry". 3 rd. ed. U .S .A Worth Publisher. Chap. 5. , pp. 120.

254 – Al– Tai, W. A.; (2000). "Bio Chemical Studies on Alfa Feto Protein (A F P) and Some Tumor Markers in Gastric Cancer". Ph. DThesis Supervised by Al – Mudhaffar S. A.; College of Science, Al – Mustansiriyah Univ.

255 – Thomas, R.; Middendorf. ; Richard, W.; Aldrich. ; et al., (2000). J. Gen. Phy. , 116 (2): 227.

256 – Edward, H.; Kunito, Y.; James, C.; John, B.; (2001). J. Cell. Scie. 114: 3035.

257 – Harsh, P. B.   ; Ramarao, V. C.; Frank R.; Jorge, M.; et al., (2003) .J. Biol. Chem., 278 (34): 32413.

258 – Klans, D. S.; Chia, H. T.; Paul, F. C.; et al. (1999). J. Biol. Chem., 274 (52): 36935.

259 – Yanari, S.; Bovey, F. A.; (1960). J. Biol. Chem., 235 (10): 2818.

260 – Silvershtien, R. M.; Bassler, G. C.; Morril, T. C.; (1981). "Spectro photo metric Identification of Organic Compounds"., New York: John Willey & Sons. Chap. 6. , pp. 305 – 331.

261 – Lakwski, M. J.; (1966). Fed. Proc., 25: 20.

262 – Singer, S. J.; (1962). Advan. Protein Chem., 17:1.

263 – Donovan, J. W.; (1969). J. Biol. Chem., 244 (8): 1691.

264 – Al – Qadi, S. Z.; (2003). "The Role of Progesterone and its Receptors in Ovarian Tumors (Benign and Malignant)". M .Sc. Thesis Supervised by Al – Mudhaffar S. A.; College of Science, Baghdad Univ.